the fundamentals of family planning

ISBN   978-1-7369-8460-4
eISBN 978-1-7369-8461-1

Library of Congress Control Number: 2021915842

Copyright © 2021 by Essential Access Health

Published September 2021

the **fundamentals** of **family planning**

A Manual for Providing Comprehensive Patient-Centered Contraceptive Counseling

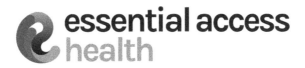

essential access health

Los Angeles | Berkeley

Table of Contents

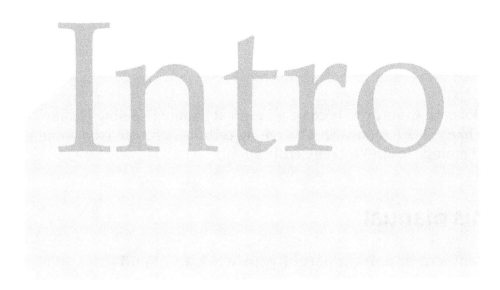

Introduction to the Fundamentals of Family Planning

Congratulations on choosing to become an informed family planning health worker! You have chosen to support people in making smart, healthy decisions about their sexual and reproductive health. This manual was written specifically to help you learn how to do that in a non-judgmental and effective way. By empowering patients to make healthy choices about when and if they want to have children and how to safely express their sexuality, you can make a very positive and lasting difference in their lives.

This manual has been designed to help you do four things:

1. Develop the skills you will need to provide effective, patient-centered contraceptive counseling in any health care setting;

2. Learn up-to-date sexual health information you can share with your patients;

3. Use easy-to-understand ways to explain family planning options to your patients;

4. Implement the recommendations in the "Providing Quality Family Planning Services: Recommendations of CDC and the U.S. Office of Population Affairs" as published in the Morbidity and Mortality Weekly Report (MMWR) on April 25, 2014.

This manual is also the main tool used to study to become a Certified Family Planning Health Worker (FPHW). If you would like to learn more about becoming certified, you can read about it the upcoming ~~section Family Planning~~ Health Worker Certification.

Topics covered in this manual

Each chapter covers a different and important part of your work as a family planning health worker.

Chapter 1: Providing Quality Sexual and Reproductive Health Care will help you understand the main principles of family planning, the importance of getting a patient's informed consent, and how to provide confidential services while complying with patient privacy and mandatory reporting laws.

Chapter 2: Patient Education will help you learn the skills needed to provide patient-centered health education and to work well with diverse patient populations.

Chapter 3: Reproduction and Puberty will help you understand how human reproductive organs work and what happens during puberty.

Chapter 4: Human Sexuality will help you understand different ways of thinking about sex and sexuality, normal sexual responses and common sexual problems patients may have.

Chapter 5: Sexually Transmitted Infections gives you basic information about the most common STIs, as well as current testing, treatment and prevention methods.

Chapter 6: Birth Control Methods has detailed information about each birth control method that you can share with your patients during contraceptive counseling sessions.

Tips for using this manual

There are many ways to use this manual. You can use it to learn what you need to know to become a Certified Family Planning Health Worker. You can use it to update your skills and knowledge if you are already an experienced health worker or health educator. And you can use it as a resource - referring to it for tips and information as you work to meet the needs of your patients every day. Below are some tips to remember as you use this manual.

Start with the basics.

You can read this manual from cover to cover. Or you may choose to read certain sections at a time.

We recommend that you read Chapters 1 and 2 before reading anything else.

Chapters 1 and 2 give you a basic understanding of the field of family planning and your role as a Family Planning Health Worker. The rest of the manual is based on these two chapters. After reading them, go to the chapters that interest you most or provide the information you need – when you need it.

Update your skills and knowledge.

Each chapter is based on up-to-date information and teaching methods. Even if you are an experienced health worker, you may find new information that will add to your skills or refresh your knowledge.

Take the quizzes.

The quizzes are in the manual for you. They will help you know if you have learned the most important points in each chapter. Take all of the quizzes. If you get an answer wrong, just review that part of the chapter again. Quizzing yourself is a great way to help you learn and remember the information. They will also help prepare you for the final exam portion of the Family Planning Health Worker certification process.

Use this manual as a resource.

Keep this book handy. If you need to know something quickly or to refresh your memory on a topic, just turn to the chapter and section that covers the information you are looking for.

Special features of the manual

This manual has special features to help you in your family planning health worker role.

It is easy to understand.

This manual was written to make information easy to understand for you and your patients. The plain language used was designed to help you explain something to a patient in a way that will help them make informed decisions.

It shows you how to "say it" to a patient.

Every chapter provides information in a way that you can use with patients. Be sure to use everyday, easy-to-understand language when you talk with your patients. When you must use a new or difficult word, be sure to explain it in a clear, simple way. Your patients will appreciate it.

It gives you practical tips.

Throughout the manual, you will find practical tips to help you work with your patients. These include suggestions for making your health education and counseling sessions work better and tips on how to handle challenging situations.

It uses inclusive language.

The manual uses gender neutral terms and inclusive language wherever possible. The language aims to help you educate patients regardless of sexual orientation or their gender identity.

NOTE: Contraceptive effectiveness rates in this manual are based on the 21st Revised Edition of Contraceptive Technology, published in 2018.

Family Planning Health Worker Certification

You may want to become a Certified Family Planning Health Worker (FPHW). Certification shows that you have the knowledge and skills needed to provide effective, high quality patient-centered contraceptive counseling. Some health care settings may require this certification for employment.

Essential Access Health has offered this certification for over 30 years, and offers it throughout the United States. The FPHW certification is valid for three years. When your certification is near expiration you will be notified of re-certification options.

Certification Options

1. Attend a FPHW training, which includes this manual.
2. Purchase this manual for self-study.

Certification Process

After attending a FPHW training and/or studying this manual, you will need to pass a final exam and video presentation to become certified.

The final exam is online and tests your knowledge of the information in the manual. It consists of 120+ questions and is time-limited. You must receive a score of 80% to pass this portion of the certification process.

For the video presentation, you will write an Education Plan and use it to create a 15-20 minute Contraceptive Counseling Session video. This portion of the certification process tests your knowledge of and comfort with contraceptive counseling. Details on education plans and birth control options for your video presentation are covered in the FPHW training and will be provided for those doing the self-study option.

To learn more about becoming certified, send an email to: learningexchange@essentialaccess. org or call the Learning Exchange at 213.386.5614, x4580 and ask about Family Planning Health Worker certification options.

About Essential Access Health

Essential Access Health champions and promotes quality sexual and reproductive health care for all. We achieve our mission through an umbrella of programs and services including health center support initiatives, advanced clinical research, provider training, and public policy and awareness campaigns. For more information visit **essentialaccess.org**

Find more Essential Access Health learning opportunities at: **essentialaccess.org/learning-exchange** and our learning portal **essentialaccesstraining.org**

Acknowledgements

All content in this issue of *Fundamentals of Family Planning* was updated in 2021 by Essential Access Health staff:

- ▸ Sandra Abarca, MS, Senior Bilingual Trainer
- ▸ Amber Eisenmann, MS, Director of Training
- ▸ Andria Hancock-Crear, MPH, Senior Trainer
- ▸ Erica Neuman, MS, Senior Trainer
- ▸ Benjamin H. Rossi, PhD, Data and Reporting Manager

The manual was updated in 2019 by staff:

- ▸ Sandra Abarca, MS, Bilingual Trainer
- ▸ Amber Eisenmann, MS, Director of Training
- ▸ Andria Hancock-Crear, MPH, Senior Trainer
- ▸ Erica Neuman, MS, Senior Trainer
- ▸ Matthew Gray Brush, BA, MPH, Intern

The manual was updated in 2017 by staff: Andria Hancock-Crear, MPH and Erica Neuman, MS

The manual was updated in 2014 by consultants and staff: Patty Cason, MS, FNP-BC, Andria Hancock-Crear, MPH, Erica Neuman, MS, and Dannelle Pietersz, NP, MSN, MPH.

The manual was updated in 2007 by: Anita Aguirre, MPH, Veronica Estrella Murillo, MPH , Shelley Marks, MPH, Chuck Marquardt, Donna Bell Sanders, MPH, Robin Lowney Lankton, MPH, Kimberly Bale, MPH, Tamara Gvozdenovic.

The original manual, *The Basic Health Worker Manual* was written in 1984 by: Phyllis Paxton, Cathy Wiley, Barbara Kass-Annese, Jo-Anne Morrison, Elisa Munoz, Rebecca Murray, Martha Torres, and Gretchen Wooden

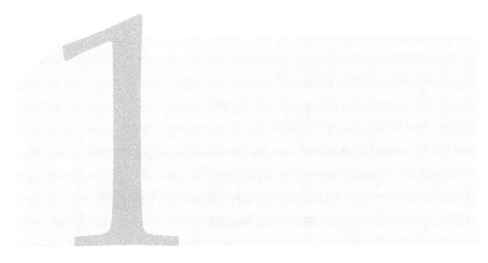

Providing Quality Sexual and Reproductive Health Care

The sexual and reproductive health services you and your team provide should be based on five principles. It is important for you to learn these principles and to know how to help your patients give informed consent.

Here are some key questions that you can help your patients think about. This is often referred to as a Reproductive Life Plan.

- ▸ How many children do I want to have in my lifetime?
- ▸ When do I want to have them?
- ▸ How do I plan to prevent pregnancy until I'm ready?

As a member of the health care team, you can help all patients develop their own Reproductive Life Plan and make the best choices for themselves.

Topics in this chapter

▶ The Principles of Quality Sexual and Reproductive Health Care

- **Principle 1:** People should be able to choose how many children to have and when to have them.

- **Principle 2:** People should be assisted in outlining a Reproductive Life Plan.

- **Principle 3:** People should receive services that are confidential.

- **Principle 4:** People should receive quality health care.

- **Principle 5:** People should receive the information they need to give informed consent.

▶ An Overview of Informed Consent

- What is informed consent?

- Why is informed consent important?

- Who can give informed consent?

- When does a patient give informed consent?

- How to make sure the patient really understands.

Objectives

After reading this chapter, you will be able to:

▶ Define the main goal of sexual and reproductive health care.

▶ List the five principles of sexual and reproductive health care.

▶ Define Reproductive Life Plan.

▶ Define informed consent.

▶ Explain why it is important to get informed consent for sexual and reproductive health services.

▶ List guidelines for making sure patients coming in for sexual and reproductive health care are giving their informed consent.

Principles of Providing Sexual and Reproductive Health Care

A key part of providing quality sexual and reproductive health care is giving your patients choices. It is important to explain that they are free to choose how many children they want to have and when to have them.

A main goal of sexual and reproductive health services is to help people plan, postpone, or prevent a pregnancy — based on each patient's own Reproductive Life Plan and family planning goals.

Another goal of sexual and reproductive health services is to improve the overall health of patients.

Sexual and reproductive health care includes many services to help patients meet their goals. These services include:

- Education about and providing birth control methods
- Pregnancy testing and counseling
- Pap tests, breast exams, and pelvic exams
- Testicular and prostate exams

Other services may include:

- Testing, treatment for, and prevention of sexually transmitted infections (STIs), including HIV
- Preconception care counseling and education
- Infertility testing, treatment, and education
- Referrals to other services, such as prenatal care, domestic violence assistance, or drug and alcohol abuse treatment, and referring for or collaborating with needed primary care services

Sexual and reproductive health services are based on five basic principles. When you understand these principles, you can provide better services to your patients. These principles guide all that is done in health care settings that include sexual and reproductive health care. Health care staff rely on these principles to help them meet the needs of their patients.

Principle 1:

People should be able to choose how many children to have and when to have them.

People have the right to choose when and if they want to have children. This means that all people should be allowed to safely and effectively plan, prevent, or end a pregnancy. And it also means everyone should have access to sexual and reproductive health services including all legal forms of birth control.

A key piece of this principle is that sexual and reproductive health decisions must be voluntary — not forced. People need to be able to make their choices freely, without pressure from friends, family members, or health care staff. Everyone has the right to make these choices for themselves, except when legally unable to make decisions. In these cases, a guardian or a court of law is allowed to make decisions for them.

Principle 2:

People should be assisted in outlining a Reproductive Life Plan.

A Reproductive Life Plan (RLP) is a person's current and/or future plan or desire for pregnancy. RLP questions are asked to find out when and if a patient might want to become a parent. This conversation may include a discussion about their education/career goals, health conditions or other life goals.

Benefits of Discussing Reproductive Goals/Pregnancy Intention

Starting a conversation about when and if a patient might want to become pregnant can be a useful way to guide the visit. This information can lead to a discussion about contraception or preconception care. For patients who want a pregnancy in the near future, it is important to address health conditions, substance use, and steps to support a healthy pregnancy. For those who do not want a pregnancy you can discuss contraceptive options. Additionally, this conversation is a patient-centered way to build rapport with patients.

Two Techniques for Discussing Reproductive Goals/Pregnancy Intention

One Key Question:

> *"Would you like to become pregnant in the next year?"*

One Key Question is a screening tool that can help identify patients in need of contraception or preconception care. You can ask patients of reproductive age who can get pregnant this question as a routine part of any health care visit.

- If the patient answers "yes", discuss preconception care, including; taking folic acid, managing medical conditions and medications, and addressing substance use.

- If the patient answers "no", discuss contraceptive methods.

- If the patient answers "unsure" or "ok either way" ask how they might feel if they became pregnant in the next year. Be prepared to discuss both contraception and preconception care.

The PATH Questions

The PATH questions can be used with patients of any gender and sexual orientation. The **PATH** acronym can help you remember the questions.

Pregnancy/Parenthood/Attitudes

"Do you think you might like to have (more) children at some point?"

Timing

"When do you think that might be?"

How important

"How important is it to you to prevent pregnancy (until then)?"

Principle 3:

People should receive services that are confidential.

Sexual and reproductive health care covers some of the most personal aspects of a person's life. Patients are often asked to talk about their sex lives or their bodies. Many patients may not feel comfortable talking about these things. Do everything you can to help your patients feel comfortable.

Patients need to know that their personal information is protected by law. Explain that almost everything shared between a patient and the health care team is confidential. That means it is *private*. It may be shared with members of the health care team who need the information. Verbal or written patient information in most cases, cannot be given to others without the patient's consent.

Tell patients that there are some limits to confidentiality. Some things a patient tells you may need to be reported to Child Protective Services (CPS) or to the police. This is especially true when someone's health or well-being is at stake.

But, in general, everything a patient tells you is confidential.

▸ **Make sure you talk with your patient in a private place.** Do not talk in hallways, in the waiting room, or in any public place. These are not confidential places to talk with patients about sexual and reproductive health issues.

▸ **Share patient information only when it is necessary for the health care of the patient.** You must inform the medical provider about patient issues such as rape, substance use, and so on. You might also need to talk with a co-worker about a patient's health care issue to provide necessary services or referrals. This is not breaking confidentiality.

▸ **Be appropriate if you need to vent about a patient.** One way to let off steam about a patient is to talk to a supervisor in a private place. Remember that there is a difference between venting and gossiping. If you need to discuss something about a patient, be professional in your choice of place and limit the number of staff members who might hear. Don't use patient names or identifying information unless there is a valid need to do so.

▸ **Think before you speak.** A patient's information may come up in a conversation in the lunchroom, lab area, or other place. Before you speak about a patient, ask yourself, "Does this member of the health care team need to know about this? Are there staff or other people who may overhear what I am saying?" If you really need to talk, but there is no privacy, set up a different time and place to talk later.

> **Limits to confidentiality**
>
> Each state and county has its own laws about what you must report. Talk to your supervisor about what laws apply to your health center. Before you ask your patients personal questions, make sure they know what you must report.

▸ **Always keep the confidentiality of patients.** Let patients know you can be trusted. When you are out in the community, always let patients greet you before you say anything to them.

Principle 4:

People should receive quality health care.

Sexual and reproductive health care services are the main source of health care for many people. Their sexual and reproductive health care visits may be the only time they see a health care provider. The regular health screening they get at their visit can help them identify or receive treatment for health problems they may not have known about.

Each health care setting has its own policies and procedures that must be followed. Programs that get government funds must also follow specific state and/or federal guidelines. These guidelines are designed to make sure that basic quality standards are met.

Whatever their cultural or language background, patients have a right to quality services. Most health care settings have policies on how to meet the special cultural or language needs of their patients. As a member of the health care team, you will want to find out how your health care site handles these special needs.

Talk to your supervisor to learn about the policies and procedures at your health care setting. Quality health care programs ensure that:

▸ Program staff have proper training and skills.

▸ Patients get comprehensive health education, prevention, and treatment services at their health care setting or by referral.

▸ Services are explained so that a patient can give informed consent.

▸ Services are given in a language that the patient understands and in a way that respects their culture and background.

Principle 5:

People should receive the information they need to give informed consent.

People need correct and complete information in a way they can understand to make wise choices. Patients can only freely consent to a medical decision (like choosing a birth control method) *after* getting the information they need. Patients also have the right not to give their consent. They can also change their minds at any time. These choices should not affect the health care services they get.

This is true for all medical services. The law requires members of the health care team to get informed consent from patients *before* the service or treatment is given.

Patient education sessions and educational materials help patients give informed consent. For example, if you are counseling your patients about their birth control options you want to help them:

▸ Find out about the many different birth control methods they can choose from.

▸ Learn about their options.

▸ Learn about the major risks and benefits of their choice.

It is important to give your patients complete and correct information in an unbiased way. Your own ideas about what might be the best method aren't as important as what patients think would be right for them. Do not pressure patients. Patients must be free to make their own choices. A patient's choice should be based on the facts and their own Reproductive Life Plan, not on your personal opinion or beliefs.

If patients don't get correct and unbiased information, they can't freely make decisions regarding their sexual and reproductive health.

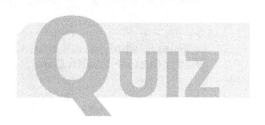

UIZ

Principles of Sexual and Reproductive Health Care

Directions: Read each of the following and write your best answer in the space below.

1. What are the main goals of sexual and reproductive health care services?

    _____

    _____

    _____

    _____

2. What are the five principles of sexual and reproductive health care?

    ▪ _____

    _____

    ▪ _____

    _____

    ▪ _____

    _____

    ▪ _____

    _____

    ▪ _____

    _____

Go on to the next page.

3. What is a Reproductive Life Plan?

_____

_____

Directions: Draw a line from the statement on the left to the principle on the right that it is based on.

Statement

4. Patients can only freely consent to a medical decision (like choosing a birth control method) *after* getting the information they need.

5. Program staff should have proper training and skills in sexual and reproductive health care.

6. Health care team members should not pressure patients to use birth control.

7. Verbal or written patient information, in most cases, cannot be given to others without the patient's consent.

8. Health care team members can help a patient think through their personal life goals about having, delaying (or not having) children.

Principle

a. **Right to choose** how many children to have and when to have them

b. **Right to get the info** they need to give informed consent

c. **Right to confidentiality**

d. **Right to quality health care**

e. **Reproductive Life Plan**

Check your answers on the next page.

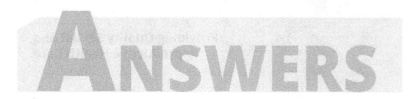
ANSWERS

Principles of Sexual and Reproductive Health Care

Check your answers.

1. The main goals of sexual and reproductive health care services are to help each patient plan, postpone, or prevent a pregnancy based on their Reproductive Life Plan.

2. The five principles of sexual and reproductive health care are:
   - People should be able to choose how many children to have and when to have them.
   - People should be assisted in outlining their Reproductive Life Plan.
   - People should receive services that are confidential.
   - People should receive quality health care.
   - People should receive the information they need to give informed consent.

3. A Reproductive Life Plan (RLP) is a set of personal goals about when or if a person wants to have children.

4. **B** **Principle 2:** "Patients can only freely consent to a medical decision (like choosing a birth control method)" *after* getting the information they need. This is based on the patient's right to get the information they need to give informed consent.

5. **D** **Principle 4:** "Program staff should have proper training and skills" is based on the patient's right to quality health care.

6. **A** **Principle 1:** "Health care team members should not pressure patients to use birth control" is based on the patient's right to choose how many children to have and when to have them.

7. **C** **Principle 3:** "Verbal or written patient information, in most cases, cannot be given to others without the patient's consent" is based on the patient's right to receive services that are confidential.

8. **E** **Principle 5:** "Health care team members can help a patient think through their personal goals about having (or not having) children" as part of discussing a Reproductive Life Plan.

An Overview of Informed Consent

In this section we focus on informed consent as it relates to birth control methods. Birth control methods, services, and treatments can only be given to patients who consent (give their permission). The law protects patients from having anything done to them without their consent. Patients must give their consent *before* they receive birth control methods, services, or treatments.

As part of the health care team, you play a key role in making sure patients get the information they need to truly give their informed consent.

What is informed consent?

When patients give their *informed consent* for a method, service, or treatment, they are saying that:

▸ They have been given the key facts needed to make an informed decision about their health care.

▸ They fully understand those facts.

▸ They freely agree to the method, service, or treatment.

To do this, patients must get all the information they need to make an educated decision.

The idea behind informed consent is that patients have the right to decide what happens to them. It is always the patient's right to *consent* to or *refuse* any method of birth control, service, or treatment.

Why is informed consent important?

A patient's informed consent is important for many reasons. Some of these reasons are legal. Others are ethical or practical reasons.

Legal Reasons

In the United States, laws protect a patient's right to make an informed choice about medical care. The laws say that health care providers must make sure that each patient makes an informed decision about their own care. If a person is harmed by a service and was not fully informed of the chances for harm (risks), the provider may be legally responsible. This can be very costly to the provider.

Age of consent

Each state has its own laws about how old a patient must be to give consent. The age a patient needs to be in order to give consent for services can vary depending on the type of services given. It can also vary depending on who funds those services.

A state or funder may have a different age requirement for each of the following types of services:

- Birth control

- STI screening and treatment

- Abortion

- Sterilization

- Rape-related services

- Drug-related services

Be sure to talk to your supervisor about the laws and rules that apply at your health care setting.

Providers need to have a signed informed consent form showing that a patient agreed to the medical care they receive after being fully informed.

Ethical Reasons

It is the right thing to do. We want patients to fully understand the kind of care they are getting.

Sexual and reproductive health services are based on patients' rights. The most important of these is the patients' right to choose what happens to their bodies. This includes the right to freely choose whether and when to have children. Patients should always be able to make their own family planning choices. To do this, they need to know the facts.

Practical Reasons

When patients fully understand and freely choose a birth control method, they are more likely to use their method well. They are also more likely to keep using it. And if their method doesn't work out, they are more likely to return to the health care site for a different one.

Who can give informed consent?

In most cases, only the person receiving services (the patient) can give consent for that service. To give informed consent, patients must make their choices without pressure from others. Patients have the right to decide for themselves.

A patient's spouse or parent *cannot* give informed consent for the patient. Neither can anyone on the health care team. Again, it is the patient's right to freely decide whether to use a birth control method and which one to use.

Many patients like to consult with other people before making decisions. Some patients want to talk with a partner or family member before giving their consent. Still others may want to talk with friends. Encourage them to get the help and support they need.

When does a patient give informed consent?

There are two rules for when a patient gives informed consent.

1. **Patients can only give informed consent after they understand the method, service, or treatment.**

   You must give your patients complete and true information in a way that they understand. You must give them a chance to ask questions and get answers. Only then can they give their informed consent.

Exceptions: Legal Guardians and Courts of Law

In rare cases, a **legal guardian** or a **court of law** can give informed consent for patients who cannot give their own consent. A legal guardian is someone who has been given the right by a court of law to handle another person's affairs. In some cases, the court makes the decision instead of a legal guardian.

2. **Patients must give their informed consent before they get the method, service, or treatment.**

Patients must give informed consent *before* they are given a method, service, or treatment. It is their right and the law.

How to make sure the patient really understands

To make sure patients understand, you need to do more than just tell or give patients information about their birth control options. You need to talk back and forth and have a conversation. You need to share information. You also need to ask questions to make sure patients understand the information. When you ask questions, it encourages patients to ask their own questions and to take part in finding out what they need to know to make an informed choice.

Here are seven guidelines for getting informed consent from your patients.

1. Make sure patients have a chance to find out basic information about all of the birth control methods.

Patients need to know their options for birth control. They also need to be able to compare the methods that are available to them. Make sure that your patients know basic information about all of the birth control methods.

Patients can get this information in many ways. You don't have to present all of it yourself. For example, patients can watch a video or read a pamphlet or an information sheet. But patients do need to have a chance to discuss their choices and questions with you.

Here are the basic facts a patient should have available for them about each method:

▸ What it is and how it works

▸ How well it works and how long it lasts

▸ Advantages and disadvantages to using the method

▸ How well it fits with the patient's Reproductive Life Plan

2. Be sure your patients *fully* understand the details of the method they choose.

Once patients understand all of their options, they can choose the method they think will be best for them. They will then need more detail about the method they choose. Here is what patients must understand about their method before they use it:

▸ What it is

▸ How it works

▸ How to use it

▸ How long it works

▸ What they need to do to have it work

▸ How well it works (how effective it is)

▸ Side effects (minor reactions or body changes that could happen because a method is used)

Patients also need to know about:

▸ Complications (rare, but serious, health problems that could happen because a method is used)

▸ Warning signs (physical signs that warn of a complication)

▸ Advantages and disadvantages of using the method

▸ What to do if they want to stop using the method

For some methods, patients must know about getting them fitted or placed. For example, a provider needs to fit the diaphragm so the patient gets the correct size. Other methods, like an intra-uterine device (IUD), need to be placed in the uterus by a trained health care provider.

About Warning Signs

Some methods have warning signs. Patients must know how to watch out for these. Warning signs are physical changes in the body that could mean the method is causing a serious health problem (a complication).

Complications are rare, but they do happen. Patients must know what to do if they have any of the warning signs. This may mean going to the health care site or getting emergency care. Tell them how, when, and where to get emergency care if they need it.

3. Make sure you give patients the information they need in a way that honors their beliefs and values.

Be aware that each person you serve is unique. Learn about the various ethnic communities your health care setting serves. Make sure that the care and information you give reflects, honors, and respects the beliefs and values of those communities.

It is important not to assume that your patients think just like you. Everyone's culture, family dynamics, religious beliefs, and educational levels are different. It is also important to realize that patients from the same ethnic group do not all think alike and that there may be important differences from one person to the next. Treat your patients with respect and as individuals.

4. Tell patients about their method and give them information in writing.

Talk with each patient about the details of their chosen method. Use plain, everyday words to explain these details. Find out what language they feel most comfortable speaking. Explain the details in that language if you can or get the help of a trained interpreter.

Also give patients the information in writing at a reading level and in a language they can understand.

Keep these things in mind when giving your patients information:

▶ It is important to give patients written information in the language they feel most comfortable reading. Even if they are speaking English with you, they may prefer to read in the language they speak at home. Ask your patients what language they would prefer reading and note it in their chart. Try to find materials that will meet their needs.

▶ Most patients appreciate having information given to them in easy-to-read, plain, everyday language. Make sure the information you give them fits their reading level. Many patients you see read comfortably at the 5th grade reading level or lower.

▶ Even if patients read very well, it does not mean that they can easily understand the vocabulary used. Most patients will appreciate getting information that is easy to read.

▶ If any of your patients have a hard time reading, you can read the printed information to them. You still need to make sure the information is written at a level they can understand.

Some patients may have special needs. Ask your supervisor how your health care team helps meet those needs. Here are some other suggestions:

▶ If a patient is deaf or hard-of-hearing, you can use pictures and printed information to share ideas. If needed, use a sign-language interpreter to translate the session.

▶ If a patient is blind or can't see well, brochures or pictures may not work. Instead, use audio or read the information to the patient. Or use models that can be touched. A magnifying glass or materials with large print may help some patients. Use Braille materials for patients who read Braille.

▶ If a patient has a learning disability, intellectual disability, head injury, mental illness, use simple language, pictures, and models.

▶ If there is a language or communication barrier, find ways to provide patients with the information they need in a way they can understand.

5. Give patients a chance to ask questions and get answers.

Encourage your patients to ask questions. Sometimes they won't know that it is okay. Or they might feel embarrassed about not knowing the answer. You can help them feel more comfortable. Always honor each patient's values, beliefs, and ways of looking at things. Tell your patients that it is good to ask questions.

Every question needs a correct answer. If you don't know the answer, tell your patient that you don't know. Refer the patient to someone who does know. Or research the answer and tell the patient later. The main thing is to only give correct information. Never guess.

Try to make sure patients get all of the correct information they need before they leave your health care site.

Sometimes information about the benefits or risks of a method changes after a patient begins using the method. Patients should be given this new information when they return for their next visit.

Keep yourself up to date on changes in birth control information. That way you can keep your patients well informed.

6. Tell your patients they can stop using their method at any time.

When you provide quality education about birth control methods, patients are more likely to choose a method they will want to keep using for a while. But patients have a right to stop or change their method at any time.

Patients may change their minds while learning how to use a chosen method. Sometimes a health care provider may find medical reasons why a patient should not use the chosen method. More often, patients may use a method for a while and then decide that it isn't right for them.

A patient's decision to stop using a method should not affect the quality of health care the health center provides. However, it is important to let them know that they can get pregnant, often immediately, if they stop using their method and do not use another one.

7. Make sure your patient signs any required consent forms.

The final step in the informed consent process is signing the consent form, if necessary. Keep the following things in mind:

▸ Consent forms should be easy to read. That way, most patients can understand them.

▸ If patients don't read well, someone must read the form to them. Or sometimes consent forms that are audio or video recorded can be used.

▸ Written consent forms should be in a language the patient understands.

▸ After a patient signs the consent form, put or scan it in to the patient's medical record. This gives you a record of the informed consent. Some health care settings also give patients a copy of the consent form.

Remember, just signing a written consent form is not the same as giving informed consent.

All seven of these guidelines must be followed to meet the standards for true informed consent. Patients must choose to give consent of their own free will.

Guidelines may differ. Check the policies at your health care setting for guidelines on informed consent and the use of consent forms.

Seven guidelines for getting a patient's informed consent

1. Make sure your patients have had a chance to find out about all of the birth control methods they can choose from.

2. Make sure your patients fully understand their chosen method.

3. Make sure you give patients the information they need in a way that honors their beliefs and values.

4. Tell your patients all about their chosen method *and* give them information about it in writing.

5. Let your patients ask questions and get answers about any of the methods, services, or treatments.

6. Tell your patients they can stop using a method at any time.

7. Make sure your patients sign any required consent form that says they understand the information described, and that they give consent to use the chosen method.

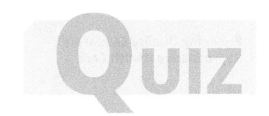

An Overview of Informed Consent

Directions: Read each of the following, and write your best answer in the space below.

1. What does informed consent mean?

    _____

    _____

    _____

2. What are three types of reasons for getting informed consent from patients? One is given to you. What are two more?

    ▪ Legal Reasons _____

    ▪ _____

    ▪ _____

Directions: Read each of the following statements. Is it true or false? Circle the best answer.

3. Patients only need to know about some birth control methods, not all of them.   **True   False**

4. Patients should fully understand the method of birth control they choose. This means they must know what it is, how it works, how to use it, how well it works, how long it works, side effects, complications, warning signs, advantages and disadvantages, and how to stop using the method.   **True   False**

Go on to the next page.

5. Individuals from the same ethnic groups all think alike about the different forms of birth control.　　True　False

6. Patients should be told in-depth information about their chosen birth control method. They should also receive this information in writing.　　True　False

7. You should encourage your patients to ask questions.　　True　False

8. Patients can only change their birth control method once a year at their annual exam.　　True　False

9. It doesn't matter if the patient really understands a method or not. As long as the patient signs a consent form, they can start using a new birth control method.　　True　False

Check your answers on the next page.

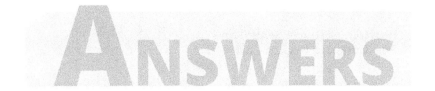

An Overview of Informed Consent

Check your answers.

1. Informed consent means patients must get all the information they need to make an educated decision. When patients give informed consent for a method, service, or treatment, it means that they know the key facts about it and that they freely agree to it.

2. Three types of reasons for getting informed consent from patients are:

   - **Legal Reasons**
     In the U.S., laws protect a patient's right to make an informed choice about medical care. The laws say that health care providers must make sure that each patient makes an informed decision about their own care.
     If a person is harmed by a service and was not fully informed of the chances for harm (risks), the provider may be legally responsible. This can be very costly to the provider. Providers need to have a signed informed consent form showing that a patient agreed to the medical care after being fully informed.

   - **Ethical Reasons**
     Sexual and reproductive health care services are based on patients' rights and the law. The most important of these is the patients' right to choose what happens to their bodies. This includes the right to freely choose whether and when to have children. Patients should always be able to make their own family planning choices. To do this, they need to know the facts.

   - **Practical Reasons**
     When patients fully understand and freely choose a birth control method, they are more likely to use their method well. They are also more likely to keep using it. And if their method doesn't work out, they are more likely to return to the health center for a different one.

Go on to the next page.

3. **False**   Make sure your patients know about *all* of their options for birth control. And they need to be able to compare all of the methods. Make sure that your patients know basic information about all of the birth control methods.

4. **True**   Be sure your patients *fully* understand the details of the method they choose.

5. **False**   All patients from the same ethnic group do *not* think alike. There may be important differences from one person to the next. Treat your patients with respect and as individuals.

6. **True**   Give your patients details about their chosen method. You should also give them information in writing.

7. **True**   Always give patients a chance to ask questions and get answers.

8. **False**   Tell your patients they can stop using their method at *any* time. It is their right to stop using a method of birth control and to start using a new method.

9. **False**   Remember, just signing a written consent form is *not* the same as giving informed consent. All seven of the informed consent guidelines *must* be followed to meet the standards for true informed consent. Patients must choose to give consent of their own free will.

Providing Quality Sexual and Reproductive Health Care

Directions: Circle the answer that best completes each sentence or fills in the blanks.

1. A main goal of sexual and reproductive health care services is to:

   a. Tell patients they shouldn't have any more children.

   b. Help patients plan, postpone, or prevent a pregnancy — based on their Reproductive Life Plan.

   c. Work with the government to limit population growth.

2. The principles of sexual and reproductive health care include the right to receive:

   a. Information needed to give informed consent

   b. Quality health care

   c. Confidential services

   d. All of the above

3. Patients can give informed consent for a medical decision _____ they get all the information about it, and _____ the service or method is given.

   a. after, after

   b. before, before

   c. after, before

   d. before, after

Go on to the next page.

4. Health care team members should not share patient information. Patient information is considered to be _____.

   a. confidential

   b. private, unless the patient's spouse wants to know

   c. public knowledge

   d. none of the above

5. _____ is when patients know the key facts about a method, service, or treatment, and they freely agree to it.

   a. Understanding

   b. Informed consent

   c. Mandatory reporting

   d. Refusal

6. In general, the _____ is the only one who can consent to or refuse any kind of birth control.

   a. patient's spouse

   b. patient's parent

   c. patient's doctor

   d. patient

7. In rare cases, a _____ or a _____ can give informed consent for patients who cannot give their own consent.

   a. friend, nurse

   b. legal guardian, court of law

   c. family planning counselor, doctor

   d. all of the above

Go on to the next page.

8. The one statement below that is not a guideline for getting a patient's informed consent is:

   a. Make sure your patients have had a chance to find out about all of the birth control methods they can choose from.

   b. Make sure your patients fully understand their chosen method.

   c. Make sure you give patients the information they need in a way that honors their beliefs and values.

   d. Tell your patients all about their chosen method and give them information about it in writing.

   e. Let your patients ask questions and get answers about any of the methods, services, or treatments.

   f. Make sure your patient's sexual partner agrees to the method, service, or treatment.

   g. Tell your patients they can stop using a method at any time.

   h. Make sure your patients sign any required form that says they understand the information described and that they give consent to use the chosen method.

Check your answers on the next page.

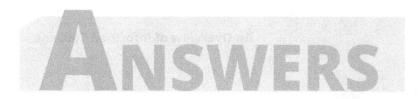
ANSWERS

Providing Quality Sexual and Reproductive Health Care

Check your answers.

1. **B** A main goal of sexual and reproductive health care is to help patients plan, postpone, or prevent a pregnancy — based on each patient's own Reproductive Life Plan.

2. **D** All of the above. The principles of sexual and reproductive health care include the right to receive:
   - Information and give informed consent
   - Quality health care
   - Confidential services

3. **C** Patients can give informed consent for a medical decision *after* they get all the information about it, but *before* the service or method is given.

4. **A** Health care team members should not share patient information. Their information is considered to be *confidential*.

5. **B** *Informed consent* is when patients know the key facts about a method, service, or treatment, and they freely agree to it.

6. **D** It is the *patient* who can consent to or refuse any kind of birth control.

7. **B** In rare cases, a *legal guardian* or a *court of law* can give informed consent for patients who cannot give their own consent.

8. **F** This is the one statement that is not a guideline for getting a patient's informed consent. A patient's sexual partner does not need to agree to the method, service, or treatment the patient chooses.

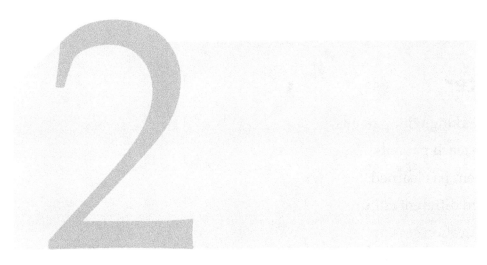

Patient Education

Helping to educate your patients is one of the most important things you will do as a member of the health care team. The good news is that there are proven ways to do this well. You will read about many of them in this chapter.

There are three basic elements to good patient education. *Giving* accurate information is one. But that is just the start. *How* you give that information is just as important. And equally important is making sure your patient really **understands** the information.

This chapter will help you build on skills you already have to become an excellent educator. It covers the basic skills you will need to communicate well. It also discusses a variety of teaching and evaluation methods you can use and hints for working with patients from different cultures. You will see these skills put to use in the overview of the four stages of a typical patient education session. Finally, you will learn how to write an education plan to prepare for your sessions.

In short, this chapter gives you a guide to the flow of a patient education session and the skills you will want to draw upon. It prepares you for later chapters where you will learn more details about the topics you will cover and how to cover them.

Patient education is about:

- Giving correct information.
- How you give the information.
- Making sure the patient understands.

Topics in this chapter

▸ Learning basic skills for working with patients

▸ Learning different ways to teach patients

▸ Evaluating what your patient has learned

▸ Working with patients from different cultures

▸ Four stages of a patient education session

- **Stage 1:** Preparing to meet your patient
- **Stage 2:** Helping your patient feel comfortable
- **Stage 3:** Sharing information so your patient can make decisions
- **Stage 4:** Wrapping up your session

▸ Four parts of an education plan

- Objectives
- Content
- Teaching methods and materials
- Evaluation questions

Objectives

By the end of this chapter, you will be able to:

▸ Show how to actively listen to patients.

▸ List three useful ways to teach patients.

▸ Describe how to evaluate the patient's learning throughout an education session.

▸ List two things you can do to work better with people from other cultures.

▸ Describe the four stages of an education session.

Learning Basic Skills for Working with Patients

Patient education is not as simple as giving the patient information. Your goal is to have your patients leave your session with the information and skills they need to make informed choices and use their birth control method successfully.

It is important to:

- Develop good listening skills.
- Ask questions.
- Talk in a way that patients understand.

Learning these basic skills will help make your job easier.

Develop good listening skills

It is important to pay attention to what patients are really saying. Actively listening to your patients is a skill that you will want to practice. Each time you work with a patient you will be learning how to do it better.

Active listening includes so much more than just hearing words. It includes paying attention to the meaning of the words you hear and to what the patient's body language is saying. It also includes using your words and body language in a way that lets the patient know you have understood.

Pay attention to non-verbal cues.

All of us use more than just words to let others know what we mean and feel. There is meaning in how we say something. There is also meaning in what we do with our bodies while we speak or while we are silent (body language).

These ways of giving meaning without words are called "non-verbal cues." People often say more with non-verbal cues than they do with their words alone. Non-verbal cues include facial expressions, eye position, posture, and body movements.

Pay attention to these cues. If a patient appears anxious or nervous, ask how they feel. You may find that they are nervous about having a pap smear. Or they may tell you that they just got a traffic ticket on the way to the health care site. Whatever it is, take a little time to talk about it. It is hard for patients to focus if their minds are on something else.

Educator Tip

The meaning of body language might change from culture to culture.

For instance, in some cultures it is rude to look someone right in the eyes. In other cultures, it is rude not to make eye contact. Try to take your cues from your patient.

Your non-verbal cues also carry a lot of meaning for patients. When you nod your head, patients may feel understood. Smiling and leaning slightly toward your patients as they talk can show warmth and caring. These non-verbal messages go a long way toward building trust with patients.

It is important to send supportive messages.

▶ **Look at your patients when they are talking and give them your full attention.** For example, if you check your watch, patients may think that you don't care about them. If you read the chart while they are talking, they may think you are not listening.

▶ **Have an interested and non-judgmental expression.** Patients may be hurt or clam up if you frown, roll your eyes in disgust, or sigh heavily as though you are bored.

▶ **Keep an open and relaxed posture.** If you cross your arms or rest your face on your hands, your patient may think you are angry or bored.

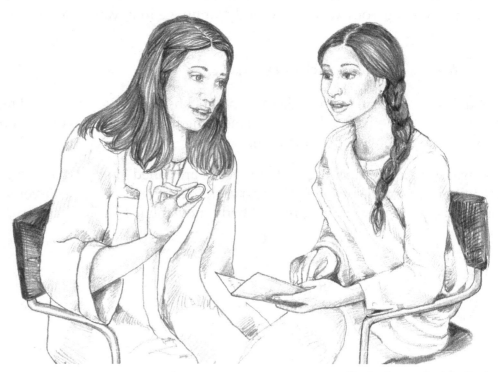

Make sure that you have understood what was said.

Tell the patient what you heard or understood. This is called active listening. This can be done in different ways:

- ▶ You might repeat what your patient said word for word.

- ▶ You might put what you heard in your own words or summarize the most important points. For example, when a patient tells you a story with lots of details, listen for the most important points of the story. Tell your patient those points. Find out if you understood correctly.

- ▶ You can reflect back your patient's feelings. For example, if the patient sighs a lot and has red-rimmed eyes, they might seem really sad. You can say that they seem sad to you. They may in fact be sad. Or may be having an allergy attack. By bringing it up, you may find out what is really happening with your patient.

Doing these things helps you know whether you have understood your patient. If you haven't understood, it gives the patient a chance to make things clearer.

> **Active Listening**
>
> To use active listening, you can:
>
> - Tell the patient exactly what you heard, word for word.
>
> - Summarize for the patient what you heard.
>
> - Reflect back the feelings you saw and heard from the patient.

Ask questions

It is important to ask questions. Questions have many uses in patient education. They help you:

- ▶ Get important information from patients.

- ▶ Find out what services patients want or what problems they are having.

- ▶ Find out how they are feeling

- ▶ Explore patients' feelings or concerns.

- ▶ Find out whether a patient has learned new information and skills during your patient education session.

Following are some basic tips that can help.

Ask only one question at a time.

If you ask more than one question at a time, the patient may not know which one to answer. And you may not know which one is being answered.

Example:

You say, "Have you decided to use the ring? Do you know anything about it?" and the patient answers, "No."

You won't know whether the patient is saying, "No, I haven't decided to use the ring" or "No, I don't know anything about it."

Ask open-ended questions.

Open-ended questions are questions that can't be answered with a "yes" or a "no" or with a few words. These kinds of questions encourage patients to give as much information as they would like to give. Open-ended questions are a great way to help you figure out a patient's needs.

Examples:

- "What brings you here today?"
- "How do you feel about being examined today?"
- "What are some ways you can protect yourself from getting a sexually transmitted infection?"

Use closed-ended questions when you need a specific answer.

Closed-ended questions can be answered with "yes" or "no" or with only one or a few words. These are often used to get specific answers.

Examples:

- "Is this the first time you've had a pelvic exam?"
- "Are you using a method of birth control?"
- "When did you start your last menstrual period?"

Both open-ended and closed-ended questions are useful.

- ▶ If you need a fact from a patient, such as the date of their last period, a closed-ended question works well.

- ▶ If you want a patient to describe a thought, feeling, or what has happened to them, open-ended questions are the best choice.

Don't ask leading questions.

Leading questions are questions asked in a way that suggests what you think the "correct" answer is. When you ask leading questions, patients will sometimes give the answer they think you want to hear.

Example:

If you say, "You only have sex with your spouse, don't you?" you are telling the patient that you think the "correct" answer is "yes." So, to please you, they might answer "yes" even if they are also having sex with someone else.

You can help prevent this by more carefully wording your questions.

Example:

You are more likely to get a truthful answer if you change your question to, "How many partners have you had sex with in the last month?"

Talk in a way that patients understand

The way you talk with patients and the words you choose are very important. To communicate well, speak in ways that patients understand. To learn, patients must understand what you are saying. Here are some tips to help you speak in a way that your patients will understand.

Take your time.

It can help to spend just a little more time with each patient. Don't be in a hurry. This will help your patients feel more relaxed and able to ask questions.

Speak the same language or find someone who can.

If you have patients who don't understand the language you speak, make sure they get help in their own languages. This could be from another health worker who speaks the language or from you with the help of a trained interpreter. To keep your patients' confidentiality, do not ask their friends or family members to interpret.

Find out your health care setting's procedure for meeting the language needs of a patient. Ideally, any special needs will be marked on the chart or electronic health record (EHR) when the patient sets up the appointment. That way, arrangements can be made to have someone who speaks their language available.

Use plain, everyday language. Try to use terms our patients know.

Try not to use technical medical words. Think about how you would explain things to your own friends or family members. When you need to use technical words or words that may be new to the patient, make sure you explain their meanings clearly. Never assume a patient knows a given term.

Listen to the words that your patient uses. This can help you learn what types of words your patient is comfortable with. Then use those words if you can.

Use familiar examples.

When you use examples, it helps your patients understand new words and concepts. Use examples that your patients can relate to or that are familiar to them. You can suggest things that may fit in with the patient's way of life.

Example:

You are talking to a patient about when to take the pill each day. Find out what your patient does at about the same time every day. If they tell you they eat breakfast at the same time every day, you could say, "You may want to take your pill with breakfast."

Use pictures or models.

It can help your patients understand what you are saying if they see it too. Use simple, uncluttered images to explain what you are trying to get across.

Example:

Use simple drawings of the anatomy of a body that can get pregnant to explain how menstruation works or pregnancy can happen. Don't use complicated drawings that show more detail than the patient needs.

Give patients small amounts of information at a time.

It is easier to remember new information when it is given in small amounts. Don't overload patients with too much information at once. Check with them often to make sure they understand. Focus the visit on the most important things the patient needs to walk away knowing.

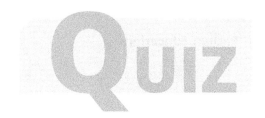

Learning Basic Skills for Working with Patients

Directions: Circle the best answer.

1. Three of these are things you should do when you are with a patient. Which one is something you should **not** do?

   a. Look at your patients when they are talking and give them your full attention.

   b. Have an interested and non-judgmental expression.

   c. Keep an open and relaxed posture.

   d. Update your paperwork while your patients speak to you.

2. How can you show your patient you are listening?

   a. Repeat what your patient just said.

   b. Put what the patient just said in your own words or summarize what was said.

   c. Reflect back to your patient what you think the patient is feeling.

   d. All of the above.

3. Which is an example of an open-ended question?

   a. What do you know about the pill?

   b. How old are you?

   c. Have you ever had an STI?

   d. When was your last menstrual period?

Go on to the next page.

4. What can you do to help your patients better understand you?

   a. Talk quickly because you have a lot of information to cover.

   b. Talk louder if the patient speaks a different language than you do.

   c. Use plain, everyday language to explain things to a patient.

   d. Tell patients only what they need to know and don't bother them with questions.

Directions: Circle all that apply.

5. What are some things that you can do to help educate and counsel your patients?

   a. Have an interested and non-judgmental expression.

   b. Keep an open and relaxed posture.

   c. Ask open-ended questions.

   d. Ask only one question at a time.

   e. Use mostly close-ended questions so you don't have to worry about getting too much information from the patient.

   f. Use a lot of technical medical words.

   g. Use familiar examples.

   h. Use pictures and models.

   i. Give patients small amounts of information at a time.

Check your answers on the next page.

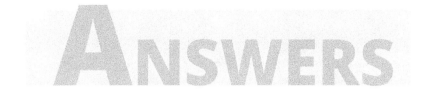
ANSWERS

Learning Basic Skills for Working with Patients

Check your answers.

1. **D**   Do not update your paperwork while your patients speak to you. When you do, it tells the patients that the paperwork is more important than they are. It could also make them feel that they are not being heard.

2. **D**   All of the above. Each of these is a form of active listening:
   - Repeat what your patient just said.
   - Put what the patient just said in your own words or summarize what was said.
   - Reflect back to your patient what you think the patient is feeling.

3. **A**   "What do you know about the pill?" is an open-ended question. It lets patients share a lot of useful information. With closed-ended questions, patients only give very short answers (often one or two words). There are times you need to use closed-ended questions, but most of the time it helps to use open-ended questions.

4. **C**   Your patients will better understand you if you use plain, everyday language to explain things.

5. **A, B, C, D, G, H, I**   You can do any of the following to help educate and counsel your patients:
   - Have an interested and non-judgmental expression.
   - Keep an open and relaxed posture.
   - Ask open-ended questions.
   - Ask only one question at a time.
   - Use familiar examples.
   - Use picture and models.
   - Give patients small amounts of information at a time.

   Using mostly closed-ended questions and a lot of technical medical words doesn't help.

Learning Different Ways to Teach Patients

You want your patients to leave your sessions with more than just information. You want them to leave with the skills they need to use their birth control method successfully.

Learning Styles

People learn best when they:

- Hear it.
- See it.
- Say it.
- Do it.

Each of us is better at some things than at others. This is true of our patients as well. Some may read well. Others may not. Some may like to hear something explained. Others may prefer to see the words written. Some can hear or see something once or twice and remember it. Many cannot.

Each of us has our own favorite learning style — our favorite way of learning. Some prefer to hear something. Others prefer to see it, say it, or do it. No matter what our favorite way of learning is, we each learn best when we do all of these things. Everyone also learns best when involved in the learning process.

To help your patients learn, allow them to use many learning styles and be involved during the session. There are many teaching methods and teaching materials to help you do this.

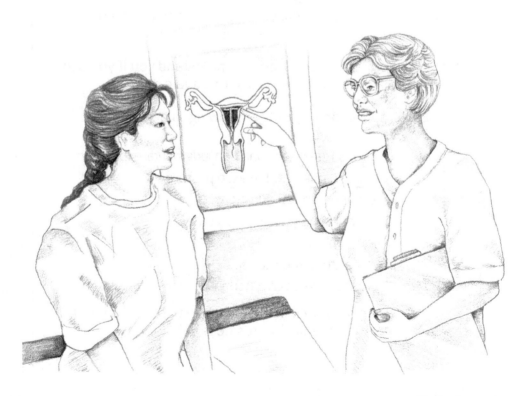

Use many teaching methods

When you use more than one teaching method during a patient education session, you help each patient get involved. You also help the patient use more than one learning style. Both of these help you reach your goal of having your patients leave with the knowledge and skills they need.

Teaching Methods
- Question and answer
- Demonstration
- Role play
- Brainstorm
- Short explanations

Ask questions.

You ask questions and the patient answers. The patient also gets to ask you questions. It is a great way to find out what patients know about a certain topic. This is also a good way to get a discussion going. You can encourage your patients' questions when you:

▸ Show you appreciate their questions. ("I'm glad you asked that.")

▸ Answer every question honestly.

▸ Make sure your patient is satisfied with your answer. ("Did that answer your question?")

If you can't answer a patient's question:

▸ Find out the answer and get back to them.

▸ Make a referral to someone who can answer the question.

Show your patient what you mean.

Show patients how to do the skill. This is called demonstration.

Examples:

- Use a model of a penis to show the patient how to put on and take off the external condom.
- Use a uterus/pelvic model to show how to put in and take out the ring, a diaphragm, the sponge and/or the internal condom.

Try doing a role play.

Doing role plays with your patients is one way to give them a chance to practice a new skill. To help a patient learn a new skill, set up a role play that you act out with them.

Let your patient practice more than once. Pay attention! As the patient practices, give feedback and support.

When you do a role play, it is best to create a situation that is close to what the patient may experience. Let your patient come up with the language or solutions that will work for them.

Example:

If the patient is having trouble talking to their partner about STIs (sexually transmitted infections), you play the partner and let them practice what they could say.

Brainstorm solutions to problems.

Brainstorming can be a useful way to find solutions to problems. When you brainstorm, you just say whatever ideas come to your mind. You don't need to worry about whether the ideas are good or not. After you come up with several ideas, you can talk about them and decide if they might work.

You can help patients plan how to solve problems they may face in the future. Think of a situation in which a problem comes up. Let the patient think out loud about ways to prevent or solve the problem. If the patient gets stuck, you can mention some ideas as well.

Example:

Your patient has chosen to use the birth control pill. Point out that one problem patients sometimes have is forgetting to take one of their pills.

You could say, "What are some ways you could prevent or solve that problem?" Ask them to come up with ideas that they think could work. Here are some suggestions you could use if they have a hard time thinking of ideas on their own:

Educator Tip
Educator Tip Practice makes perfect. We all know it is not always easy to learn new skills. The more we practice, the better. ■ Give your patients a chance to practice their new skills. ■ Always have patients practice their new skills in front of you.

- If you eat breakfast at the same time every day, you could plan to take your pill then.

- Put a note on your bathroom mirror.

- Put a recurring reminder/alarm in your phone.

- Ask your partner to text you a reminder.

- Sign up for a free reminder web or mobile app notification service.

- Find out what to do if you forget to take a pill or call your health care provider for advice.

Give short explanations.

When you explain something to a patient, keep it short. It is best to involve the patient in discussion or demonstrations as much as you can.

Use different kinds of teaching materials

You can also help patients become involved by using different teaching materials. Pictures, brochures, samples of birth control methods, models of the human body, or internet tools can help patients learn new information. You can use these to explain new ideas or to reinforce learning. There are many kinds of teaching materials to choose from. Try to use more than one type of teaching material in each session.

Print materials

Print materials include things like booklets, pamphlets, information sheets, charts, and wallet cards. You can use written information like these as discussion tools with your patients. Choose materials that are accurate, easy to read, appealing to your patients, attractive, and respectful.

Personalize the written material for your patient. You can:

> Refer to it while talking to your patient.

> Circle or highlight important sections.

> Write special instructions or the date of a follow-up appointment on it.

> Put your health care site's telephone number on it.

Encourage your patients to take the material home.

> Ask patients to re-read the material at home to help them remember what you have talked about.

> You might suggest that patients share the information with family members or loved ones.

> You could mention that some patients use the materials to help them talk to their partners.

> Encourage your patient to call if they have any other questions after re-reading it.

Educator Tip

Don't wait until the end of the session to give a pamphlet.

Use the pamphlet during your session. That way you can:

- Personalize the pamphlet.

- Show patients how to find information in the pamphlet.

- Help patients to see the pamphlet as useful.

Visual aids

Remember that people learn best when they use more than one learning style. Visual aids can help with this. Visual aids include brochures, posters, and drawings. You can use visual aids to:

▸ Help patients know what you are talking about.

▸ Reinforce the most important information.

Visual aids let you *say it* and *show it*. When you say **and** show something, the patient is more likely to understand you and remember the information.

> **Use a variety of teaching materials.**
> - Pamphlets or booklets
> - Fact sheets or wallet cards
> - Pictures
> - Flip charts
> - Posters
> - Samples of birth control
> - Models of the human body
> - Video Clips
> - Calendars
> - Smartphones
> - Websites or Apps

Example:

You might need to talk to a patient about their uterus (womb). If you have a drawing of internal reproductive organs, you can point to the uterus. Even if the patient doesn't understand the word you are using, they might recognize it in the drawing. Or perhaps they have heard the word before but thought it was something else. Now when they hear the word, they may think of the drawing you showed them.

Audiovisuals

Many people really like audiovisuals (AVs). These include videos, DVDs, slide shows, mobile applications and websites.

When using audiovisuals:

▸ Always watch the AV before you share it with patients. Make sure it says or shows what you think it should.

▸ Introduce the AV to patients before you show it to them. Explain why you are having them watch it.

▸ Discuss the AV after showing it.

Samples and models

Samples are products that patients can see and touch. For example, a pack of birth control pills or a sample IUD.

Models are copies of things that patients can see and use to practice skills. For example, a model of a uterus or of a penis.

You can use samples and models to:

- ▸ Help patients develop skills.
- ▸ Help patients feel comfortable by allowing them to touch and hold the product.
- ▸ Show patients how to do something.
- ▸ Give patients a chance to practice with your support.

> ### Educator Tip
>
> Have patients use their chosen birth control method with a model. Have them remove it too. Knowing how to remove a birth control method is often as important as learning how to put it on or in.

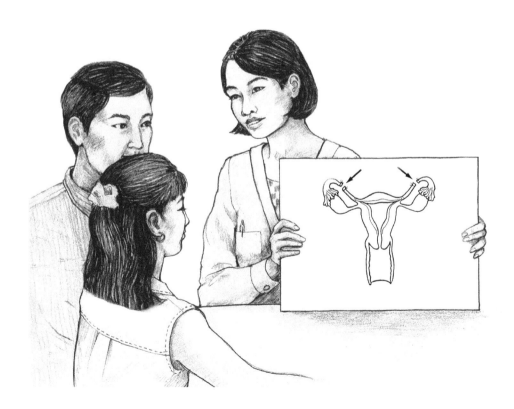

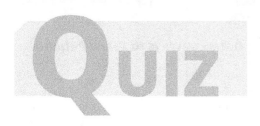

Learning Different Ways to Teach Patients

Directions: Read each of the following statements.
Is it true or false? Circle the best answer.

1. Patients learn best when they use many learning styles and are involved in a session. True False

2. Showing the patient how to do something (demonstration) is a bad way to teach patients. True False

3. If you don't know the answer to a question, make a good guess and tell the patient that. True False

4. Role plays can help your patient practice a new skill. True False

5. Brainstorming is not a good way to find solutions to problems. True False

6. When you explain something to a patient, keep it short. True False

Directions: Write your best answer in the spaces below.

7. List four different types of teaching materials that you could use to help your patients learn.

   - _____

   - _____

   - _____

   - _____

Check your answers on the next page.

Learning Different Ways to Teach Patients

Check your answers.

1. **True**   Patients learn best when they use many learning styles and are involved in a session. There are many teaching methods and teaching materials to help you do this.

2. **False**   Showing the patient how to do something is a very *good* way to teach patients.

3. **False**   If you can't answer a patient's question, ***don't guess.*** Instead:
   - Find out the answer and get back to them.
   - Refer the patient to someone who can answer the question.

4. **True**   Role plays can help your patient practice a new skill.

5. **False**   Brainstorming can be a *good* way to find solutions to problems.

6. **True**   When you explain something to a patient, keep it short. It is best to spend more time involving the patient in discussion or demonstrations when you can.

7. Here are some types of teaching materials you can use to help your patient learn:

   - Pamphlets and booklets
   - Fact sheets and wallet cards
   - Pictures
   - Flip charts
   - Calendars
   - Websites
   - Posters
   - Samples of birth control methods
   - Models of the human body
   - Video Clips
   - Mobile Apps

Evaluating What Your Patient Has Learned

The goal of health education is for patients to be able to keep or improve their health. It is not enough to simply go over the information with your patients. You need to make sure they have understood it. To do this, you evaluate.

This section talks about when and how to evaluate what your patients have learned. It also gives you some simple suggestions for finding out from the patient how well you communicated that information.

When should you evaluate what your patients have learned?

Evaluate your patients' knowledge and skills throughout the patient education session — at the beginning, in the middle, and at the end.

Many patients already know a lot before your session starts. Finding out what patients already know is the first part of evaluation. Then, throughout the session, make sure they understand any new information you give them. Finally, find out what information they know at the end of the session.

At the beginning

Find out what the patient already knows at the beginning of the session.

- Ask what they know about whatever issue they are there for.
- Ask this question *before* you start giving patients any information.

Then build your session around what they still need to learn.

Example:

A patient tells you they want to start using the implant. You need to ask, "What do you know about the implant?"

Maybe the patient knows almost everything they need to know. In that case, you can adjust your teaching plan. You can have the patient tell you about the implant through questions and discussion. You may just need to fill in the gaps and correct any misinformation.

Or maybe the patient has never used the implant before and doesn't know much about it. In this case, you will need to cover more details.

During the session

Evaluate the patient's knowledge and skills many times throughout the session.

- ▶ Find out if the patient understands you.

- ▶ Adjust to the patient's needs. Some patients are quick learners. Others may need extra help learning the main points.

If a patient is unclear about something, make sure they understand it before you give more information. You can repeat what you have said or shown but in a new way. Try using a different teaching method.

Once you know the patient understands that information well, you can go on to the next point.

At the end

Make sure patients know everything they need to know before they leave your session. Review all of the key points even if you checked on those points earlier in the session. Repeating the information can help patients remember it.

> **When to Evaluate**
>
> Evaluate what your patient knows throughout the session:
>
> - At the beginning
> - During
> - At the end

How do you evaluate what your patient has learned?

For you to evaluate what your patients have learned, they need to tell or show you the main points of the session.

There are different ways to find out what patients know or have learned. You can:

- ▶ Ask questions.

- ▶ Have patients show what they have learned.

> **Educator Tip**
>
> Have the patient *tell* you or show you something they need to know.

Ask questions.

Ask questions and listen to the patient's answers. This helps you know what the patient knows or has learned from the session. When you ask evaluation questions, it is usually best to ask open-ended questions. This lets patients give the answers in their own words.

Examples:

Here are some questions you can ask to find out what a patient has learned about birth control pills:

- What is one of the ways the pill works to keep you from getting pregnant?
- What would you do if you forgot to take a pill?
- What are warning signs of serious health problems for the pill?
- If you have any of these warning signs, what should you do?

Do not simply ask, "Do you understand?" Most patients will politely answer "yes" whether they really do or not.

Asking evaluation questions

Instead of asking, "Do you understand?" ask your patients to explain or show you how they will do what they need to do.

If you find they have a hard time doing this, you will know that you need to do more to get the idea across to them.

Try sharing the information again in a different way.

Have patients show you what they have learned.

If patients are already familiar with a skill, ask them to show you how it is done.

Example:

Your patient tells you they know how to use condoms. Give them a new condom and a model of a penis. Ask the patient to show you and tell you how to put on and take off a condom. Watch how they do it. You can let them know if there are any steps they may have missed.

Whenever you demonstrate a new skill, it is important to give your patients a chance to do it themselves. Ask them to show you what they have learned.

Example:

You show a patient how to put in a ring using a pelvic model. After you show them, give them the model and a ring. Ask the patient to tell and show you all the steps for putting a ring in the vagina and taking it out.

Ask your patients for their opinions

At the end of an education session, you can ask patients to talk about how they think you did. Ask them for ideas and suggestions to improve your teaching skills. You might ask, "How could this session have been better for you?"

It is important to:

▸ Welcome and encourage feedback.

▸ Learn ways to improve from the people you are teaching.

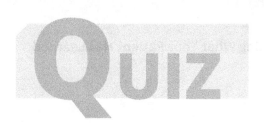

Evaluating What Your Patient Has Learned

Directions: Circle the best answer.

1. When do you evaluate what a patient has learned?
   a. At the beginning of a session
   b. During a session
   c. At the end of a session
   d. All of the above

2. What are good ways to evaluate what patients have learned?
   a. Ask them questions.
   b. Have them tell you what they have just learned.
   c. Have them show you a skill that they have just learned.
   d. All of the above

3. Which question will help you evaluate what the patient has learned?
   a. Do you understand?
   b. Do you have any questions?
   c. How will you use the condom?
   d. Have I explained everything okay?

4. It is important to ask your patient for their opinions because:
   a. It helps you evaluate what the patient has learned.
   b. It can help you improve your teaching skills.
   c. It helps you understand how the patient will use a birth control method.
   d. None of the above

Check your answers on the next page.

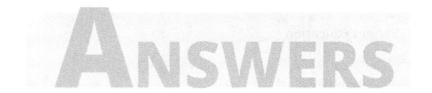

Evaluating What Your Patient Has Learned

Check your answers.

1. **D**   All of the above. Evaluate your patient's knowledge and skills throughout the patient education session: at the beginning, in the middle, and at the end.

   Many patients already know a lot before your session begins. Finding out what patients already know is the first part of evaluation. Then, throughout the session, make sure they understand any new information you give them. Finally, find out what they know at the end of the session.

2. **D**   All of the above. Asking questions and having patients tell or show you what they have learned are good ways to evaluate what the patient knows.

3. **C**   "How will you use the condom?" is a good evaluation question.

   When you ask evaluation questions, it is usually best to ask open-ended questions. This lets patients give answers in their own words. Do not simply ask "Do you understand?" or "Have I explained everything?" Most patients will politely answer "yes" whether they really do or not.

   Likewise, if you ask "Do you have any questions?" they may just say "no." You might try asking, "What other questions do you have?"

4. **B**   Feedback from your patients can help you improve your teaching skills. Always encourage and welcome feedback.

Working with People from Different Cultures

As a member of the health care team, you have the opportunity to work with patients who come from a rich variety of cultures, ethnic groups, and backgrounds. To work with these patients, you will want to:

- Learn about the patients your health care site serves.

- Develop good communication skills.

- Be respectful and non-judgmental.

Culture is made up of the beliefs, values, attitudes, and customs a group of people shares.

An **ethnic group** is a group of people with a common racial, national, or language background.

A person's **background** includes all the things that have influenced them — like culture, gender, economics, education, religion and family interactions.

Learn about the community you serve

Learn as much as you can about the patients your health care site serves. The more you know and understand, the better prepared you will be to meet their needs in a respectful way. And the better your education sessions will be.

You may be surprised by the variety of backgrounds and life experiences your patients bring.

- Some patients may be older and others quite young.

- Your patients may be married, single, monogamous, or have many partners.

- They may be straight, gay, bisexual, or pansexual.

- They may identify as transgender. They may identify as a gender that is different from their sex assigned at birth.

- They may identify as non-binary or non-confirming. Their gender identity falls outside of the male-female binary.

- Some patients may have a physical, visual, hearing, intellectual, or learning disability.

- Your patients may come from many different ethnic, racial, and religious groups.

- Some may have lived in the U.S. their whole lives; others may have been here only a short time.

Your patients may also have had different opportunities for education. Their levels of income may differ as well. Each of these things affects the way your patients may look at the world and approach life.

Working with patients who have different backgrounds offers you a wonderful opportunity to learn about them and the world. One way to learn about patients is to pay attention to what you see and hear when you work with them. Another way is to watch other health workers as they work with their patients. Think about what you notice.

Be sensitive to different communication styles

Good communication is at the center of patient education. It involves more than just talking to patients. It includes listening to and being respectful of their thoughts, feelings, needs, and desires. To do this and to avoid misunderstandings, it helps to be aware of different communication styles.

Everyone's communication style is influenced by their culture and life experiences. For example, your own communication style may be influenced by your family members. But it may also be influenced by your friends, teachers, and coworkers.

When you work with patients, pay attention to all levels of communication — including body language. You may notice many things your patients do that are the result of their culture or life experience.

Examples:

- In some cultures, making eye contact shows interest and caring. In other cultures, eye contact may be seen as a lack of respect. In these cultures, it is more polite not to look directly at a person's eyes.

- How close people stand to one another is also affected by culture. Some patients feel comfortable when you stand close to them. They may even touch you kindly on the arm. Others prefer to keep a physical distance. They may think it is rude to stand too close to or touch a person they don't know well.

Pay attention to different communication styles and behaviors. As you become more aware, you will be better able to understand your patients — and make yourself understood. The more you learn and practice, the easier it will become.

Don't worry. Even when your communication style is different from your patient's, you can probably make yourself understood. The more you learn and practice, the easier it will become. If you make a mistake, relax. When you are sincere in what you say and do, most people will understand.

Educator Tip

Don't be afraid of making mistakes. Everyone makes them. You can learn from your mistakes. And that learning will make you a better health worker.

So find out as much as you can. Observe and ask questions. And enjoy this opportunity to learn about and appreciate the many ways people communicate.

Be respectful and non-judgmental

Our personal backgrounds influence our values and the choices we make. There will be times when you don't share the same values as your patient. That is okay. Always remember that patients have the right to make different choices from the ones you would make. Respect their choices and their views. Don't try to change their views to match your own.

To communicate with respect and in a non-judgmental way, you should:

- ▸ Use words and gestures that show respect for each patient.

- ▸ Try to understand each patient's point of view. Be careful not to judge what a patient says, thinks, or does.

- ▸ Present information and options honestly and fairly so patients can make their own choices.

Example:

A 36-year-old patient wants to use the ring as their birth control method. But they tell you that they feel uncomfortable touching their vagina.

You can say, "Some patients feel uncomfortable at the beginning. But once you learn how to put it in and take it out and practice doing so, it may no longer bother you. If this is the method you really want to use, let's talk about ways to make it easier for you to use it."

Also remind them that if it still bothers them, there are many other methods they can choose from.

Realize that each patient is unique.

Be aware that all members of a group are not alike. Don't assume all patients will be or think a certain way just because of their culture or group. That is stereotyping. Though we are all influenced by our culture and family upbringing, we each have unique values and beliefs. It is important to treat each patient as an individual with their own values, beliefs, issues, and concerns. Appreciate and respect the differences between you and your patients. Communicate in a non-judgmental way. This will improve the quality of service you give.

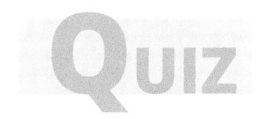

Working with People from Different Cultures

Directions: Read each of following statements. Is it true or false? Circle the best answer.

1. The more you know and understand about the patients your health care site serves, the better prepared you will be to meet their needs in a respectful way. **True   False**

2. Good communication depends only on the way you talk to your patients. **True   False**

3. You should tell your patients which birth control method would be best for them. **True   False**

4. All members of a culture or ethnic group think alike. **True   False**

5. Learning from your mistakes can help you become a better patient educator. **True   False**

Check your answers on the next page.

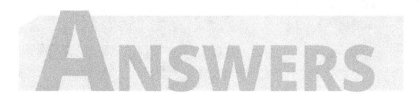
ANSWERS

Working with People from Different Cultures

Check your answers.

1. **True**   Learn as much as you can about the patients your health care site serves.

2. **False**   Good communication is at the center of patient education. It involves more than just talking to patients. It includes listening to and being respectful of their thoughts, feelings, needs, and desires. To do this and to avoid misunderstandings, it helps to be aware of different communication styles.

3. **False**   Our personal backgrounds influence our values and the choices we make. There will be times when you don't share the same values as your patient. That is okay. Always remember that patients have the right to make a different choice from the one you would make. Respect their choices and their views. ***Don't*** try to change their views to match your own.

4. **False**   All members of a culture or ethnic group do not think alike. Believing that they do is stereotyping. Though we are all influenced by our culture and family upbringing, we each have unique values and beliefs.

5. **True**   Learning from your mistakes can help you become a better patient educator. So, if you make a mistake, relax. Learn from it. And know that when you are sincere in what you say and do, most of your patients will understand.

The Four Stages of a Patient Education Session

There are many ways to plan a session. One way is to think about a session in four stages. This can help you be more organized. The four stages are:

Stage 1: Preparing to meet your patient

Stage 2: Helping your patient feel comfortable

Stage 3: Sharing information so your patient can make decisions

Stage 4: Wrapping up the session

Stage 1: Preparing to meet your patient

You need to be ready *before* you meet your patient. To prepare, ask yourself these questions:

▸ How can I make the room we meet in comfortable?

▸ What do I know about why the patient has come in?

▸ If I talk to the patient about that issue, what will I need to help me get information and skills across to them?

Each health care setting has its own way of doing things. Here are some basic guidelines. Talk to your supervisor about how to do things in your health care setting.

Prepare the room you will be using

The room can tell patients many key things:

▸ The conversation they have with you is private.

▸ You care about them.

▸ The staff members are prepared to give good health care.

Here are some things you can do to help send the right message to your patients.

Make sure you have a room with a door.

Patients should receive services that are confidential. Your patients will need to talk about some of the most private things in their lives. Speaking to them in a room with a door can help them feel comfortable. If patients feel they can talk to you, they will share the information you need. That information allows you to give them quality health care.

Take away any barriers between you and the patient.

When you sit behind a table or desk, it may tell the patient you feel distant and removed. It is a good idea to sit on the same side of the desk or table as your patient. You will want to face your patients. This helps them know that you will listen and that you care.

Keep the room neat.

Many health care settings have little space to work with. But you can still try to keep rooms clean and user-friendly.

Keep a supply of health education materials in the room.

These could be easy-to-read pamphlets on sexually transmitted infections. Or they could be fact sheets on birth control methods in the languages your patients most often speak. Posters of reproductive anatomy can help during patient education sessions. Penis models or uterus pelvic models can also be useful. Having these items in the room tells the patient that you are ready to talk about their sexual and reproductive health care.

Find out what you can about your patient

Knowing something about your patients before you meet them helps patients feel you see them as individuals. Here are some of the basic things you should know before you meet each patient.

Know your patient's name.

It is important to call patients by their accurate names. You want them to feel welcomed and comfortable. If it is a difficult name, try to find out how to pronounce it ahead of time.

Note: When you meet your patients, you may ask them how they would like to be addressed. When you find out, write it down in the chart. It is also a good idea to write down how to pronounce a patient's name.

Know your patient's pronouns.

Pronouns are words that refer to people who are being talked about. They replace a person's name in a statement. Some common pronouns include: she, he, they, ze, and zir. Gender neutral pronouns can be used to avoid assuming a patient's gender identity.

> *Example:*
>
> Chris has some questions about *their* symptoms.

When you meet your patients, you may share your pronouns with them and then ask them what their pronouns are. Use them and make note of them in the patient's chart. If you make a mistake and use a pronoun your patient does not identify with, correct yourself, briefly apologize, and move on. Be sure to use the correct pronoun the next time.

Know why your patient came in for health care.

Patients usually make appointments for specific reasons. They may want a new birth control method. Or they may want a physical exam. They may just want information.

Note: There will be times when it is not that simple. A patient might say they are coming for one reason. But, the real reason may be something that is hard for them to talk about. Or they may have changed their mind about the service they want. Often you won't know the reason until you meet the patient and begin asking questions. They may recognize their need for emergency contraception and/or STI testing at this visit as well.

Find out if your patient has any special language needs.

Check patients' charts to find out if they have any special language needs. Then follow your health care setting's procedures for meeting those needs. You may need to find materials in the patient's language. If you don't speak the patient's language, you may need to switch the patient to a different staff member. Or you may need to arrange for an interpreter to assist you either in person or by phone.

Find out what materials you will need to have in the room.

Once you know why the patient came to your health care site, think about what teaching materials you will want to use. Make sure you have them in the room before you bring the patient in. That way you won't need to leave your patient to get something.

> *Example:*
>
> A patient is coming to your health care site for an IUD. Make sure you have fact sheets on all IUDs in the room you will be meeting in. It is very helpful to give an IUD sample to the patient to hold and touch while you are counseling about IUDs.

Stage 2: Helping your patient feel comfortable

Patients need to feel comfortable talking to you and sharing private information about their lives. There are many things you can do to make them feel at ease. You should:

- ▶ Greet them and introduce yourself.
- ▶ Talk about confidentiality and mandatory reporting.
- ▶ Find out the reason for their health care visit.
- ▶ Ask about their pregnancy intentions or reproductive life plan.
- ▶ Review birth control method and emergency contraception options.
- ▶ Find out what the patients need and want to know.
- ▶ Discuss the session objectives and encourage them to ask questions.

Think about what it is like for your patients.

You were probably once a patient in a health care setting. Think about what you liked to have happen when you were there.

- ▶ What is the first thing you liked health workers to do when they called you from the waiting room?

- ▶ What did you want them to tell you about themselves and their role?

Greet your patient and introduce yourself and your role

This is the first thing you will do with patients. It is both simple and important. It can help put the patient at ease and set the tone for the entire session. Share your name and pronouns and ask what pronouns the patient uses. Be sure to tell patients what your position is at the health care site and what they can expect during this visit. When they know who you are and what to expect, it is easier for them to share information with you.

This is also a good time to start connecting with your patients and building a climate of trust.

Connect with your patient.

Patients can feel more comfortable with you if they feel a connection. To connect with your patients, try to:

- ▶ **Use the patient's name.** If it is a hard name for you to pronounce, you can say, "Could you please repeat your name so I can say it correctly?" In the chart, write down how the name sounds so other staff members can see it. Also, find out how the patient would like to be addressed (by first name, Mr., Mrs., Ms., nickname and pronouns). Do not assume the patient's name on the chart or health insurance card is the one they are currently using and do not assume a patient's pronouns based on gender or sex.

▸ **Notice something positive about each of your patients.** When you say something nice about your patients, it shows that you are paying attention to them personally.

▸ **Validate their feelings, worries, or opinions.** You can let them know that their concerns are understandable. You can say, "I can see why you are upset about that."

▸ **Be encouraging.** Praise them for coming to the health care site and taking care of their health. Give your patients credit for the healthy choices they are making.

Build a climate of trust.

Patients need to trust you to feel comfortable talking with you. When you are with your patients, be sure to:

▸ **Be professional.** Keep a balance between caring about your patients and trusting them to take care of their own problems. Don't share personal experiences.

▸ **Be accepting of the patient.** Each patient will be different. Try to find out what is important to your patient and build on that. Don't try to change them to match your idea of what they should be.

▸ **Talk in a way that doesn't judge them.** Always be respectful. Never criticize or put down your patients.

Talk about confidentiality and mandatory reporting

Tell patients that what they share with you will be kept private and confidential.

▸ Explain that you will not tell it to anyone outside of their health care team, including their parents, partners, or friends. If there are things the law makes you report (like sexual abuse of a minor), explain this to patients before you begin asking personal questions.

▸ **Sample Confidentiality Statement**: "Everything that we discuss will remain between us and the health care team unless you tell me that you have been hurt, you plan to hurt yourself or you plan to hurt someone else. Then I will have to speak to someone else to get you the support that you may need. Is that okay with you?"

Mandatory Reporting

Each state and/or county has its own laws about what you must report. Talk to your supervisor about what laws apply to your health care setting.

Find out what your patient needs and wants to know

When you are aware of what a patient needs and wants to know, it helps you meet the patient's needs and use your time wisely. That will make your education session more successful.

Ask patients why they came in to your health care site.

This is a key question. Before you meet with patients, look at their chart to learn the reason they gave for coming to your health care site. But be aware that sometimes the real reason for their visit may be something else. Or maybe they have changed their minds about what they want. To better know what patients need from the education session, ask them why they came in.

> **Find out what your patient needs and wants to know**
>
> Always ask patients the reason they came to see a health care provider.
>
> If for birth control, then ask, "What are you looking for in a birth control method?" or "What is important to you about your birth control method?" When you do an overview of all the methods you can highlight which methods fit with their preferences.

Assessing Pregnancy Intention – Reproductive Life Plan

Finding out if or when a patient would like to become pregnant is important information that can help guide the patient education session. We want to know if they want birth control or if they need preconception care because they are seeking pregnancy. One way to assess this is by asking the One Key Question **"Do you want to be pregnant in the next year?"** along with additional follow up questions to get a picture of what they want.

Or, ask the PATH questions:

> Pregnancy / Parenthood Attitudes: **"Do you think you might like to have (more) children at some point?"**
> Timing: **"When do you think that might be?"**
> How important: **"How important is it to you to prevent pregnancy (until then)?"**

Hearing their thoughts can help you personalize the information that you discuss with your patient as you conduct your patient education session.

Be sure your patient has basic information about every method

To make sure your patients know what their choices are, they must have basic information about every method of birth control and emergency contraception. This allows them to see all the birth control methods available and to compare the methods.

Find out what method your patient would like to learn more about

Once you are sure the patient has basic information about every method, you can ask which method the patient would like to learn more about. You can then give the patient detailed information about that method.

Note about Reviewing Method Precautions

Now would be a good time to discuss any precautions for their chosen method. If the patient has a condition that would keep them from being able to use that method, they can choose another one before you continue with the patient education session.

Ask patients what they already know

This is where you find out exactly what the patient does and does not know about the topic they are there to discuss. You may find that the patient has some misinformation. The answer to this question will tell you what information or skills you will need to teach.

Example:

Marisa has told you that they came for birth control and that they want the birth control shot. But before you start talking about the shot, you could also ask:

- What do you already know about the shot? How do you feel about getting shots?
- Do you know anyone who has used the shot? What did they tell you about it?

Dispel myths or wrong information the patient provides. Validate any part of it that is correct or "find the yes" and then add the correct information. Use "Yes, and…" Avoid "No, but…"

Example: "Yes, you are right it's generally not normal to miss periods, AND it is perfectly healthy to not have a period if you ARE using a hormonal method".

Discuss the objectives for the session with your patient

The objectives for your session are statements about what the patient will be able to do or say by the end of the session. They are not what you, the health worker, will do or say. They cover the most important points the patient will learn.

> **Objectives**
>
> Objectives are what the *patient* will be able to say or do by the end of the session.

> *Example:* "At the end of our session, you will be able to tell me what the depo shot is, how the shot works, how effective it is, how to use it and stop using it, what to do if you make mistakes, common side effects, rare complications and warning signs and we will discuss advantages and disadvantages."

When patients know the objectives for their session, it helps them focus on the key things they need to know or do.

Encourage your patient to ask questions

Tell patients that they can ask questions at any time. Then be sure to invite them to ask their questions throughout the session. You can do this by asking, "Please stop me throughout the session to ask questions or ask me to repeat anything." This shows that you expect them to ask questions and are eager to provide them with the information they need.

Helping the patient feel comfortable

▶ **Introduce yourself** (give your name, title, pronouns). **Ask the patient their pronouns.**

▶ **Talk about confidentiality.** State what information is private and what is not.

▶ Find out the **reason for their health care visit** or confirm the reason if already known.

▶ **Ask about their pregnancy intention** using PATH Questions or One Key Question.

▶ **Review birth control method and emergency contraception options.**

▶ Find out **what they already know.** And **correct any misinformation** they may have.

▶ **List the session objectives** once you know which method they want to learn more about.

▶ **Encourage the patient to ask questions** throughout the counseling/education session.

Stage 3: Sharing information so your patient can make decisions

You have created a good environment for learning. Now you can begin to cover the information about birth control methods and other topics that the patient needs in order to make a choice and give informed consent. This includes detailed information about the birth control method they have chosen. As you read through the rest of this section on Stage 3, you will learn which topics you need to cover. You will also find tips and examples for talking about each of them.

When you think about providing this information to patients, remember that *how* you provide the information is as important as the information itself. As you read through what you need to cover in an education session, think about these questions:

> ‣ How can I say this in a way that is easy for patients to understand?

> ‣ What can I do to make things clearer for my patients?

> ‣ How can I make sure my patients have really understood the information?

Reading through the following tips on providing basic and detailed information should help you answer those questions.

Note: Throughout the session, check to make sure your patient understands with evaluation questions.

Describe what the method is

You need to talk about:

> ‣ How it looks

> ‣ The different forms the method might come in

> ‣ What it is made of

> ‣ How to get it

Example:

For the external condom you might say:

External condoms are thin coverings that fit over an erect penis or sex toy. They come in three kinds of materials:

> ▪ Latex, which is a kind of rubber

> ▪ Polyurethane, which is a thin plastic

> ▪ Animal membranes, like sheepskin or lambskin

External condoms come in different sizes, colors, textures, and even flavors. You can buy them at drugstores, grocery stores and online. You can get them in many clubs and restaurants. You can also get them here.

Tell how the method works

Patients need to know how their method works to prevent pregnancy. This is very important. If they know how it works, they can help make sure it will work for them.

To understand how a method works, patients must know the basics of how pregnancy happens. Never just assume they know.

You can do a quick quiz to help find out how much they know. You might say to your patients, "Tell me what you know about how pregnancy happens." Then listen to their answers and correct any misinformation they have.

Once it is clear that they know the basics of how someone gets pregnant, ask what they've heard about how their chosen method works. Make sure they know the basics of how it works to keep sperm from meeting with an egg. As you go along, explain any words or concepts your patient may not be familiar with. Use some of the teaching methods discussed earlier in this chapter.

What patients need to know

Patients need to know as much as they can about their chosen method.

They need to know:

- What it is
- How it works
- How well it works
- How to use it and stop using it
- Side effects
- Complications and warning signs
- Advantages and disadvantages

Let your patient know how well the method works

All methods help prevent pregnancy. But no method is perfect. Each method can fail even if it is used perfectly. Patients need to know how well their method works. This is called the effectiveness rate.

The effectiveness rate is given in percentages. It lets you know how many users out of 100 who use the method may get pregnant the first year they use the method.

How well each method works depends a lot on how well it is used. There are two effectiveness rates for each method. One is for *perfect use.* The other is for *typical use.*

- **Perfect use:** This lets you know how many users out of 100 might get pregnant in a year if they use the method in exactly the right way.

- **Typical use:** This lets you know how many users out of 100 might get pregnant in a year if they do not use their method in exactly the right way. Most users are typical -- this means they may make mistakes.

You should tell patients the rates for perfect use and for typical use.

Example: Here are the two effectiveness rates for the patch:

Perfect use: 99% effective. This means that 1 out of 100 patients who use the patch perfectly may get pregnant in a year.

Typical use: 93% effective. This means that about 7 out of 100 patients who use the patch may get pregnant in a year if they don't use it exactly the right way.

Here is what you can say to a patient:

> Jordan, the patch works well to prevent pregnancy. But some users may still get pregnant while using it.
>
> - If 100 people use the patch perfectly during a year, 1 of them may get pregnant. Using the patch perfectly means using it exactly the right way (changing it on time, wearing it in the correct locations, replacing immediately if it falls off, etc.).
> - Some people may not use the patch exactly the right way. If 100 people don't always use the patch the right way, 7 of them may get pregnant in a year.

Let your patients know that:

- If they use their method correctly all the time, their chances of getting pregnant would be closer to the "perfect use" rates.
- If they don't use the method correctly all the time, they have a much higher chance of pregnancy.

You can help your patients compare choices by telling them:

- If 100 patients who can get pregnant have reproductive sex using no birth control method at all, 85 of them might get pregnant in a year.

Also talk to your patients about:

- Any reasons a method might fail.
- Things they can do to prevent or solve that problem.
- What to do if the method fails or if they forget to use it.

Talk to patients about Emergency Contraception (EC).

Let your patients know that they can take a pill or combination of pills (oral EC) or have an Intra-uterine Device (IUD) placed to help prevent pregnancy *AFTER* unprotected sex. You can learn more about Emergency Contractiption options at the end of Chapter 6.

Explain how to use the method

When you teach patients how to use a method, teach all of the steps clearly. Be logical. Start at the very beginning. Think about the first thing patients will need to do to start a method when they leave your session:

- ▸ Will the patient need to have an exam first?
- ▸ Will the patient need to come back at a different time?
- ▸ When will the patient start the method?

Tell and show your patient how to use the method.

Tell patients how to use the method and show them how. Then have them tell and show you.

Example:

For the internal condom, you might explain each step as you show them how to use it. You could say:

- ▪ Let me show you how to use the internal condom. First, carefully take it out of its package. Squeeze the smaller ring together and slip it into your vagina. The outer ring will hang out. You can use lube with it which may make it easier to put in.
- ▪ Here is a model of the vagina. I will use it to show you how to put the internal condom into your vagina and how to remove it.
- ▪ Now you try and tell me the steps as you do them.

Make sure your patient understands.

Ask questions to make sure patients know how to make the method work in their own lives. Ask patients to describe what they can do to make the method work for them.

Example:

You might say to the patient:

- ▪ You need to put a new condom in your vagina every time you have sex.
- ▪ Where will you keep new condoms so that you can get to one when you want to have sex?

Also make sure you tell patients what to do if they want to stop using the method. They need to be told that they can stop a method whenever they want to. You should also let them know if their method takes some time to leave the body (like the birth control shot). And, in the case of all other methods, tell them that their fertility returns quickly and they can get pregnant right away.

Tell your patient about the method's common side effects

Side effects are minor reactions people might get when they use a method. Side effects are common. They can be unpleasant or annoying, but they are not life threatening. Some patients will have side effects. Other patients may not.

When you talk about side effects, it helps patients know what to expect. If patients know about a side effect in advance, they are more likely to deal with it well if they get it. They will be less likely to become scared or angry.

> **Educator Tip**
>
> Ask your patients which side effects they are most worried about. Then talk to them about how they can make those side effects less of a problem.
>
> Patients are more likely to keep using a method if side effects don't come as a surprise to them.

Example:

Most people who use the birth control pill will have less bleeding during their periods. Their periods may be lighter and shorter. Both of these side effects are normal for patients using this type of birth control pill.

If you tell a patient to expect these changes, they are less likely to become frightened if it happens to them. And they are more likely to keep using the pill.

Here are some things to do when you talk to patients about side effects:

- First, ask if they have heard anything about the side effects of the method and dispel any myths.

- Correct any misinformation they have.

- Discuss possible side effects.

- Tell patients whether the side effects are common or unusual.

- Find out how patients feel about the side effects.

- Explain what they should or can do if they get a side effect.

Examples:

For the birth control shot, you might say:

A very common side effect of using the shot is having changes in menstrual bleeding. When you first start the shot, you might have spotting between periods. You may also have heavier periods. But most likely you will have lighter periods. After using the shot for one year, some patients stop getting their periods while using it. This is normal. How do you think you would feel about not having a period?

For spermicidal cream or jelly you might say:

One side effect is an allergic reaction, such as itching or a rash. You may be able to find a different spermicide that you are not allergic to if you experience these side effects.

Discuss possible complications and warning signs

You must discuss the possible complications of any method or procedure with patients. You must also tell them what the warning signs of each complication are so they can know when to get help.

Complications

Complications are serious health problems that are caused by a medication or procedure. **Complications are rare.** Some complications can be life threatening.

Tell your patients what the complications of their chosen method could be. Also tell them that most patients don't get complications.

If a method has no complications, say so. You could say, "This method causes no serious health problems."

Warning signs

When you talk about complications, you must also talk about **warning signs.**

Warning signs are changes in the body that could be a sign of a serious health problem. Tell your patients what the warning signs are for each complication.

> *Example:*
>
> For the oral combined pill (or any of the methods containing estrogen) you might say:
>
> Here is a list of the warning signs for the pill you will be taking. One way to remember these warning signs is to think of the word **A-C-H-E-S.**
>
> - **A** stands for "Abdominal pain that is severe." That could be a sign of a liver tumor, gall bladder disease, blood clot, or pregnancy in your tubes.
> - **C** stands for "Chest pain that is severe with shortness of breath." These could be signs of a heart attack or blood clot.
> - **H** is for "Headache that is severe and includes dizziness, weakness, or numbness anywhere in the body." Extreme headache may be a sign of high blood pressure or a stroke.
> - **E** is for "Eye problems that are severe." Pressure behind the eyes or sudden blurry vision may be a sign of a stroke, blood clot, or high blood pressure.
> - **S** stands for "Severe leg pain in the calf or thigh." This could be a sign of a blood clot.

Then ask, "What should you do if you get any of these warning signs?"

Be sure patients understand that they must immediately tell a health care provider about any warning signs they have. Say, **"If you experience any of these warning sings at any time, go to your health care provider or the emergency room right away."**

Discuss the advantages and disadvantages of the method

By now you have covered a lot of information. This is a good time to find out how the patient is feeling about the method.

Advantages

First, find out what the patient likes about the method (its advantages). Ask each patient: "What do you think you might like about this method?"

Once the patient tells you a few things they like, you can share things some other people like about it.

Benefits

Some of the methods have other benefits besides preventing pregnancy.

For example,

- Some patients use hormonal methods to have a more regular bleeding pattern.

- Some birth control pills can help clear up acne.

Everybody is different.

Keep in mind that what one person likes might be just what another person doesn't like. Be careful not to make too many assumptions about what is "good" or "bad."

For example, many users will not have periods after a year of using the birth control shot. Some may feel this is a good thing. Others may not like this side effect at all.

Disadvantages

Each method may have problems and concerns. Find out what concerns your patient may have about the method. Ask each patient: "Is there anything you may dislike about this method?" Be sure to listen to any cultural, social, or personal concerns they may have. These may include:

▶ Cultural beliefs that would keep them from using the method the right way.

▶ A partner who doesn't like the idea of using the method.

▶ A feeling that using the method could show a lack of trust in their partner.

Help patients find ways to overcome these problems so they can use the method successfully.

Example:

Angel wants to use the birth control shot. You ask them, "Do you have any concerns about using the shot?"

Angel answers, "I'm really not happy that I could gain weight on the shot."

You can now help them problem-solve. You could ask, "What do you think you could do to help keep you from gaining weight?"

Hopefully, Angel will start thinking about how to make sure they eat healthy foods. They might think about getting more exercise. They may also need to get comfortable with the idea that they might gain 2 to 5 pounds. If Angel is not able to come up with solutions on their own, offer some suggestions.

- Give your patients time to come up with their own answers.
- Talk about other ideas for solving the problem.

Example:

A couple has chosen to use the condom. You point out that one of the problems people sometimes have is running out of condoms.

You could ask them, "What could you do to prevent or solve the problem?"

Let them come up with their own solutions. Here are some examples:

- Carry extra condoms in my bag or pockets.
- Have extra condoms stored nearby.
- Go to the store for more.
- Decide to wait until another time to have sex.

Share information about other topics of interest

You will need to talk about more than just birth control methods. You may need to talk about any of the following:

▸ Breast self-examination

▸ Human sexuality

▸ Sexually transmitted infections (STIs)

▸ Health care site-specific procedures

▸ Other topics

No matter what topic you discuss, the process is about the same. First, you meet the patient and make them feel comfortable. As you do this, you find out what the patient needs and wants to know about the topic. You then start teaching about the topic. You will need to cover the most important information about the topic. Always be sure to give patients enough information so they can do what they need to do to keep healthy.

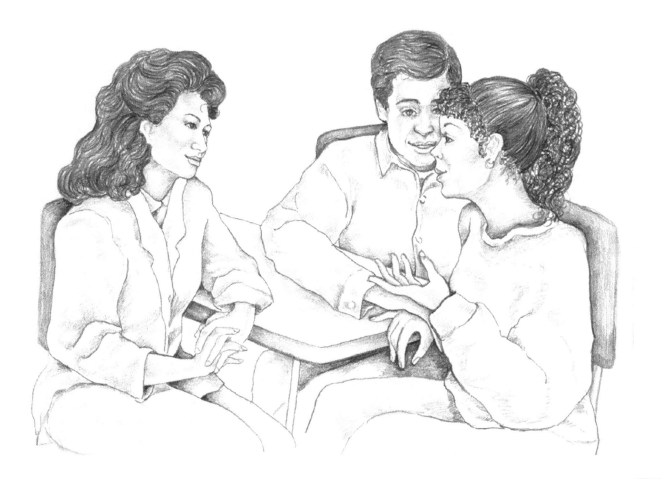

Stage 4: Wrapping up your session

There are a few things you will need to do to wrap up a session. Though each health care setting may differ, keep the following things in mind:

- ▸ Evaluate your patient on the key points covered in the session.
- ▸ Make sure your patient has written information to take home.
- ▸ Give your patient information on who to contact in case of problems or questions.

Evaluate your patient on the key points

Find out how well the patient knows the key points of the session. Even though you evaluate the patient's understanding throughout the session, you need to do it again at the end. Focus on the basic steps the patient will need to follow to use a method.

Make sure the objectives of the session have been met.

Example:

Michael is going to use the external condom. Here are some of the questions you can ask to make sure they understand the key points:

- ▪ What do you look for on the condom package before you open it?
- ▪ What do you do with the condom right after you are done having sex or using a sex toy?

Make sure your patient has written information to take home

Give patients something on the birth control method you discussed.

Example: You may have a patient starting the ring. Give them a pamphlet about using the ring. It is also a good idea to give them a pamphlet on preventing STIs.

Give your patient contact information

Patients may think of questions after they leave the education session. Or they may have problems using their method or side effects they want to talk about.

Make sure they know who to contact to get answers. This may be you or another health care provider. Give them phone numbers, web addresses, or e-mail addresses that will help them get the answers they need.

The Four Parts of an Education Plan

The four parts of an education plan are **1) Objectives 2) Content 3) Teaching Methods and Materials** and **4) Evaluation.**

Your education plan provides a guide for how you proceed through your patient education session. It is recommended that you complete a plan for each method. For each part, fill in the information that you will cover. Refer to this during your session.

Objectives: State the objectives that you want to accomplish by the end of your education session. This will help your patient know what to listen for and what is important to remember.

Content: Include the content that you will share about the method. This includes all of the information covered in Stages 2, 3, and 4 of the patient education session.

Teaching Methods and Materials: Think about the teaching methods and materials (and visual aids) that you want to use for each content area to increase learning. List them in this section.

Evaluation: Include how you will evaluate that learning has taken place. Add quality, open-ended questions at key points in your education plan so that you can create a dialogue with your patient. As they answer your questions, you will know if they understand the material you have covered.

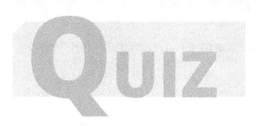

The Four Stages of a Patient Education Session

Directions: Read each of the following and write your best answer in the space below.

1. What are the four stages of a patient education session?

   Stage 1: _____

   Stage 2: _____

   Stage 3: _____

   Stage 4: _____

2. List two things a health care worker can do to prepare to meet with a patient.

   _____

   _____

   _____

   _____

3. A patient tells you they want to start using the Birth Control Pill. What question could you ask them to find out what they already know about the Pill?

   _____

   _____

   _____

   _____

Go on to the next page.

4. There are seven topics about a birth control method that you must cover with your patients. One topic is "How it works." What are the other six?

   • _____

   _____

   • _____

   _____

   • _____

   _____

   • _____

   _____

   • _____

   _____

   • _____

   _____

5. What are three things a health worker should be sure to do when wrapping up a session?

   • _____

   • _____

   • _____

Check your answers on the next page.

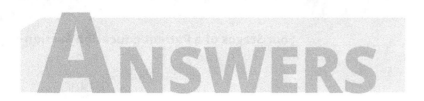
ANSWERS

The Four Stages of a Patient Education Session

Check your answers.

1. The four stages of a patient education session are:

   Stage 1: Preparing to meet your patient

   Stage 2: Helping your patient feel comfortable

   Stage 3: Sharing information so your patient can make informed decisions

   Stage 4: Wrapping up the session

2. Here are eight things a health worker can do to prepare to meet a patient:

   - Make sure you have a room with a door.
   - Take away any barriers between you and the patient.
   - Keep the room neat.
   - Keep a supply of health education materials in the room.
   - Know your patient's name and pronouns.
   - Know why your patient made an appointment at your health care setting.
   - Find out if your patient has any special language needs.
   - Find out what materials you will need to have in the room.

3. If you want to know what a patient already knows about something, be direct. In this case, you could ask, "What do you already know about the Birth Control Pill?"

4. "How it works" is one of the seven topics about a birth control method that you must cover with your patients. The other six are:
   - What it is
   - How well it works
   - How to use it
   - Side effects
   - Complications and warning signs
   - Advantages and disadvantages

5. The three things a health worker should do when wrapping up a session are:
   - Evaluate the patient on the key points covered in the session.
   - Make sure the patient has written information to take home.
   - Give the patient information on who to contact in case of problems or questions.

Chapter Quiz

Patient Education

Directions: Read each of the following statements. Is it true or false? Circle the best answer.

1. Active listening includes paying attention to the meaning of the words you hear and to what the patient's body language is saying. **True** **False**

2. Open-ended questions are a great way to help you figure out a patient's needs. **True** **False**

3. Using technical medical words that your patients don't know will help them use their birth control methods better. **True** **False**

4. It is **not** a good idea to use pictures or models to help explain some things to your patient. **True** **False**

5. Examples can help your patient understand new words and ideas. **True** **False**

Directions: Read each of the following and write your best answer in the space below.

6. List two teaching methods that you could use to help your patients learn.

   - _____

   - _____

7. List four types of teaching materials that you could use to help your patients learn.

   - _____

   - _____

   - _____

   - _____

Go on to the next page.

8. When do you need to evaluate what your patient knows?

_____

_____

_____

9. What kind of question should you ask when you want your patient to give more than a simple yes-or-no or very short answer?

_____

_____

_____

Directions: Circle the best answer.

10. What can you do to help yourself work better with patients from different cultures, ethnic groups, or backgrounds?

    a. Learn about the patients your health care site serves.

    b. Be respectful and non-judgmental.

    c. Realize that each patient is one of a kind.

    d. All of the above.

11. Which is not a good thing to do when you work with patients?

    a. Pay attention to the patient's body language.

    b. Be judgmental about their decisions.

    c. Use words and gestures that show respect for the patient.

    d. All of the above.

12. When you prepare to meet patients, you should make sure to:

    a. Have a private place to speak with them.

    b. Know the name of each patient before you greet them.

    c. Have health education materials in the room to use during the session.

    d. All of the above

Go on to the next page.

13. The first thing you should do when you greet patients is:

    a. Say hello, and tell them your name and your position at the health care setting.

    b. Tell them to follow you. Don't introduce yourself.

    c. Grab them by the arm and pull them out of the waiting room.

    d. None of the above

14. Your patient has told you they want to start using the Birth Control Shot. Which question should you ask to find out what they already know about the shot?

    a. Do you know that the shot works for 12 weeks?

    b. What do you already know about the shot?

    c. You know the shot is given in the arm or hip, right?

    d. None of the above

Directions: Read each of the following statements.
Fill in the blanks with a word or words from this list.

Hormones	Warning signs
Complications	Effectiveness rates
Side effects	Birth control methods

15. _____ are minor reactions people might get when they use a method. They are common. They can be unpleasant or annoying, but they are not life threatening.

16. _____ are serious health problems that can be caused by a medication or procedure. Some can be life threatening. But they are rare.

17. _____ are changes in the body that could be a sign of a serious health problem.

Go on to the next page.

Directions: *Read each of the following and write your best answer in the spaces below.*

18. What are the seven topics patients must understand about a birth control method before they can give their informed consent? (We've given you the first one.)

    What it is
    - _____

    - _____

    - _____

    - _____

    - _____

    - _____

    - _____

19. What are the four parts of an education plan?

    - _____

    - _____

    - _____

    - _____

Check your answers on the next page.

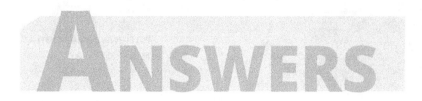

Patient Education

Check your answers.

1. **True** Active listening includes much more than just hearing words. It does include paying attention to the meaning of the words you hear and to what the patient's body language is saying. It also includes using your words and body language in a way that lets the patient know you have understood.

2. **True** Open-ended questions are a great way to help you figure out a patient's needs. Open-ended questions encourage patients to give as much information as they would like to give.

3. **False** Using technical medical words that your patients don't know makes it ***hard*** for them to understand how to use their birth control methods. Try not to use those words. Think about how you would explain things to your own friends or family members. When you need to use technical words or words that may be new to the patient, make sure you explain their meanings clearly. Never assume a patient knows a given term.

4. **False** It is always a ***good*** idea to use pictures or models to help explain some things to your patient. When patients see something, they often better understand what is being said. This can also help them remember it.

5. **True** Examples can help your patient understand new words and ideas.

6. Here are five of the teaching methods you could use to help your patients learn:
   - Question and answer
   - Demonstration
   - Role play
   - Brainstorm solutions to problems
   - Short explanations

Go on to the next page.

7. Here are nine types of teaching materials that you could use to help your patients learn:
   - Pamphlets or booklets
   - Fact sheets or wallet cards
   - Pictures
   - Flip charts
   - Posters
   - Samples of birth control
   - Models of the human body
   - Internet tools/Apps
   - Calendars

8. You need to evaluate what your patient knows at the *beginning* of a session, *during* the session, and at the *end* of the session.

9. Ask open-ended questions when you want your patient to give more than a simple yes-or-no or very short answer. Open-ended questions allow patients to tell you as much information as they would like to.

10. **D** All of the above. You can do any of these to help yourself work better with patients from different cultures, ethnic groups, or backgrounds:
    - Learn about the patients your health care site serves.
    - Be respectful and non-judgmental.
    - Realize that each patient is one of a kind.

11. **B** It is not good to be judgmental about a patient's decisions. Always remember that patients have the right to make a different choice from the one you might make. Respect their choices and their views. Don't try to change their views to match your own.

12. **D** All of the above. When you prepare to meet a patient, you should make sure to:
    - Have a private place to speak with them.
    - Know the name of each patient before you greet them.
    - Have health education materials in the room to use during the session.

13. **A**   The first thing you should do when you greet patients is tell them your name and your position at the health care site. It is both simple and important. It can help put the patient at ease and set the tone for the entire session. Besides telling them what your position is, also tell them what your role is and what they can expect during this visit. When they know who you are and what to expect, it is easier for them to share information with you.

14. **B**   "What do you already know about the shot?" This is a good open-ended question to ask. It's important to ask what the patient already knows about the shot. It gives the patient a chance to tell you any information or misinformation they might have.

15. *Side effects* are common, minor reactions people might get when they use a method.

16. *Complications* are serious health problems that are caused by a medication or procedure. Some can be life threatening. But they are rare. Be sure to say they are *rare*.

17. *Warning signs* are rare changes in the body that could be a sign of a serious health problem.

18. The seven topics patients must understand about a birth control method before they can give their informed consent are:
    - What it is
    - How it works
    - How well it works
    - How to use it
    - Side effects
    - Complications and warning signs
    - Advantages and disadvantages

19. The four parts of an education plan are:
    - Objectives
    - Content
    - Teaching methods and materials
    - Evaluation questions

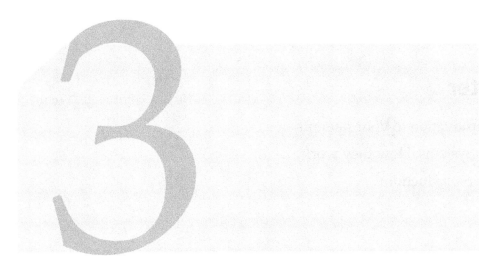

Reproduction and Puberty

Human Reproduction is how bodies work together to cause pregnancy. The parts of the body that make this happen are called *reproductive organs*. Together all these organs are called the *reproductive system*.

Puberty is a period of time when young bodies change as they are growing up. These changes make it possible for most of them to *reproduce*.

It is important that your patients understand the basics of both reproduction and puberty. If patients don't have this important information, they may feel afraid, embarrassed, or confused about their bodies and reproduction. They may make mistakes when they use birth control and have an unplanned pregnancy. They may get a disease or infection. You can help your patients avoid these problems by helping them understand how their bodies work. This chapter explains the basic facts about reproduction. You can share this with your patients. It will also give you, the health worker, more details that you may find helpful in your work.

Topics in this chapter

▸ The Basics: Explaining reproduction to your patients

▸ The Human Reproductive Systems: How they work

▸ Puberty: Getting ready for reproduction

Objectives

After reading this chapter, you will be able to:

▸ Explain reproduction in a simple way to your patients.

▸ Identify the main human reproductive organs.

▸ Explain how the reproductive systems work.

▸ Explain when a person can and cannot get pregnant during the menstrual cycle.

You will also be able to:

▸ Define puberty.

▸ State the ages at which puberty begins.

▸ Describe the physical body changes that typically happen during puberty.

Words to know

Words	Definition
Fertility and being fertile	Being able to get pregnant or get someone else pregnant.
Fertility awareness	Knowing when a person can get pregnant during the menstrual cycle.
Fertile days	The days of the cycle that a person **can** get pregnant.
Infertile days	Those days of the cycle that a person **cannot** get pregnant.
Fertile mucus	The thin, slippery mucus made by the cervix that helps sperm stay alive around the time an egg leaves an ovary.
Infertile mucus	The thick, sticky mucus made by the cervix that helps prevent sperm and germs from getting into the uterus.
Menstrual cycle	The time between the start of a menstrual period and the beginning of the next period. A normal cycle can be from 22 to 36 days long.
Menstrual period	The time when the uterus sheds its blood filled lining each month. A period usually lasts 4-7 days.
Hormones	A hormone is a chemical messenger. Everyone has many hormones that are made in different parts of the body. Each hormone is responsible for carrying messages to other parts of the body to help them work in healthy ways.

The Basics: Explaining Reproduction to Your Patients

People may think getting pregnant is easy. Two people just have sex, right? But it is not that simple. It is important to understand how human bodies work together to make pregnancy happen.

When you know the basics, you can help patients learn about their bodies and reproduction. By doing this, you can help patients take good care of themselves. Your patients will be able to use birth control methods well and be better able to plan if and when they have children.

When you talk with your patients, it is best to start with the basics:

▸ Sperm are made every day in the testicles.

▸ An egg is released from an ovary about once a month.

> These basics are explained here in a simple way that you could use with your patients. Later in this chapter you will be given more details to help you better understand these basics and answer questions you may be asked.
>
> As you explain the basics, use a drawing that shows the different parts of the human reproductive systems. Remember to keep it simple. Using what is written here can help.

Sperm are made every day in the testicles.

Millions of sperm are made in the testicles every day. The testicles are held away from the body in a sac called the scrotum. Sperm are stored and kept cool and healthy there.

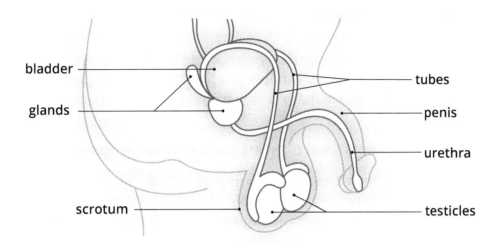

Here is what happens to the sperm when a person with testicles has reproductive sex (i.e., sex that can cause a pregnancy):

▶ The body has two **tubes**, one tube coming from each testicle. During sex, **sperm** may travel from the testicles through one of these tubes.

▶ The tube carries the sperm past special **glands** that make liquid. This fluid joins the sperm to help the sperm travel and stay healthy. This fluid is now called **semen**.

▶ The semen then flows into another tube that is in the middle of the **penis**. This tube is called the **urethra**.

▶ During ejaculation ("coming"), the semen moves through this tube, out of the penis, and into the vagina.

▶ The sperm travel through the vagina, into the uterus, and up the fallopian tubes where there may be an egg. Sperm can live inside a body that ovulates for up to 5 days. If an egg is in the tube or travels there within 5 days, the egg may become fertilized. If so, it may then travel and implant in the uterus causing a pregnancy.

▶ **If sperm are in or near the outside of the vaginal opening, they can still cause a pregnancy.**

  ▪ Many birth control methods, like the external and internal condoms, work by keeping the sperm from getting into the uterus and tubes.

  ▪ If sperm can't enter the tubes, it can't meet the egg, so fertilization and pregnancy cannot happen.

An egg is ready once a month.

An egg is ready about once a month. After the egg goes into a fallopian tube, it only lives and can be fertilized for about one day. Sperm can live in a body that can get pregnant for up to 5 days. That means that a person who ovulates is able to get pregnant only about one week out of each menstrual cycle.

Menstrual "Cycle" vs. Menstrual "Period"

A menstrual cycle begins on the day the period starts. It ends on the day before the next period starts. Cycles are typically 22-36 days long.

A menstrual period is the time frame of when bleeding starts to when it stops. A period is typically 4-7 days long.

Here is what happens in a body that can get pregnant.

A menstrual cycle starts on the first day of a menstrual period. During a period, the blood from the lining of the **uterus** leaves the body through the **vagina**. The body then starts to get ready for a possible pregnancy:

▸ An egg gets ready to leave one of the **ovaries**.

▸ The uterus makes a special lining where a fertilized egg can grow.

▸ The **cervix** makes special fertile mucus. This mucus helps sperm travel into the uterus.

About once a month, an egg leaves one of the ovaries.

▸ It goes into one of the **tubes**.

▸ The egg lives about 12-24 hours.

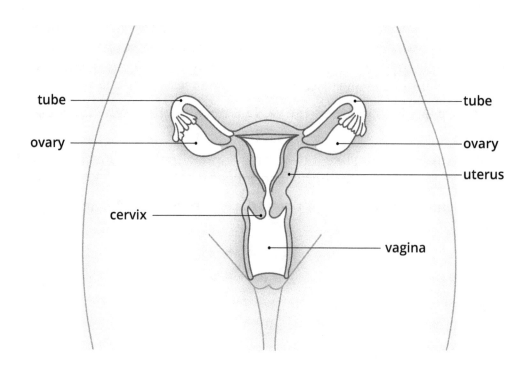

tube — ovary — cervix

tube — ovary — uterus — vagina

If sperm are already in the tube, or travel there while an egg is in the tube, a pregnancy can happen.

- ▸ Some birth control methods, like the birth control pill and the birth control shot, stop the egg from leaving the ovary. Since there is no egg for the sperm to meet, pregnancy does not happen.

- ▸ Other birth control methods, like the external or internal condoms, stop sperm from getting into the uterus to meet the egg. Since the sperm and egg do not meet, pregnancy does not happen.

Fertility

- ▸ A body with testicles may make millions of sperm every day. This means a person who makes sperm is **fertile every day**.

- ▸ A person who ovulates can become pregnant only about 5-7 days each cycle. This means they are **fertile about 1 week** each cycle.

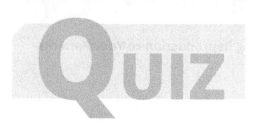

The Basics: Explaining Reproduction to Your Patients

Directions: Circle the best answer.

1. What are the fertile days of a person who ovulates?

   a. Any day from their first menstrual period until they reach menopause.

   b. Those days of the cycle when they could get pregnant.

   c. Those days of the cycle when they cannot get pregnant.

   d. The time when they bleed each month.

2. How long can sperm live inside the body of a person who can get pregnant?

   a. No longer than 1 day

   b. No longer than 5 hours

   c. Up to 5 days

   d. None of the above

3. The first day of a menstrual *cycle* starts when?

   a. When the ovary releases an egg

   b. On the last day of a menstrual period

   c. On the first day of a menstrual period

   d. None of the above

Go on to the next page.

4. What does a body that can get pregnant make to help sperm travel into the uterus?

    a. A special mucus made by the cervix

    b. A special lining in the uterus

    c. Nothing, sperm can travel on its own

    d. Eggs

5. When is a person who makes sperm fertile?

    a. Every day, starting during puberty when they first begin making sperm

    b. Only 7 days each month

    c. 21 days each month

    d. None of the above

Check your answers on the next page.

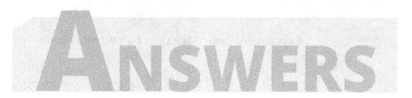

The Basics: Explaining Reproduction to Your Patients

Check your answers.

1. **B**   The fertile days are the days of the cycle when a person who ovulates could get pregnant.

2. **C**   Sperm can live inside the body of a person who can get pregnant for as long as 5 days.

3. **C**   The first day of a menstrual *cycle* starts on the first day of the menstrual period.

4. **A**   The cervix makes a special mucus to help sperm travel into the uterus. This is called fertile mucus.

5. **A**   A person who makes sperm is fertile every day starting during puberty.

The Reproductive System of Bodies that Make Sperm

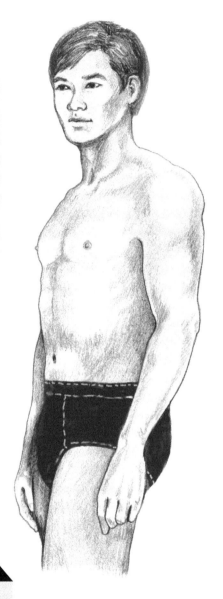

This section gives you some of the details that you, the health worker, may need to know about the reproductive system of bodies that make sperm and how it works. These details can help you better understand the basics you will explain to your patients. They can also help you answer questions you may be asked. You don't need to use all of these words when you talk with your patients. Using too many medical terms can make it hard for patients to understand and learn about reproduction.

The reproductive organs

Brain. Two parts of the brain are responsible for making the testicles work: the hypothalamus and the pituitary gland. These glands make hormones that travel through the bloodstream to the testicles and tell them to start making sperm and the hormone, testosterone. Without help from the brain, testosterone and sperm would never be made and this person would also not be able to get sexually excited and have sex.

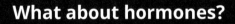

What about hormones?

Hormones: A hormone is a chemical messenger. Everyone has many hormones that are made in different parts of the body. Each hormone is responsible for carrying messages to other parts of the body to help them work in healthy ways.

Testosterone: This is the hormone that tells the testicles to make sperm. It also controls other secondary sex characteristics, such as growth of body and facial hair. It also causes a person to want to have/desire sex.

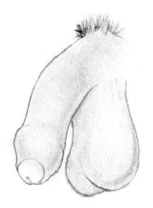

with foreskin

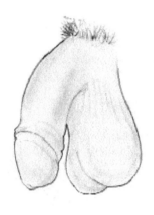

without foreskin

Penis. The penis is an organ made of tissue and blood vessels. It has many nerve endings. When a person with a penis gets sexually excited, the tissue in the penis fills with blood. This makes it get longer and wider. It also gets firm (erect, hard).

Glans. The glans is the head of the penis. When a baby with a penis is born, the glans is covered by loose skin called foreskin. Some parents have this foreskin cut away in an operation called circumcision. When a baby has been circumcised, they have no foreskin and the glans always shows. If someone has not been circumcised, the loose skin covers the glans and naturally pulls back when the penis is erect.

Testicles. Sperm are made in the testicles (also called testes). A person born with a penis typically also has two testicles — one on each side of the penis. Testicles are sex glands. They make sperm and the hormone testosterone. Sperm cannot be made without testosterone.

Scrotum. The testicles are protected by a pouch of skin called the scrotum. The scrotum, which is outside the body, keeps the testicles cooler than the temperature inside the body. The temperature inside the body is too warm for sperm to be made.

Epididymis. Inside the scrotum, there is one epididymis on top of each testicle. The sperm finish maturing and are stored there until they are able to travel up the tubes and out the penis.

Vas deferens. The vas deferens are two tubes — one leading from each epididymis. Sperm leave each epididymis through these tubes.

Seminal vesicles. Glands called seminal vesicles are connected to each tube. These glands make a thick fluid that flows into the tubes and mixes with the sperm as they travel through the tubes. This fluid helps sperm move through the tubes. It also keeps the sperm healthy.

Prostate gland. The sperm in the tubes then pass through the prostate gland. This gland makes a thin, milky fluid that mixes with the sperm. This fluid helps the sperm move and keeps them healthy.

Urethra. The urethra is a thin tube that goes down the center of the penis. Once the sperm travel through the prostate gland, they move into the urethra. During an ejaculation, the sperm travels out of the penis through this tube.

Urine (pee) also comes out of the urethra, but this cannot happen at the same time ejaculation is taking place.

Cowper's glands. Next to the urethra, there are two Cowper's glands. Like the other glands, these glands make a fluid. This fluid, often called pre-come or pre-ejaculatory fluid, flows into the urethra and prepares the way for the sperm. During sexual excitement, this clear, slippery fluid starts to be released. This happens before ejaculation. This fluid is important because it helps sperm stay healthy.

Urinary opening. This is the opening at the end of the penis. During an orgasm, semen leaves the urethra through the urinary opening. This is called ejaculation.

Anus. This is the opening where the bowel movement leaves the body.

What is ejaculation?

Semen

- When the sperm is mixed with the fluids from the seminal vesicles, and the prostate gland, it is called semen.

- This white fluid is what leaves the penis during ejaculation ("coming").

Ejaculation

- When semen leaves the penis during an orgasm this is called ejaculation.

- During ejaculation, only semen can go through the tube.

- Urination (peeing) cannot happen at the same time as ejaculation.

The Reproductive System of Bodies That Make Sperm
Front View

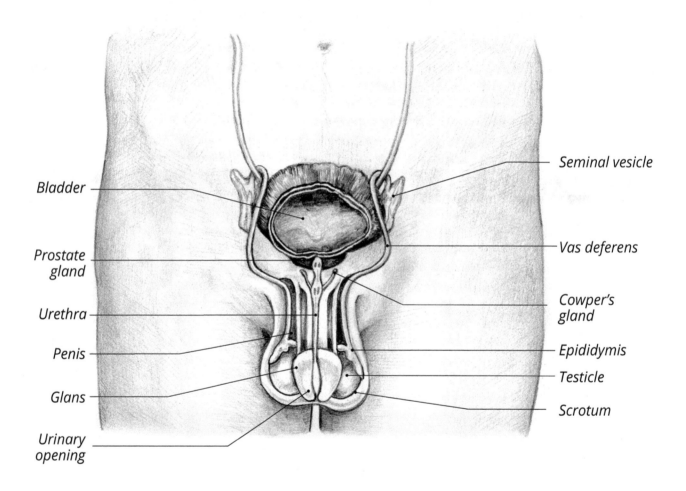

Bladder

Prostate gland

Urethra

Penis

Glans

Urinary opening

Seminal vesicle

Vas deferens

Cowper's gland

Epididymis

Testicle

Scrotum

The Reproductive System of Bodies That Make Sperm
Side View

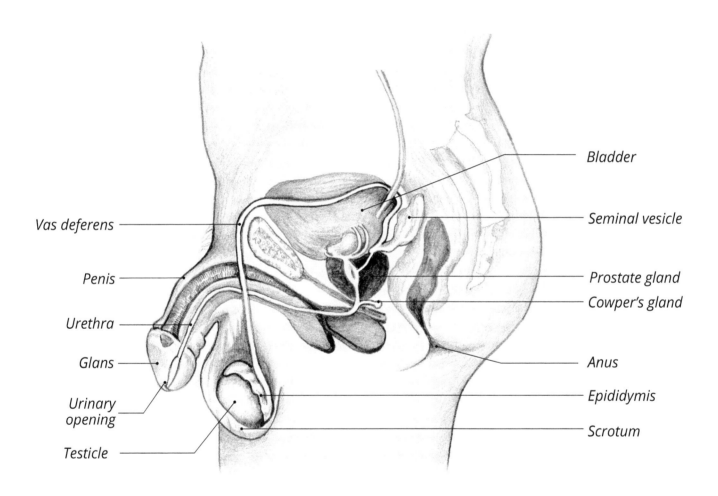

Vas deferens

Penis

Urethra

Glans

Urinary opening

Testicle

Bladder

Seminal vesicle

Prostate gland

Cowper's gland

Anus

Epididymis

Scrotum

The life cycle of sperm

1. Sperm are made in the testicles.

2. They are stored in the epididymis until they are ready to move on their own.

3. When a person with a penis gets sexually excited, their penis gets hard and their Cowper's glands start to release a fluid to prepare the way for sperm.

4. Sperm leave the epididymis and move into one of the two tubes called the vas deferens.

   ▶ The sperm keep traveling and mix with fluid from the seminal vesicles.

   ▶ The sperm then pass through the prostate gland and mix with fluid made by the prostate gland.

   ▶ Once sperm is mixed with fluid from the seminal vesicles and the prostate gland, the mixture is called semen.

5. Next, the semen travel through the tube in the center of the penis called the urethra.

   ▶ The Cowper's glands make a fluid that cleans out the urethra shortly before ejaculation takes place. It helps sperm live as it travels through the urethra and out of the body.

6. During orgasm, the penis ejaculates semen, which includes sperm.

   ▶ During ejaculation, the semen travels through the urethra. It leaves the penis through the urinary opening.

   ▶ If the semen enters a vagina, the sperm move up to the uterus and into the fallopian tubes.

   ▶ Sperm can live in the body of person who ovulates for up to 5 days.

   ▶ If sperm are in the tubes when the egg leaves one of the ovaries or soon after, a pregnancy can happen.

Infertility

Sometimes a person with testicles may not be able to cause a pregnancy. This means they are infertile. This problem can happen for many reasons. It can often be treated.

There are many causes of infertility in a person with a penis. Some of the causes are listed here:

- ▸ Alcohol and drugs
- ▸ Diabetes, thyroid and other health problems
- ▸ Some prescription medicines
- ▸ Testicle crush injury
- ▸ Untreated infections such as chlamydia and gonorrhea
- ▸ Poor nutrition
- ▸ Stress

How long can a person keep making sperm?

Once a person starts making sperm they typically do so their entire lives.

- Bodies that make sperm usually start around age 11 to 13.

- Bodies that make sperm can make about 250 million to 1 billion sperm every day.

As they age, they will make fewer sperm and be less fertile.

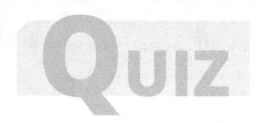

Reproductive System of Bodies that Make Sperm

Directions: Draw a line from the description on the left to the word on the right that it describes.

Description	Word
1. Sperm are made in these two sex glands.	Epididymis
2. Testicles are protected by this pouch of skin.	Prostate gland
3. This is where sperm are stored after they are made. This is also where they mature and become able to swim.	Seminal vesicles
4. These two tubes carry sperm from each epididymis.	Semen
5. These two glands are connected to the vas deferens. They make a thick fluid that flows into the tubes and mixes with the sperm. It keeps them moving and healthy.	Testicles
6. This gland produces a thin, milky fluid that helps sperm move and keeps it healthy.	Scrotum
7. This is a thin tube which goes down the center of the penis. Both sperm and urine travel through this tube (but not at the same time).	Cowper's glands
8. These two glands are attached to the urethra. They make a fluid that prepares the way for sperm. This fluid is released before ejaculation.	Vas deferens
9. When sperm and fluids from the seminal vesicles and prostate gland are mixed, it is called this.	Urethra

Check your answers on the next page.

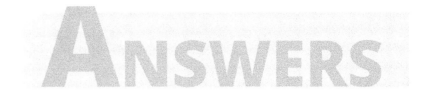

Reproductive System of Bodies that Make Sperm

Check your answers.

1. **Testicles** Sperm are made in the two testicles.

2. **Scrotum** Testicles are protected by the scrotum.

3. **Epididymis** The epididymis is where sperm are stored after they are made. This is also where they mature and become able to swim.

4. **Vas deferens** The vas deferens carry sperm from the epididymis.

5. **Seminal vesicles** Seminal vesicles are connected to the vas deferens. They make a thick fluid that flows into the tubes and mixes with any sperm. This fluid keeps them moving and healthy.

6. **Prostate gland** The prostate gland produces a thin, milky fluid that helps sperm move and keeps it healthy.

7. **Urethra** The urethra is a thin tube which goes down the center of the penis. Both sperm and urine travel through this tube.

8. **Cowper's glands** The Cowper's glands are attached to the urethra. They make a fluid that prepares the way for sperm. This fluid is released before ejaculation.

9. **Semen** When sperm and fluids from the seminal vesicles and prostate gland are combined, it is called semen.

The Reproductive System of Bodies that Ovulate

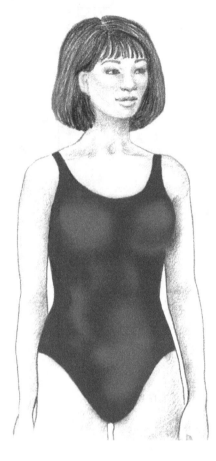

This section gives you some details that you, the health worker, may need to know about the reproductive system of bodies that ovulate. These details can help you better understand the basics that you will explain to your patients. They can also help you answer questions you may be asked. You don't need to use all of these words when you talk with your patients.

The reproductive organs (inside the body)

A person who ovulates has many special organs that work together so that they can have sex and get pregnant. Here are the reproductive organs inside a body that ovulates.

Brain. Two parts of the brain are responsible for making the ovaries work: the **hypothalamus** and the **pituitary gland**. These parts make hormones that travel through the bloodstream to the ovaries. They tell the ovaries to grow eggs and when to let an egg leave the ovary.

Uterus. The uterus (also called the **womb**) is a hollow, flexible, muscular organ about the size and shape of a pear. The uterus is where a pregnancy begins if a fertilized egg implants into it and starts to grow.

Endometrium. The lining of the uterus is called the endometrium. This lining changes during a menstrual cycle so that a pregnancy is possible.

▸ If an egg is fertilized by a sperm, the fertilized egg may attach to this lining and keep on growing. If this happens, there is a pregnancy. After about 9 months, a baby is born.

▸ If the egg does not meet with sperm, it is not fertilized. Pregnancy does not happen. Several days later, the blood from the lining of the uterus leaves the body through the vagina. This is called menstruation, or a period.

Ovaries. There are typically two ovaries. This is where the eggs (also called ova) are developed. A baby is born with about one million potential eggs called follicles already in their ovaries. After puberty, the ovaries start to make the hormones **estrogen** and **progesterone**. These hormones help people with uteruses become pregnant and have a healthy pregnancy. Every cycle, these hormones activate hundreds of follicles. But most of the time, only one of these follicles will mature into an egg and leave the ovary. This is called **ovulation**.

Fallopian tubes. A person with a uterus typically has two fallopian tubes, one next to each ovary. When an egg leaves an ovary, it travels through one of these thin tubes and moves toward the uterus. An egg can live for only 12-24 hours. If it does not meet with sperm during this time, the egg is absorbed in the tube.

Can more than one egg leave the ovaries at a time?

Sometimes more than one egg can leave the ovaries.

- The second egg will leave an ovary within 1 day after the first egg.

- When more than one egg leaves the ovary, fraternal twins (or triplets!) can happen.

If there are sperm in the fallopian tubes when the egg leaves the ovary, the egg can be fertilized.

Cervix. The cervix is the opening of the uterus. Sperm must go through it to get to the fallopian tubes. During the fertile days, the cervix opens a little more to let sperm through.

During birth, the cervix flattens and opens wide to let the baby leave the uterus.

The Reproductive System of Bodies that Ovulate Front View

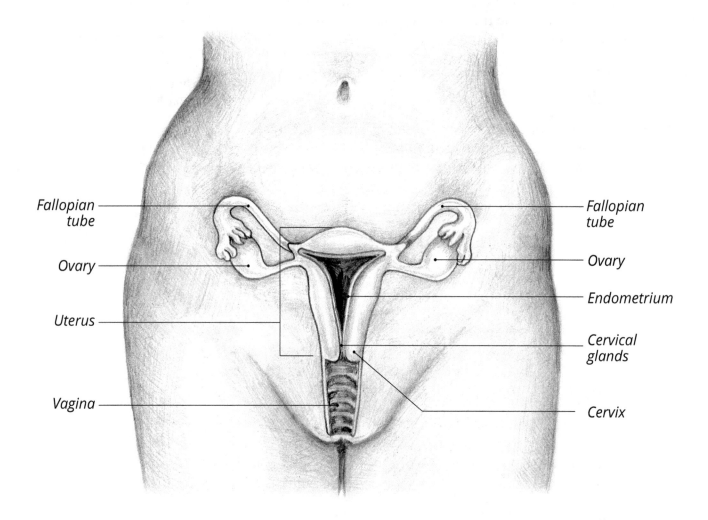

Fallopian tube

Ovary

Uterus

Vagina

Fallopian tube

Ovary

Endometrium

Cervical glands

Cervix

The Reproductive System of Bodies that Ovulate
Side View

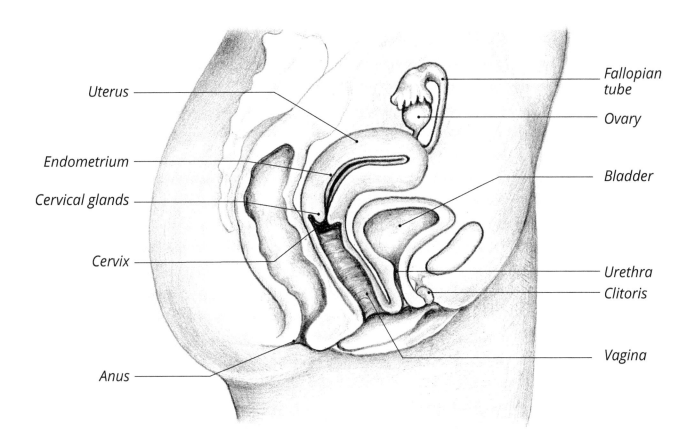

Uterus

Endometrium

Cervical glands

Cervix

Anus

Fallopian tube

Ovary

Bladder

Urethra

Clitoris

Vagina

Cervical glands. The cervical glands are in the cervix. These glands make cervical mucus, which changes during the menstrual cycle. For some days of the cycle, the mucus can be thick, dry or sticky. This is infertile mucus. This kind of mucus helps prevent sperm from traveling through the cervix.

As the time of ovulation nears, the mucus changes so that it can help sperm live and travel into the uterus. This is called fertile mucus. When fertile mucus is there, sperm can easily travel through the cervix. Sperm can then live in the vagina, uterus and fallopian tubes for up to 5 days.

Fertile mucus lets sperm live and travel easily. If semen is anywhere near the vaginal opening, sperm can get into the fertile mucus. The sperm can travel up into the vagina and into the tubes.

Vagina. The vagina is a muscular tube. Mucus, menstrual blood, and the baby pass from the uterus through the vagina. Semen from the penis goes into the uterus through the vagina.

When sexually aroused, more blood goes into the muscles in the vagina. This causes the vagina to get wider and longer. When the muscles get swollen with blood, a wet fluid that covers the vaginal walls is created. This change is also important for comfortable sex.

During birth, the baby comes out of the uterus and cervix through the vagina.

Why does Rose have a discharge?

Rose is 16 and has noticed a discharge on her underwear that she didn't have when she was younger. Sometimes it is wet and changes in color. She has never had sex, but worries that she may have a medical problem.

Rose is most likely seeing the cervical mucus that her body naturally makes. You can describe cervical mucus and the changes it makes through the cycle. Encourage Rose to ask the health care provider about it to make sure that it isn't something else.

The external reproductive organs (outside the body)

The parts of the reproductive system of bodies that ovulate that are on the outside of the body are all part of the **vulva**. They are described below.

Vaginal opening. The vaginal opening is at the outside of the vagina. During vaginal sex, this is where a penis can be inserted. This opening expands during birth for the baby to come out of the vagina. Some people like to have their vagina touched by a finger, tongue or sex toy.

Hymen. The hymen is a thin piece of tissue that partly covers the vaginal opening. It may be widened during exercise, masturbation, tampon use, or sex. Some people with vaginas may be born with no hymen at all.

Urinary opening. This is where urine (pee) leaves the body. It is just above the vaginal opening.

Clitoris. The clitoris is just above the urinary opening and extends inside the body. Its purpose is to give sexual pleasure. It is made of tissue and nerve endings. During sexual arousal, the tissue becomes swollen with blood. This makes it get larger and firm during sexual excitement.

> **Educator Tip**
>
> Talk about different ways people get sexual pleasure.
>
> This will help your patient understand that you are a safe person to talk to.

Labia minora. The labia minora (small lips) are folds of skin on each side of the opening to the vagina. These folds can meet at the top of the clitoris to help cover, and protect it.

Labia majora. The labia majora (large lips) are folds of skin and fat around the inner lips. There are oil and sweat glands in the labia majora to keep the area moist and healthy.

Mons pubis. The mons pubis is a pad of protective fat over the pubic bone.

Anus. This is the opening where the bowel movement leaves the body.

The Reproductive System of Bodies that Ovulate
The Vulva

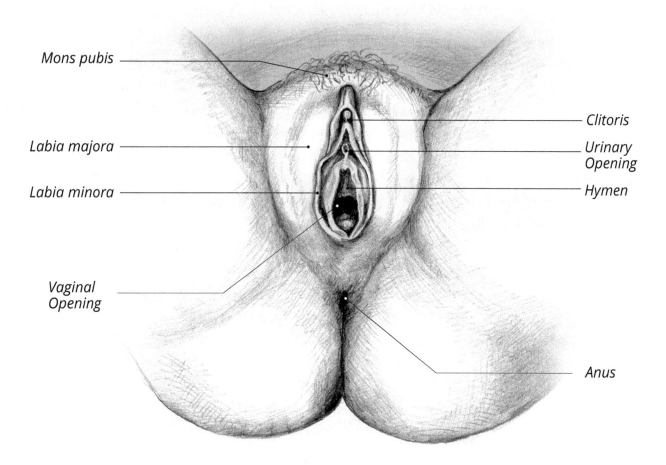

Mons pubis

Labia majora

Labia minora

Vaginal
Opening

Clitoris

Urinary
Opening

Hymen

Anus

What happens during the menstrual cycle?

During each menstrual cycle, the body gets ready to be pregnant. This is the reason for having a menstrual cycle.

Each cycle *begins* on the first day of a period and *ends* the day before the next period starts. A menstrual **period** can be 2 to 7 days long, but most have periods that are 4 to 5 days long. Most *cycles* are 22 to 36 days long. Some people normally have longer cycles and some have shorter cycles. A menstrual cycle can be a different length each month.

Cycle vs. Period

A menstrual cycle is *not* the same as a period.

The menstrual cycle has three stages:

▸ The time *before* an egg leaves one of the ovaries

▸ The time *when* the egg leaves the ovary

▸ The time *after* the egg leaves the ovary

Before the egg leaves the ovary

This part of a menstrual cycle starts on the day the period begins. At this time, the brain sends a message to the ovaries. This message causes eggs to start growing. Anywhere from 100 to 1,000 eggs start to grow. Each egg grows in its own body called a **follicle**. The follicles make the hormones needed to become pregnant. Though hundreds of eggs may start to grow, only one or two eggs completely mature and leave the ovary during each cycle. The rest of the eggs stop growing.

As the egg inside the follicle is growing, the follicle makes the hormone **estrogen**. The estrogen tells the body to:

▸ Start to make a new lining in the uterus so a fertilized egg can have a place to grow.

▸ Make a special kind of mucus in the cervix so sperm can live longer and travel to the egg.

▸ Make the opening of the cervix soften so that it can open enough to let sperm travel through it.

What are hormones?

Hormones are the messengers of the body.

- Chemical signals from one part of the body tell another part of the body what to do.

- The brain signals the ovaries, telling them when to start growing eggs and when to let an egg leave the ovaries.

- The ovaries make their own hormones.

- Two of these hormones are estrogen and progesterone.

Lining of the uterus

When the egg is ready to leave one of the ovaries, the lining of the uterus keeps on getting ready for pregnancy. Blood and nutrients keep going into the lining to allow a pregnancy to grow.

Special kind of mucus

After a period ends, the cervix makes mucus that is thick, somewhat white to yellow, and doesn't feel wet. This kind of mucus keeps the sperm out of the uterus. This is called **infertile mucus.** Sperm can only live in this mucus for a few minutes to a couple of hours.

Then, a few days before an egg leaves one of the ovaries, the cervix makes a special mucus called **fertile mucus.** The mucus starts to feel wet and there is more of it. It can be creamy white at first and will get cloudy or clear. Then the mucus changes and gets very wet, slippery, and stretchy. This special mucus helps sperm in two ways:

What is Fertile Mucus like?

Fertile mucus usually looks and feels like raw egg whites (before they are cooked). If you were to pinch fertile mucus between your finger and thumb, and then slowly spread them apart, the mucus would not break. It would stretch just like raw egg whites.

> ▸ Fertile mucus helps the sperm swim through the cervix and into the uterus and fallopian tube to meet the egg.
>
> ▸ Fertile mucus helps sperm live up to 5 days inside the vagina, uterus and fallopian tubes.

That means that after sex, sperm have up to 5 days to find and fertilize an egg. So if someone has sex on Monday night, they can become pregnant even if their egg doesn't leave their ovary until the next Saturday.

Changes in the cervix

A day or two before an egg leaves an ovary, the cervix changes. It gently rises or moves to the back of the vagina. A person with a uterus can't feel this happening but when it does, it may be hard for a them to feel their cervix with a finger during this time in their cycle.

The cervix also softens and becomes more open. This makes it easier for sperm to get to the egg.

The time *when* the egg leaves the ovary

If a person that ovulates is not on a hormonal method of birth control, one egg usually leaves an ovary each cycle. It then travels into one of the fallopian tubes. The egg is only about the size of a grain of sand. It can live for 12- 24 hours. If sperm is not already in the tube to meet it, or does not meet with it soon, the egg will be absorbed in the tube.

Around the time that the egg leaves the ovary:

- ▸ Their body temperature changes.
- ▸ The mucus made by the cervix changes.
- ▸ The cervix changes.

Other Fertility Signs

There are other fertility signs that can happen one or two days before ovulation or during ovulation:

- Aching or pain in the lower belly
- Spotting or light bleeding
- More energy, clearer skin, tender breasts
- Increase in sexual feelings

Pregnancy is possible about 1 week of per cycle.

Even though an egg can only live about one day, sperm can live in the vagina, uterus, and tubes for up to five days. Because of this, a person that ovulates can get pregnant for only 6 or 7 days during their cycle.

Example: If someone has sex on Monday and their egg doesn't leave one of their ovaries until Friday, they could still get pregnant. The sperm can stay alive and wait for the egg to leave the ovary.

Changes in body temperature

A person's **basal body temperature** (BBT) is the temperature of their body at rest. This means the temperature of the body right after they wake up and before they get out of bed.

A person's BBT changes in a special way during their cycle. Seeing the changes in their BBT can help someone know when their fertile days end.

- ▸ During their period and for a few days afterwards, a person's BBT is at its lowest.
- ▸ Shortly before, during, or just after the egg leaves the ovary, the BBT gets higher. It can go up anywhere from 0.3 degrees to 1.0 degree Fahrenheit. It should stay that high until that menstrual cycle ends.
- ▸ After the BBT goes up and stays up for a few days, it means the egg has left the ovary and is no longer in the tube to meet with the sperm. That means that they are not able to get pregnant until their next cycle.

When a person charts their BBT, they can tell when their fertile days end and when during their cycle they can no longer get pregnant. Those are called infertile days.

Note: Natural Family Planning (NFP) and the Fertility Awareness Method (FAM) are two birth control methods that use BBT. By taking their BBT a few days a month, someone can know that the egg has left the ovary and is no longer in the tube to be fertilized. They will then know when they cannot get pregnant for the rest of the days of their cycle.

Changes in cervical mucus

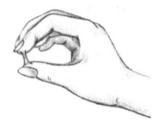 As a person gets close to the time when they will release an egg, their cervical mucus changes from infertile mucus to fertile mucus. Fertile mucus is wetter, thinner, and more slippery to the touch than infertile mucus. Fertile mucus keeps sperm healthy and alive and helps it travel to the egg. Without fertile mucus, sperm cannot live very long.

A person who ovulates can learn to track the changes in their mucus on a chart or app. They can use this information to help them use NFP or FAM, which are methods of birth control. They can also use it to help plan a pregnancy.

The time *after* the egg leaves the ovary

Once the egg leaves the ovary, the follicle the egg was growing in changes into a special gland called a **corpus luteum**. The corpus luteum makes the hormone **progesterone**. Progesterone's job is to protect pregnancy. It tells the body to make changes in the:

▸ Lining of the uterus

▸ Cervical mucus

▸ Cervix

These are the changes progesterone makes.

Changes in the lining of the uterus

The lining becomes thicker and fuller with blood and nutrients. The corpus luteum will keep making hormones for about 12 to 16 days.

▸ If the corpus luteum does **not** get a signal that pregnancy has occurred, it will stop making progesterone. Without progesterone, the lining stops growing. The blood in the lining will start to leave the uterus and travel through the cervical opening and down the vagina. This is the beginning of the **menstrual bleeding** (their period) and the start of a new menstrual cycle.

▸ If the corpus luteum **does** get a signal that pregnancy has occurred, it will keep making progesterone and estrogen. The lining will then keep the blood and nutrients needed to support the pregnancy.

Changes in the cervical mucus

Right after the egg leaves the ovary, the cervical mucus changes to infertile mucus again. There is less mucus than before and it no longer feels wet. It is often sticky and white or yellowish. Sperm can't live or travel in this thick and clumpy mucus. The infertile mucus also blocks the opening of the cervix. This helps keep sperm and germs out of the uterus. By keeping germs out of the uterus, if there is a pregnancy, infertile mucus will help protect it from infections.

Changes in the cervix

When the cervix starts to make infertile mucus, the cervix gets firmer, and its opening is closed. The changes also help keep sperm and germs out of the uterus. These changes also help protect pregnancy.

Educator Tip

To remember what progesterone does, try this: "PROgesterone PROtects pregnancy."

What if the egg is fertilized?

An egg waits in the fallopian tube for about a day to meet with sperm. If the egg is fertilized, it travels down into the uterus and attaches to the lining of the uterus. It takes about four to five days for it to travel through the tube, into the uterus, and then to become attached to the lining of the uterus.

When the fertilized egg attaches to the lining of the uterus, it sends out another hormone. This hormone is called HCG (human chorianic gonadatropin). Pregnancy tests measure this hormone. When it is present, the person is pregnant.

Remember

Pregnancy can happen even if a person's periods are not regular.

HCG tells the corpus luteum that pregnancy has occurred. This signals the corpus luteum to keep making progesterone and estrogen. Progesterone keeps the lining of the uterus full of blood and nutrients to support the pregnancy. It also keeps the cervical mucus thick and the cervix firm and closed to keep out germs and sperm. During the nine months of pregnancy, the cervix stays closed and the mucus stays infertile.

How could Alex get pregnant during their period?

Alex had sex only during their period. But still got pregnant. How could that happen?

An egg cannot leave the ovaries while someone is on their period. But the egg can leave within a few days after the bleeding stops or during the last days of the period. This is what happens when a cycle is 25 days or less.

If a menstrual cycle is 25 days or less, they can start making fertile mucus during their period. If there is fertile mucus, sperm could then live inside their body for up to 5 days. If an egg is released after or near the end of their period, the sperm could still be alive to fertilize it.

This is how Alex got pregnant when they only had sex during their period.

The life cycle of the egg

1. Eggs are stored in the ovaries.

2. Each month, the ovaries release hormones. These hormones are called estrogen and progesterone.

   Estrogen helps the body get ready for a possible pregnancy. These changes take place:

   ▸ The lining of the uterus gets thicker.

   ▸ The cervix makes fertile mucus which helps sperm live as long as 5 days in the vagina, uterus or fallopian tubes.

   ▸ The cervix gets soft, lifted, and its opening widens.

   During this time, the temperature of the body at rest stays low.

3. One egg fully matures and leaves the ovary. It travels through a fallopian tube and lives in the tube for only about 12-24 hours unless it is fertilized.

4. After the egg leaves the ovary, the ovary starts to make both estrogen and progesterone.

   The progesterone helps the body get ready for pregnancy. This is what happens:

   ▸ The lining of the uterus stays in place.

   ▸ The cervix makes infertile mucus to help keep sperm and germs from getting into the uterus.

   ▸ The cervix becomes firmer, lower in the vagina, and more closed.

   During this time, the temperature of the body at rest is high, and stays high until the next period starts.

5. If the egg is not fertilized, the body makes less estrogen and progesterone. This is a signal for the blood in the lining of the uterus to come out and the period starts.

   If the egg is fertilized and attaches to the lining of the uterus, the fertilized egg is now a pregnancy.

Why does the length of menstrual cycle change from cycle to cycle?

The average length of an entire menstrual cycle is 28 days. Many people have shorter cycles. Some have longer ones. And many cycles are a different length every cycle.

To understand why many people have cycles that vary in length from cycle to cycle, think of the menstrual cycle as being in two parts:

    Part 1: The number of days from the *first day of their period* until an egg is released.

    Part 2: The number of days from the *day an egg is released* to the first day of their next period.

Part 2 is usually the same. A period will typically start about 14 days after ovulation. (It is normal for this to be anywhere from 12 to 16 days). So once a period starts, you can figure out when they last ovulated. But Part 1 can change.

Someone can never know for sure when they will ovulate. Some months, a person may ovulate 8 days after their period starts. Other months, it may be as long as 20 days. Why? It is the brain that tells the ovaries to grow eggs and release an egg. That means that anything that affects the brain can change when the eggs are growing. Things that may affect the brain include:

- Poor diet or change in diet
- Changes in life situation
- Alcohol
- Drugs
- Illness
- Vacation or travel
- Relationships
- Anything that causes stress (good stress or bad stress)

Some bodies that ovulate are more sensitive to these things than others. For these people, the number of days before they ovulate may change often. That could mean that each of their cycles may be a different length.

To summarize:

The number of days between the first day of a period and ovulation can be:

- Shorter (like 6 to 8 days)
- Longer (like 20 to 23 days)
- Different each cycle.

That is all normal.

But the number of days between the time an egg is released and the day the next period starts will usually be **12 to 16 days**. A person can find out when they ovulated by counting back 12 to 16 days from the day their period starts.

What this means is:

- We can usually know when someone last ovulated.
- We can only guess when the next egg will leave an ovary.

> **Educator Tip**
>
> Transgender patients taking testosterone may experience changes in their periods. Periods may also stop or become irregular.

> **How long does someone have periods?**
>
> Periods usually start at about 12 years of age. But it is normal for them to start earlier or later. For the first two or three years, periods may not be regular. As people who menstruate get older, their periods become more regular.
>
> Ovulation happens about once every month until the age of 45. At about this age, many may stop having regular periods. After a while, between the ages of about 50 to 55, most people will stop ovulating and stop having periods.
>
> Once someone has not had a period for 12 months in a row, they have reached **menopause**. After that, they can no longer get pregnant.

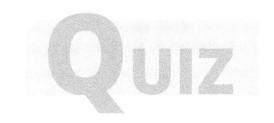# Quiz

The Reproductive System of Bodies that Ovulate

Directions: Circle the best answer to each question.

1. A menstrual cycle lasts this long.
    a. 2 to 7 days
    b. 22 days
    c. 22 to 36 days
    d. 36 days

2. When an egg leaves an ovaries, it is called:
    a. Ovulation
    b. Menses
    c. Ejaculation
    d. Pregnancy

3. Before ovulation, the egg follicles release estrogen. Estrogen tells the body to do which of the following?
    a. The cervical glands produce thin and stretchy, or wet, mucus called fertile mucus.
    b. The cervix softens and opens. It also rises or moves to the back of the vagina.
    c. The lining of the uterus gets thicker with blood and nutrients.
    d. All of the above

4. How many days during a cycle is a person that ovulates fertile?
    a. Up to 7 days
    b. 2 days
    c. 28 days
    d. None of the above

5. After ovulation, the corpus luteum releases progesterone. Progesterone tells the body to do which of the following?

   a. The cervical glands make thick and clumpy mucus to keep sperm and germs out of the uterus.

   b. The cervix will get more firm and closed and lower in the vagina.

   c. The lining of the uterus still gets thicker with blood and nutrients, just in case an egg was fertilized and needs to be nourished.

   d. All of the above

6. If someone is not pregnant, the time from when they releases an egg to when they start their next period is:

   a. 12 to 16 days

   b. 2 to 7 days

   c. 6 to 7 days

   d. No one can say.

7. When a fertilized egg attaches to the uterus, it sends out a hormone that lets the body know it is pregnant. This hormone is called:

   a. Testosterone

   b. Estrogen

   c. Progesterone

   d. hCG (Human Chorionic Gonadatropin)

8. Which of the following can affect the brain and might cause the release of an egg earlier or later than expected?

   a. Alcohol and drugs

   b. Relationship stress

   c. Work stress

   d. All of the above

Check your answers on the next page.

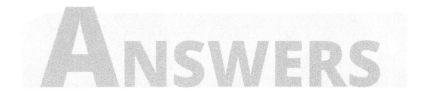

The Reproductive System of Bodies that Ovulate

Check your answers.

1. **C**   The menstrual cycle lasts from *22 to 36 days*. A cycle begins on the first day of the period and ends on the day before the next period starts.

2. **A**   When an egg leaves one of the ovaries, this is called *ovulation.*

3. **D**   All of the above. Estrogen is the signal from the follicles that tells the body to get ready for a pregnancy. It causes the cervical glands to make a thin and stretchy mucus called fertile mucus. It also causes the cervix to get softer and to open and move to the back of the vagina. And it causes the lining of the uterus to fill with blood and nutrients. This lining will nourish the egg, if they get pregnant.

4. **A**   A person that ovulates is only fertile for *up to 7 days* out of each cycle.

5. **D**   All of the above. Progesterone is the signal from the corpus luteum that tells the body to protect a possible pregnancy. It causes the cervical glands to make a thick and clumpy mucus. It also causes the cervix to get firm and close. And it tells the uterus to keep the lining full of blood and nutrients.

6. **A**   If pregnancy does not happen, the time between they release of an egg to the start of the next menstrual period is usually *12 to 16 days*.

7. **D**   When a fertilized egg attaches to the uterus, it sends out a hormone that lets the body know it is pregnant. This hormone is called *hCG.*

8. **D**   All of the above. Anything that causes stress, good or bad, could affect when ovulation happens. Stress could be caused by a poor diet, alcohol or drug use, major changes at school or work, vacation/travel, children, or relationships.

Puberty

Puberty is a time of major physical and emotional growth and development for every person.

For people assigned female at birth:

- ▸ Puberty usually begins around age 10.
- ▸ It usually ends around age 16.
- ▸ The first menstrual period often starts around age 12.

For people assigned male at birth:

- ▸ Puberty usually begins around age 11.
- ▸ It usually ends around age 18.
- ▸ The first ejaculation (release of semen) often starts around the ages 10 to 13.

During puberty, the reproductive system matures. At some point during puberty, people become able to reproduce. That means that bodies that ovulate can get pregnant and bodies that make sperm can cause pregnancies.

Puberty is also a time when sexual feelings increase.

Every person goes through the same process of physical development during the years of puberty. But the experience is different for each person. Some people develop quickly. Others change more slowly.

What are the changes that happen?

Many changes happen during puberty. Those changes are caused by an increase in certain hormones. Some of these hormones come from the brain. Others come from the sex glands (the ovaries and the testicles).

When it is time for puberty, the brain signals the sex glands to make more hormones:

- ▸ The signal makes the ovaries make more of the hormone **estrogen**.
- ▸ The signal makes the testicles make more of the hormone **testosterone**.

These two hormones cause the many changes of puberty.

Changes in those assigned female at birth

The hormone **estrogen** causes bodies with a uterus and ovaries to change in the following ways:

- ▸ Breasts begin to grow. This is one of the first signs of puberty. It is common for one breast to be a little larger than the other breast. Breasts may feel tender as they grow.

- ▸ Hair starts to grow on parts of the vulva (external genitalia) and in the armpits.

- ▸ They get taller.

- ▸ Their hips get broader.

- ▸ They start having more sexual feelings.

- ▸ First menstrual period typically happens 1 to 2 years after puberty starts. The first menstrual period is called menarche (MEN-ar-kee).

A body that ovulates can get pregnant as soon as the first egg leaves their ovary. This happens about 2 weeks before the first period. That means that they can become pregnant even *before* they get their first period. Even some 10-year-olds can get pregnant before they have their first period.

Many people have irregular periods for the first year or so. That is often because their bodies have not matured enough to make an egg come out of the ovaries on a regular basis.

Educator Tip

Be sure your patients know that a person who ovulates can get pregnant if they have unprotected sex, even if their periods are not regular yet.

Should Sage be worried?

Your 13-year-old patient, Sage, had their first period at age 12. They get a period every 2 to 4 months and want to know why they don't have periods every month like their friend Sarah. Sage is worried something is wrong with them. What could you say?

"Periods are irregular when you first start having them. This is totally normal. With time, your periods will get more regular and happen about once every month like your friend."

Changes in those assigned male at birth

The hormone **testosterone** causes bodies with testicles to change in the following ways:

> Masturbation is
> normal and healthy.
>
> During puberty,
> adolescents start to
> have more sexual
> feelings. They may
> start to masturbate or
> masturbate more.
> This is a normal part
> of puberty.
>
> Masturbating is a
> healthy way for people
> to learn how their
> bodies work. And, they
> find pleasure doing
> something that is safe
> and risk free.

- Shoulders and chest get bigger.
- They get more breast tissue. This can make breasts feel tender.
- The scrotum and penis grow.
- They get taller.
- Hair begins to grow in the armpits, on the chest, and around the penis and scrotum.
- Their voice changes.
- The body begins to make mature sperm and seminal fluid.
- They start having more sexual feelings.
- First ejaculation typically happens around ages 10 to 13. This is called semenarche (SEE-men-ar-kee).

First ejaculation often happens during sleep. This is normal. It can be caused by a sexual dream. But it can also be caused by the penis rubbing against clothing or sheets. Testosterone makes the penis more sensitive. The dream or rubbing makes the penis firm and larger. The semen can then be released. This is called a **wet dream** or a **nocturnal emission**. The person does not usually wake up when this happens.

As soon as bodies with testicles start to ejaculate, they can cause a pregnancy. Even 10-year-olds have caused pregnancies.

Each person is different.

While all adolescents go through puberty, it is different for each person. Some people start at age 10 or 11. Others don't start until the middle of their teen years. You can help your teen patients by letting them know it is normal for each of them to develop at different rates.

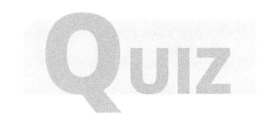

Puberty

Directions: Read each of the following statements.
Is it true or false? Circle the best answer.

1. Puberty is a time of major physical and emotional growth and development.   **True   False**

2. First menstrual period often starts around age 12.   **True   False**

3. Bodies with testicles usually start puberty around age 11.   **True   False**

4. Some adolescents develop quickly in puberty. Others change more slowly.   **True   False**

5. Estrogen is the hormone that causes the many changes of puberty in bodies with testicles.   **True   False**

Directions: Circle all that apply.

6. What puberty changes happen to bodies with a uterus?

    a.   Breasts begin to grow.
    b.   Hair starts to grow in the armpits and around the vulva.
    c.   They get taller.
    d.   Hips get broader.
    e.   Increase in sexual feelings
    f.   Menstrual period begins 1 to 2 years after puberty starts

7. What puberty changes happen to bodies with testicles?

    a.   Shoulders and chest get bigger.
    b.   Scrotum and penis grow.
    c.   They get taller.
    d.   Hair starts to grow in the armpits and around the penis and scrotum.
    e.   Increase in sexual feelings.
    f.   They start to make mature sperm and seminal fluid.

Check your answers on the next page.

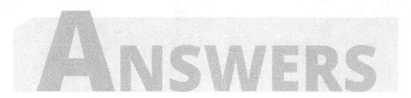

Puberty

Check your answers.

1. **True**   Puberty is a time of major physical and emotional growth and development for adolescents.

2. **True**   The first menstrual period often starts around **age 12**.

3. **True**   Bodies with testicles usually start puberty around **age 11**.

4. **True**   Some adolescents develop quickly in puberty. Others change more slowly.

5. **False**   ***Estrogen*** is the hormone that causes the many changes of puberty in ***bodies with a uterus and ovaries***. ***Testosterone*** is the hormone that causes the many changes of puberty in ***bodies with testicles***.

6. All of the changes listed are things that happen to bodies with a uterus during puberty.
   - Breasts begin to grow
   - Hair starts to grow in the armpits and around the vulva
   - They get taller
   - Hips get broader
   - Increase in sexual feelings
   - Menstrual period begins 1 to 2 years after puberty starts

7. All of the changes listed are things that happen to bodies with testicles during puberty.
   - Shoulders and chest get bigger
   - Scrotum and penis grow
   - They get taller
   - Hair starts to grow in the armpits and around the penis and scrotum
   - Increase in sexual feelings
   - The body starts to make mature sperm and seminal fluid

Reproduction and Puberty

Directions: Next to each number, write out the name of the reproductive organ that the line points to. Choose from the words listed below.

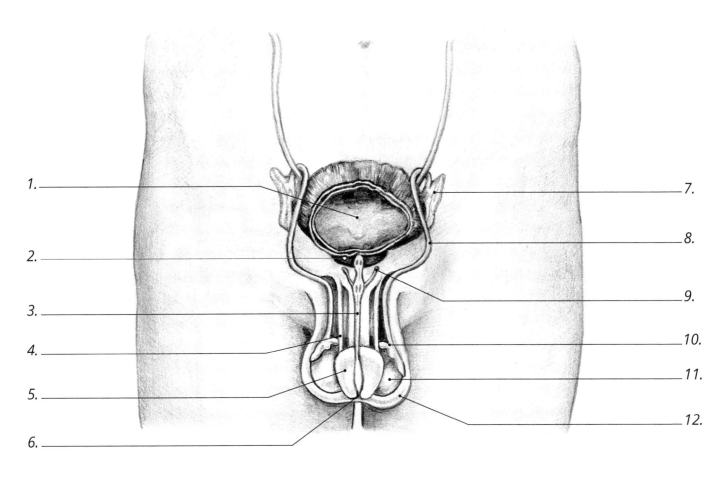

1. _____
2. _____
3. _____
4. _____
5. _____
6. _____

7. _____
8. _____
9. _____
10. _____
11. _____
12. _____

Bladder

Cowper's gland

Epididymis

Glans

Penis

Prostate gland

Scrotum

Seminal vesicle

Testicle

Urethra

Urinary opening

Vas deferens

Go on to the next page.

Directions: Next to each number, write out the name of the reproductive organ that the line points to. Choose from the words listed below.

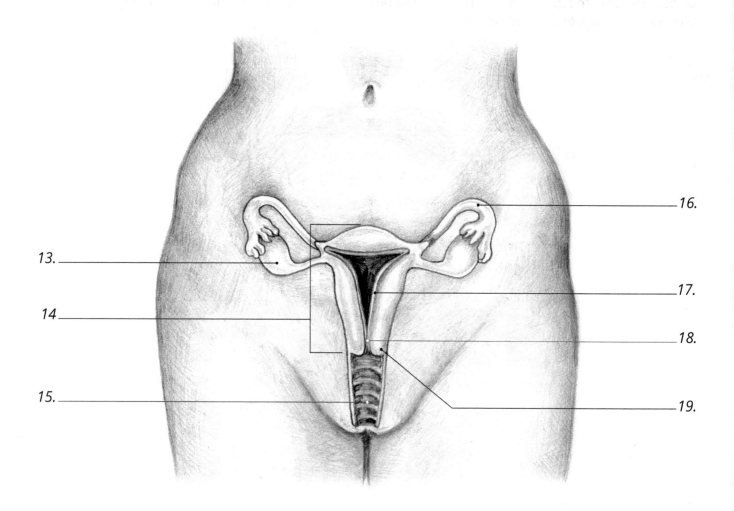

Cervical gland   Ovary

Cervix   Uterus

Endometrium   Vagina

Fallopian tube

Go on to the next page.

Directions: Next to each number, write out the name of the reproductive organs that are outside of the body. Choose from the words listed below.

20. _____

21. _____

22. _____

23. _____

24. _____

25. _____

26. _____

27. _____

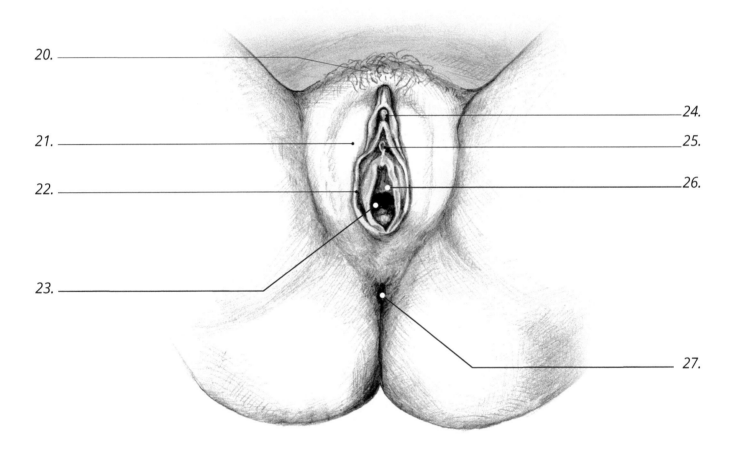

Anus   Labia minora

Clitoris   Mons pubis

Hymen   Vaginal opening

Labia majora   Urinary opening

Go on to the next page.

Directions: Circle the best answer.

28. The testicles make these two very important things:

    a. Semen and estrogen

    b. Progesterone and testosterone

    c. Sperm and testosterone

    d. Urine and pre-ejaculatory fluid

29. Which of the following are signs that a body that ovulates is in their fertile days?

    a. They have a thin, slippery mucus or wetness in the vagina.

    b. Their cervix has moved to the back of the vagina or is harder to reach.

    c. There is a rise in their BBT of 0.3 to 1.0 degree Fahrenheit.

    d. All of the above

30. When the egg leaves an ovary, it is called
    _____.

    a. Ovulation

    b. Menstruation

    c. Menarche

    d. Menopause

31. Which hormone do the follicles release *before* ovulation to help someone get pregnant?

    a. Estrogen

    b. Progesterone

    c. Testosterone

    d. hCG

Go on to the next page.

32. Which hormone does the corpus luteum release *after* ovulation to help protect a pregnancy?

    a. Estrogen

    b. Progesterone

    c. Testosterone

    d. hCG

Directions: Read the following statements and fill in the blanks.

33. Sperm can live up to ___ days in a body that is making fertile cervical mucus.

34. A pregnancy can happen if _____fertilizes an _____ in a fallopian tube first.

35. For people with a uterus, puberty usually starts around age _____ and ends around age _____.

36. For people with testicles, puberty usually starts around age _____ and ends around age _____.

Check your answers on the next page.

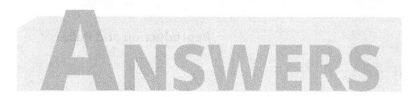

Reproduction and Puberty

Check your answers.

Reproductive System of Bodies that Make Sperm

1. Bladder
2. Prostate gland
3. Urethra
4. Penis
5. Glans
6. Urinary opening
7. Seminal vesicle
8. Vas deferens
9. Cowper's glands
10. Epididymis
11. Testicle
12. Scrotum

Reproductive System of Bodies that Ovulate (inside)

13. Ovary
14. Uterus
15. Vagina
16. Fallopian tube
17. Endometrium
18. Cervical glands
19. Cervix

Reproductive System of Bodies that Ovulate (outside)

20. Mons pubis
21. Labia majora
22. Labia minora
23. Vaginal opening
24. Clitoris
25. Urinary opening
26. Hymen
27. Anus

28. **C**   The testicles make *sperm* and *testosterone.*

29. **D**   All of the above. Cervical mucus will become thin, stretchy or feel like wetness in the vagina, the cervix will become harder to reach because it has moved farther to the back of the vagina, or higher in the vagina, and their BBT will rise slightly.

30. **A**   *Ovulation* is when an egg leaves the ovary.

31. **A**   Before ovulation, follicles release *estrogen* to help a person get pregnant.

32. **B**   After ovulation, the corpus luteum releases *progesterone* to help protect a pregnancy.

33. **5**   Sperm can live up to *5* days in a body that is making fertile cervical mucus.

34. **Sperm, egg**   A pregnancy can happen if *sperm* fertilizes an *egg* in a fallopian tube first.

35. **10, 16**   For people with a uterus, puberty usually starts around age *10* and ends around age *16.*

36. **11, 18**   For people with testicles, puberty usually starts around age *11* and ends around age *18.*

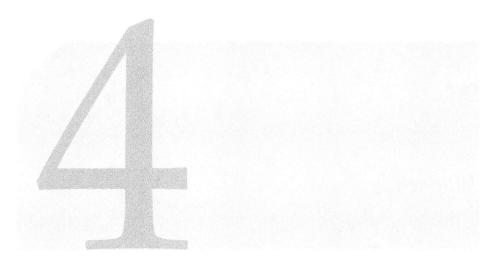

Human Sexuality

Much like your personality, sexuality is something you are born with and that is influenced by your life experiences. It is an important part of being human. Because sexuality education and counseling is an important part of sexual and reproductive health care services, it is something you will want to feel comfortable talking about.

You will need to ask your patients many questions about their sexual lives. These questions help you gather important information about your patients. For example, you learn about their risk of infection and pregnancy. You might also find out about their history or risk of sexual abuse.

Relax

If talking about sexuality is hard for you, relax. It takes practice and will get easier with time.

Let your patients know that sex is a safe topic to discuss. Help them feel free to talk with you about their sexual issues, questions, and concerns. You can also refer them to someone else when they have questions you can't answer.

The more you understand about sexuality, the easier it will be for you to talk with your patients about it. The more comfortable you are talking with your patients about sexuality, the more comfortable they will be talking with you. The information in this chapter should help.

Topics in this chapter

▸ Sexuality

▸ Sexual Expression

▸ The Body's Physical Sexual Response

▸ Common Sexual Problems

Objectives

After reading this chapter, you will be able to:

▸ Explain what human sexuality is.

▸ List five things that affect sexuality.

▸ Describe five ways that people express their sexuality.

▸ Describe a human sexual response cycle.

▸ Explain how a health worker can help a patient with sexual problems and concerns.

Sexuality

We are all sexual beings. So what a person thinks about sex and sexuality is important. It affects many things in life — including the need for family planning. Though everyone is born with sexuality, their thoughts about it are influenced by the world around them.

Sexuality Definitions

▶ Sex (a persons' traits that include, hormones, chromosomes and internal and external reproductive organs)

▶ Gender roles (learned behaviors associated with a particular gender in a culture)

▶ Gender identity (a person's internal sense of gender as a man, woman or something else)

▶ Gender expression (the way a person expresses their gender identity, often by their appearance, the way they dress and/or their behaviors)

▶ Sexual orientation:

  ▪ Straight – attracted to the opposite sex/gender

  ▪ Gay – attracted to the same sex/gender

  ▪ Bisexual – attracted to two sexes/genders

  ▪ Pansexual – attracted to all sexes/genders

▶ Sexual expression (all the ways people show their sexual feelings, including, hugs, kisses, oral sex, anal sex, masturbation, sexual intercourse, or even abstinence).

▶ Human Growth and Development (physical changes that happen during puberty, pregnancy, menopause, aging, etc.)

▶ Body image (how you see and think about your body)

As you can see, sexuality is much more than just "having sex" or "feeling sexy."

Every person is a sexual being. It doesn't matter whether we are young or old, married or single, with or without disabilities.

What influences a person's sexuality?

Many factors influence how we feel and think about our sexuality and how we act sexually. Here are a few of them.

Transgender and Intersex persons

A person can be assigned male or female at birth.

An intersex person may be born with genitals that make it hard to assign them a sex at birth.

Learn more about intersex persons at: www.isna.org

A transgender person is someone who does not identify with the sex they were assigned at birth.

Gender roles

▶ Most people are assigned male or female at birth based on their external genitalia (sex organs). This is called their sex. Someone's sex may or may not match their gender identity.

▶ Gender roles are what it means to be "masculine" or "feminine." Gender roles refer to the attitudes and behaviors our society expects us to act out. We are not born knowing what men and women are "supposed" to do. We learn these roles. Gender roles are different in each culture and can vary from family to family.

▶ How we feel about our assigned sex, or what things we should or should not do because of our gender, influence how we behave. For example, in some cultures women are allowed to cry in public, but men are not.

▶ Gender roles can lead to stereotypes about sexuality. For example, people may think that "a man should always want sex and be ready for it" or that "women shouldn't talk about sex." These stereotypes can be damaging and affect the way people relate.

Family

▶ What families do or don't do and what they say or don't say about sex shapes what a child thinks is right.

▶ The way parents treat children helps form the way children feel about themselves and their bodies.

Culture and religion

▶ All cultures and religions have certain beliefs about sexuality and when and how it should be expressed.

▶ Some of these beliefs are clearly stated and others may be unspoken.

▶ These beliefs influence people whether or not they agree with the ideas.

Media

▸ What people see and hear on TV, in the movies, in music, on the Internet, and in print affects their sexuality and their feelings about it.

▸ The media often gives sensational or unrealistic images of people's sexual lives and bodies. For example, couples in movies and TV often have sex, but rarely deal with consent, birth control, pregnancy, or sexually transmitted infections (STIs).

Past sexual experiences

▸ A person's sexual experiences often have a lasting impact on their sexuality.

▸ Being physically forced to have sex or being hurt emotionally can be very harmful to one's sexuality.

▸ Feeling respected and loved can lead to a more positive sense of sexuality.

Knowledge about sexuality

▸ People who are informed about sexuality can make healthier choices about their lives.

▸ For example, an adolescent may think they cannot get pregnant the first time they have sex. They may not think they need to use a birth control method or protect themselves from sexually transmitted infections.

Peers

▸ Friends can play a large role in shaping sexuality.

▸ If a friend acts a certain way, you may be more likely to act that way. For example, young people can feel pressure to have sex if they think all of their friends are having sex.

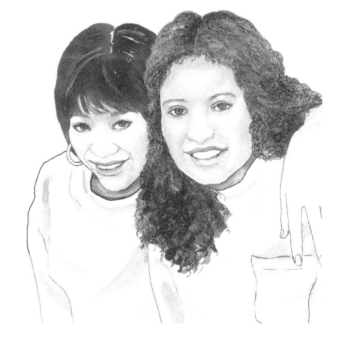

Values and attitudes

▸ The way you think, feel, and act shapes your values and attitudes about sex.

▸ These values and attitudes can be very important to people.

Body image

▸ The way you feel about your own body — how it looks, feels, smells, and even tastes — is called your body image. And your body image affects your sexuality.

▸ If you don't feel good about your body, you may feel uncomfortable with your sexuality.

▸ How you feel about your body is affected by the media (Internet, TV, movies, magazine ads). The media present a certain body type as normal, attractive, and sexy. But every body is different. Very few people in real life match the media's image.

Respect each patient's values.

Patients may talk with you about how they feel about sex. A patient's values may be similar to your own. Or they may be very different. As a health worker, you should always respect your patients' values and choices — even when they are different from your own. Focus on helping patients make the best choices for *their* lives.

Sexual orientation

▸ "Sexual orientation" refers to who you find yourself attracted to. Everyone is different. Some are attracted to the opposite sex/gender (heterosexual or "straight"). Others are attracted to the same sex/gender ("gay" or "lesbian"). And still others are attracted to two (bisexual) or all sexes/genders (pansexual).

▸ How you feel about different sexual orientations is affected by the media, by religion, by culture, and by the values and attitudes of the people around you.

▸ How you feel about your own sexual orientation can affect how you feel about sex. It can also affect how you express your sexuality.

▸ People who identify as lesbian, gay, bisexual or pansexual may find it hard to feel comfortable about their sexuality in certain cultures or situations. They may feel more comfortable if the people they are around support them.

Sexuality throughout life

We are sexual beings from the day we are born until we die. We are built to enjoy the touch and closeness of other people. As we grow up, we need to be able to love and to feel loved. In different ways, we all can feel sexual pleasure throughout our lives, no matter what our age. How a person experiences sexual feelings will change throughout life.

Here is an overview of sexuality throughout life.

Everyone is sexual.

Everyone, young and old, healthy or ill, can experience sexual pleasure. This includes people who have physical or mental disabilities.

Babies

Babies are born with the need to be touched and cuddled. They cannot thrive without touch. Babies enjoy touches, kisses, cuddles, massages, and baths. Babies like learning about their bodies and enjoy putting fingers and toes into their mouths and touching their genitals (the area around the penis or the area around the vulva).

Babies are learning how to feel about their bodies. It is important that babies are treated with tenderness. For example, it is not a good idea for someone to spank a baby's hand away when a baby touches their own genitals, or to frown when changing a diaper. The baby may think that the body and genitals are something to be ashamed of.

Children (ages 3 through 7)

From 3 through 7 years of age, all children are curious about their bodies and the bodies of thers. In addition to looking at or touching their own genitals, they may also be curious about the genitals of other children of the same age.

At this age, it is good to teach their children the names of their body parts and to talk to them in a way that does not bring guilt or shame. Parents can help their children feel comfortable about their bodies. They should express affection by hugging, kissing, and giving back rubs. Children this age love to sit right next to their caregivers or in their laps.

It is important that children of this age are taught that NO one has the right to touch them in any way that makes them uncomfortable. This is good age-appropriate practice for talking about consent with children.

Preteens (ages 8 through 12)

When children begin their preteen years, around the age of 8, they often begin to play separately. Preteens may have crushes on older people or on other children their own age. Kissing games are normal as puberty nears.

Preteens are curious about their own sexuality. They may also be curious about other's sexuality and have many questions. They may masturbate (rubbing their own genitals). They may have orgasms. Some may explore the genitals of a friend their own age.

Some children become more modest as they get older. Their need for privacy should be respected. Parents should talk to their children about reproduction and puberty so that they will be prepared for the changes they will go through. It is also important for children to feel that they have someone they can talk to about this important topic.

Teens (ages 13 through 19)

Many major physical changes take place as the teen's body starts to develop into the body of an adult. Feelings of being sexual and wanting sexual activity usually get stronger. It is common for teens to have sexual experiences, like kissing or fondling, with people whose gender is the same or different from their own. They may be experimenting with their sexuality. Or they may be physically and emotionally attracted to people of the same sex or gender.

At some point, many teens have sexual intercourse or other forms of sexual activity. It is important that teens have the information they need to protect themselves if they do choose to have sex. They need to know about birth control, STI prevention, and how to talk about what they really want.

They should not feel pressured into having sex if they are not really ready for it. Talking with peers, parents, and other trusted adults can help teens through this challenging and sometimes confusing time of life. So can taking classes in sexuality education.

Young adults (20s and 30s)

By age 21, most people (but not all) have had one or more sexual partners. As they leave the teen years, young adults are exploring what it means to be intimate and what kind of relationships will work best for them. For some people this means finding a long-term partner and perhaps starting a family. It may mean exploring their sexuality as a single person.

Sometimes it involves working through problems they have had that make it difficult for them to have the type of healthy relationships they want. Some people, whether they are in a long term relationship or not, may benefit from counseling. It can help them learn more about how to express their needs as well as how to support others in loving, healthy ways.

Adults (40s and 50s)

People in the middle years of their lives are still very interested in sexual activity. But there may be some changes in the way they feel and function during sex.

For example, it may take more time for a penis to get erect or the penis may not get as hard. Some vaginas may become dryer and may need to use lubricant during sexual intercourse.

All people may benefit from learning new ways of giving and getting sexual pleasure.

Older Adults (60s and older)

Throughout our lifespan, people are sexual beings. Most people keep wanting to be close, loving, and sexual with another person all their lives. This is true into the 80s and 90s and beyond. People with testicles in their 80s are sometimes still fertile and able to cause a pregnancy.

Older people can fall in love just as intensely as young teenagers do. While people are able to have sex throughout their lives, it is more common for older people to have medical problems. Some medical issues have an effect on the ways that older people can express their sexuality.

Families and health care providers should support older people's sexual needs and desires, not dismiss them.

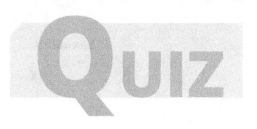

SEXUALITY

Directions: Circle the best answer.

1. Sexuality is a person's feelings, thoughts, and actions around which of the following?

    a. Gender roles and body image

    b. Human growth and development

    c. Sexual orientation and sexual expression

    d. All of the above

2. Which of the following influences our sexuality?

    a. Family and peers

    b. Culture and religion

    c. Knowledge about sexuality

    d. All of the above

3. We are sexual beings from the time we are born until when?

    a. Puberty

    b. Menopause

    c. We die

    d. None of the above

4. We are sexual beings at which of the following stage or stages of our lives?

    a. When we are babies

    b. When we are teens and young adults

    c. When we are older adults (60 years of age and older)

    d. All of the above

Check your answers on the next page.

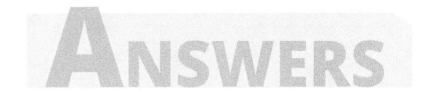

SEXUALITY

Check your answers.

1. **D**   All of the above. Sexuality is a person's feelings, thoughts, and actions around gender roles, body image, human growth and development, sexual orientation, and sexual expression. It also includes a person's feelings, thoughts, and actions around their family and relationships.

2. **D**   All of the above. Each of the following influences our sexuality:
    - Family and peers
    - Culture and religion
    - Knowledge about sexuality

    Our sexuality is also influenced by:
    - Gender roles
    - Media
    - Past sexual experiences
    - Values and attitudes
    - Body image
    - Sexual orientation

3. **C**   We are sexual beings from the time we are born until we die.

4. **D**   All of the above. We are sexual beings our whole lives long.

Sexual Expression

There are many ways to express sexuality. Some think they need to have sex to give or receive love and affection. But people can enjoy a wide range of sexual expression without intercourse. They can hold hands, hug, kiss, massage, dance, touch, and more. All forms of sexual expression are normal and okay — as long as the people involved agree.

People have a right to:

- Express their sexuality in different ways.
- Refuse to do anything they don't want to do.

People do *not* have a right to:

- Express their sexuality in ways that cause harm.
- Force someone to do something.
- Tell others how to express their sexuality.

If a patient feels pressured by a sex partner

If one of your patients feel pressured into having any sexual contact that they do not want, they may want to talk to someone about it.

- You can talk to them about ways to talk to their partners.
- You can also refer them to someone else who is specially trained to help them.

This section describes some of the many ways people can express their sexuality. Different people enjoy different forms of expression. No one choice is right for everyone or for all times in someone's life.

Abstinence

Abstinence means different things to different people. It basically means choosing not to have certain kinds of sexual contact. For example, for some people abstinence means not having any kind of sex. For others it may mean just not having vaginal sex. Find out what abstinence means to your patient.

There are many reasons that people choose abstinence:

- To prevent pregnancy.
- To prevent STIs.
- To follow their personal beliefs.
- To respect their family or cultural values.

Abstinence can refer to the *postponement* or *delay* of having sex. This means choosing to wait to have sex. For example, your patient may be waiting:

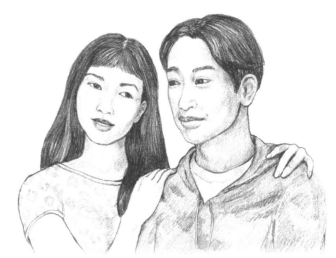

▶ Until they get married.

▶ Until they have a birth control method.

▶ Until they get condoms.

▶ Until they both feel ready.

▶ Until they are in a stable and committed relationship.

You can talk to your patients about whatever abstinence means to them. Read more about it in Chapter 6.

Fantasies

People can feel sexually aroused just by thoughts, dreams, or images.

▶ Fantasies can be a way to think about and imagine many sexual choices.

▶ People can choose to share their fantasies with a partner or not. A person can have a fantasy without wanting to act out that fantasy in real life.

Touching

Touching can be a full sexual experience.

▶ It can include cuddling, kissing, biting, licking, fingering, or mutual masturbation.

▶ Massages, back rubs, foot rubs, or shared showers or baths can feel wonderful.

▶ Some parts of the body are more sensitive than others. But the whole body can be a source of pleasure.

Masturbation

This means touching your own body (often the genitals) to get sexual pleasure. It can also be a way for people to learn more about their own bodies.

▶ People cannot become pregnant or get an STI when they masturbate.

▶ Most people masturbate at some time. Masturbation is normal and does not harm a person's health.

▶ Masturbation is a way for someone to celebrate their sexuality in a healthy way.

▶ Many people learn how to have an orgasm by masturbating.

Oral sex

▸ When a person uses their mouth to stimulate the partner's external sex organs, it is called oral sex.

▸ When it is done on a vulva/clitoris, it is called "cunnilingus."

▸ When done on a penis/testicles, it is called "fellatio."

▸ People can't get pregnant or cause pregnancy through oral sex.

▸ You can give and get an STI through oral sex if one of the partners is infected. But the risk of some STIs may be less with oral sex than with vaginal or anal sex.

Vaginal sex

Vaginal sex (sexual intercourse) is when the penis is put inside the vagina. The vagina can also be penetrated by fingers and sex toys.

▸ There are many different positions that a couple can use. What matters is what feels good to each partner.

▸ With vaginal sex, a person with a uterus who ovulates can get pregnant. If they do not want to get pregnant, a birth control method must be used.

▸ With vaginal sex, either partner could get HIV or another STI. Using external or internal condoms can help prevent this. There are gloves and finger condoms that can be used for protection when fingers or hands are in contact with another person's genitals. Sex toys should be cleaned between uses.

Anal sex

Anal sex means penetrating the anus with the penis, sex toys or fingers.

▸ Both opposite sex and same sex couples may have anal sex.

▸ Some people like to have their anus touched with a finger or the tongue.

▸ A person can get pregnant even when having anal sex. This is because of the cervical mucus that can come out of the vagina. This mucus can be found in the area between the vagina and anus. After anal sex with ejaculation, sperm can flow out of the anus into this mucus. They can then swim into the vagina and may fertilize an egg. A pregnancy can happen if the fertilized egg implants into the uterus. This is why you need to use a birth control method even when you have anal sex.

▸ People can get HIV and other STIs by having anal sex. Using condoms can help protect against these infections.

Making decisions about sex

Each person needs to decide how and when to express themselves sexually.

▶ Some people follow rules taught by their parents, spiritual or religious leaders, or peers. Others are not given rules or do not agree with the rules.

▶ It is important for people to understand their values and make their own decisions.

You can support patients as they think through their choices. You can also encourage them to make sure that their choices are the right ones for them.

Sexual Orientation and Family Planning

It is easy to assume that everyone who comes into a birth control clinic is heterosexual and only concerned about birth control. But remember that family planning clinics provide many services that are good for **anybody** who is sexually active. You will find your patients have a variety of gender identities, gender expressions and sexual orientations. Some patients may participate in behavior you identify as "same sex," but they may not identify as gay or lesbian or bisexual.

Try not to label your patients as gay, straight or bi. Instead, think of how specific sexual behaviors can affect their health and their goals for coming to the clinic. Then do your best to meet their needs.

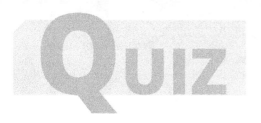

SEXUAL EXPRESSION

Directions: Read each of the following statements.
Is it true or false? Circle the best answer.

1. People have a right to express their sexuality in different ways. **True   False**

2. People have a right to refuse to do anything sexual that they don't want to do. **True   False**

3. People don't have a right to force someone to do something sexual. **True   False**

4. There is only one way to define "abstinence." **True   False**

5. You can't get an STI by having oral sex. **True   False**

6. Family planning patients may be gay, lesbian, bisexual, or heterosexual. **True   False**

Directions: Write your answer on the space below.

7. List four different ways that patients might express their sexuality.

   ▪ _____

   ▪ _____

   ▪ _____

   ▪ _____

Check your answers on the next page.

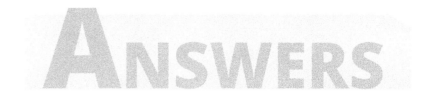

SEXUAL EXPRESSION

Check your answers.

1. **True** People do have a right to express their sexuality in different ways.

2. **True** People do have a right to refuse to do anything sexual that they don't want to do.

3. **True** People don't have a right to force someone to do something sexual.

4. **False** There is more than one way to define abstinence. Abstinence means different things to different people. It basically means choosing *not* to have certain kinds of sexual contact. For example, for some people abstinence means not having *any* kind of sex. Others may feel it means just not having *vaginal* sex.

5. **False** You *can* get an STI by having oral sex. You can give and get an STI through oral sex if one of the partners is infected. But the risk of some STIs may be less with oral sex than with vaginal or anal sex.

6. **True** Family planning patients may be gay, lesbian, bisexual, or heterosexual. It is easy to assume that everyone who comes into a birth control clinic is heterosexual and only concerned about birth control. But remember that family planning clinics provide many services that are good for *anybody* who is sexually active.

7. Some ways to express sexuality are:
   - Abstinence
   - Fantasy
   - Touching
   - Masturbation
   - Oral sex
   - Anal sex
   - Vaginal sex

   There are many other forms of sexual expression, including holding hands, hugging, kissing, dancing, and massage. All forms are normal and okay — as long as the people involved agree.

The Body's Sexual Response

Our bodies go through physical changes when we have a sexual experience. This is called the **sexual response**.

The body is able to have a sexual response throughout life. It may change as we grow older, but most of the time it is very pleasurable.

There are things that can interfere with our sexual response. Physical problems such as illness or drug use can change it. Feelings such as guilt, confusion, or fear can also affect it. You can read more about this later in this chapter under "Common Sexual Problems."

People can be sexually excited (sexually aroused) by many things. For example, people may be aroused when they:

- ▸ Are touched.
- ▸ Listen to music.
- ▸ Think about a special person.
- ▸ Think about having sex.

Thoughts, feelings, sights, smells, sounds, and touches are all things that can make someone sexually excited. What excites one person may or may not excite someone else.

The sexual response cycle

When people become sexually aroused, their bodies start to go through specific physical changes. These same changes happen no matter how or why a person has become sexually aroused.

The purpose of these changes is to prepare our bodies for further arousal and intercourse. If arousal continues and orgasm takes place, there will be more physical changes.

The series of changes that occur is called the **sexual response cycle**. The sexual response cycle has four phases (according to the original Masters and Johnson model of sexual response):

1. Excitement phase (becoming aroused)

2. Plateau phase (preparing for orgasm)

3. Orgasm phase (climaxing or "coming")

4. Resolution phase (returning to normal, unaroused state)

Knowing these phases gives you a good idea of what happens in the body when a person is sexually aroused. But the exact response in each person is different. And it never feels exactly the same each time a person has sex.

Be aware that not everyone has an orgasm every time they have sex. And know that a person can stop the cycle at any point. Once stopped, the body will return to its unaroused state.

Sexual response cycle for a person with a penis and testicles

Here are the physical changes that happen during their sexual response cycle.

1. **Excitement phase (becoming aroused)**

    As they start to feel excited:

    ▸ More blood flows to the penis.

    ▸ The penis gets longer, wider, and hard (erect). This allows the penis to enter the vagina or anus easily.

    ▸ The skin of the scrotum thickens. The scrotum pulls up and lifts the testicles closer to the body.

    ▸ Muscles in other parts of the body become tense.

    ▸ The heart beats faster and blood pressure goes up.

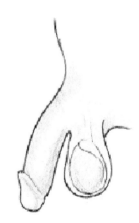

Penis before blood flows in

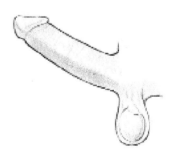

Erect Penis

2. **Plateau phase (preparing for orgasm)**

   As the feelings grow stronger, the body prepares for orgasm.

   ▸ The penis lengthens and widens to its full size.

   ▸ The testicles rise to a point where they press against the body. They also get much larger as they become filled with blood.

   ▸ The Cowper's glands send clear fluid (pre-come) to the tip of the penis.

   ▸ More blood flows to the skin at the center of the lower chest and changes its color. This change in skin color is called the "sex flush."

   ▸ The heart beats faster and blood pressure goes up.

   ▸ Breathing is also faster and deeper.

   ▸ Muscles become more tense.

3. **Orgasm phase (climaxing or "coming")**

   Orgasm is the peak of intense pleasure during sexual activity. It can feel different at different times. People with a penis and testicles often have an orgasm and ejaculate at the same time.

   ▸ **Orgasm** is the peak pleasure response during sex.

   ▸ **Ejaculation** ("coming") is when semen comes out of the penis.

   During the orgasm phase:

   ▸ The vas deferens, prostate gland, and seminal vesicles contract.

   ▸ Muscles contract in other parts of the body.

   ▸ The heart beats more quickly.

   ▸ Breathing becomes irregular and fast.

   ▸ Semen goes into the urethra and out of the penis.

4. **Resolution phase (returning to normal)**

   After orgasm and ejaculation, the body goes back to its relaxed, unaroused state:

   ▸ Blood flows away from the penis.

   ▸ Breathing, heart rate, and blood pressure return to normal.

   Many people with a penis and testicles are not able to have another full erection and ejaculation for some time. The amount of time needed is different for each person. Once this time has passed, they can be sexually aroused again.

Sexual response cycle for a person with a vagina and clitoris

Here are the physical changes that happen during their sexual response cycle.

1. **Excitement phase (becoming aroused)**

   As they start to feel excited:

   ▸ More blood flows to the vagina and other sex organs.

   ▸ The vagina gets moist and lubricated.

   ▸ The vagina lengthens and widens. This also makes intercourse more comfortable.

   ▸ The clitoris gets bigger and becomes erect.

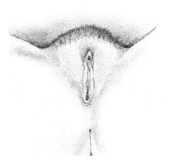

Labia before the excitement phase

   During this phase:

   ▸ The labia majora flatten and open away from the vagina.

   ▸ The labia minora swell. They may triple in size.

   ▸ The breasts swell and nipples may get hard.

   ▸ The uterus grows larger and lifts up a bit. This pulls the cervix upward in the vaginal canal.

   ▸ Muscles in other parts of the body become tense.

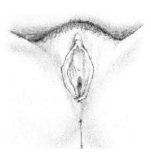

Labia during the excitement phase

2. **Plateau phase (preparing for orgasm)**

   As feelings grow stronger, the body prepares for orgasm:

   ▸ More blood flows to the vagina and muscles become more tense.

   ▸ The tissue in the outer part of the vagina becomes filled with blood. This narrows the vaginal opening.

   ▸ Vaginal lubrication may slow.

   ▸ The clitoris becomes more swollen and is pulled back.

   Other changes can be noticed:

   ▸ The breasts swell more. This makes the nipples seem smaller.

   ▸ A "sex flush" can spread over the stomach, chest, and neck.

   ▸ The heart beats faster and blood pressure goes up.

   ▸ Breathing gets faster and deeper.

3. **Orgasm phase (climaxing or "coming")**

   Orgasm is the peak of intense pleasure during sexual activity. All the muscles that were tightened during sexual arousal first tense and then relax, causing a very pleasurable feeling.

   During the orgasm phase:

   ▸ The heart may beat faster and blood pressure may go up.

   ▸ Breathing is faster.

   ▸ Muscles throughout the body quickly tense and relax, but mostly those around the vagina, uterus, and anus.

   ▸ Some people with vaginas may also ejaculate a fluid during orgasm.

   Orgasms may feel different at different times.

4. **Resolution phase (returning to normal)**

   After orgasm, the body goes back to its relaxed, unaroused state.

   ▸ Blood flows away from sex organs.

   ▸ Breathing, heart rate, and blood pressure return to normal.

   Some changes happen quickly. Others can take more than an hour.

   Many people with a vagina and clitoris can have more than one orgasm in a short time.

A note about orgasm in a body with a clitoris

The clitoris, the vagina, or both can be stimulated by being touched, rubbed, or caressed. This stimulation can lead to an orgasm. Most orgasms come from direct or indirect stimulation of the clitoris. Every body responds a different way to various kinds of touch. Each person has their own likes and dislikes for how their clitoris is touched. With practice alone or with a partner, each person can decide what works best for them.

About the G-Spot

There is a place inside the vagina called the **G-Spot** (short for the Grafenberg spot). It can become very sensitive during sex play. Some feel greater pleasure when the G-Spot area is stimulated. There is some controversy about the size and exact location of the G-Spot, most agree that this area is about an inch or two inside the vagina on the side closest to the navel. Multiple studies have shown that this area is not the same for all people with a vagina and that some do not experience heightened sensitivity when this area is stimulated.

If you have a patient that thinks something is wrong with them because they cannot find this spot during sex or they do not feel increased pleasure when this area is stimulated, assure them that if they have an otherwise enjoyable sex life they shouldn't worry.

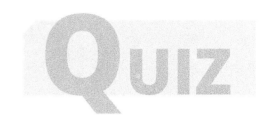

THE BODY'S SEXUAL RESPONSE

Directions: Circle the best answer.

1. Which of the following can excite people sexually?

    a. Being touched

    b. Listening to music

    c. Thinking about a special person

    d. All of the above

2. The first three stages of the sexual response cycle are the excitement phase, the plateau phase, and the orgasm phase. What is the fourth phase?

    a. The resolution phase

    b. The anti-climax phase

    c. The pre-ejaculatory phase

    d. None of the above

3. Which of the following happens during the excitement phase?

    a. Blood rushes to the genitals

    b. Muscles in other parts of the body become tense

    c. Blood rushes away from the genitals

    d. Both A and B

4. Which of the following happens during the orgasm phase?

    a. Muscles throughout the body quickly tense and relax, but mostly those around the vagina, uterus, and anus.

    b. Semen goes into the urethra and out of the penis.

    c. Breathing is faster.

    d. All of the above

Check your answers on the next page.

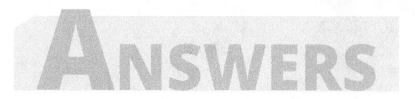

THE BODY'S SEXUAL RESPONSE

Directions: *Check your answers.*

1. **D**   All of the above. Some of the things that can sexually excite (sexually arouse) a person include being touched, listening to music, and thinking about a special person. Thoughts, feelings, sights, smells, sounds, and touches are all things that can make someone sexually excited. What excites one person may or may not excite someone else.

2. **A**   The fourth phase of the sexual response cycle is the ***resolution phase***.

3. **D**   Both A and B. During the excitement phase, blood rushes to the genitals and muscles in other parts of the body become tense.

4. **D**   All of the above. During the orgasm phase, each of the following happens:

   - In people with a vagina and clitoris, the muscles throughout the body quickly tense and relax, but mostly those around the vagina, uterus, and anus.
   - In people with a penis and testicles, semen goes into the urethra and out of the penis.
   - Breathing is faster.

Common Sexual Problems

Most people have sexual concerns or problems at one time or another. Some problems fix themselves. Others, people can solve on their own. But there are some problems people might need or want help with.

The type of help a patient needs depends on the problem. Sometimes, people need counseling from a trained sex therapist. It is important to offer referrals to patients who need that kind of help. But often you can help patients just by talking things through with them. You can also help them learn more about their bodies and how they work. Sometimes the problem can be related to their health. Encourage your patients to tell the health care provider what is going on.

Many people have a hard time talking about sex with a partner. You can encourage them to share their feelings and sexual needs with their partners. You may be able to suggest ways your patients can start talking about these things.

Common sexual problems

All patients may have questions and concerns about sex. Here are some common problems your patients may have:

- The vagina may not have enough lubrication.
- They may feel pain during sex.
- The penis may not be able to become erect.
- The person with a penis may ejaculate sooner than they or their partner would like.
- They may not have much desire for sex.
- They may not have orgasms with partner sex.

If your patient tells you about any of these problems, be sure to make a note of it for the health care provider. Encourage your patient to talk with the provider about what can be done to help.

Sexual lubrication of vaginas

One common sexual problem patients with vaginas may have is not having enough vaginal moistness during sex. You can help your patients find out what to do if that is happening to them.

It can be very helpful to use personal lubricant (lube) products. It's good to tell them that needing to use lube doesn't mean that they are not aroused (or turned on). It just means that they need more lube for sex to feel even better.

- Lubricant can be found in any drug store.

- Lube can be placed inside the internal condom or on the outside of the external condom. If using an external latex condom, the lube should be water-based.

- Anyone can use the lube. It can be put on the skin of the penis, at the opening of the vagina, or inside the vagina or anus.

Some facts about sexual abuse

- About 1 in 5 women will be a victim of rape or attempted rape in their lifetime.

- About 1 in 3 girls under age 18 has been a victim of sexual abuse.

- 75% of women over 18 were raped by a husband, partner, or date.

- 1 in 5 males under age 18 has been sexually abused.

- 4 in 10 gay men and 1 in 2 bisexual men experience sexual violence in their lifetime.

- 1 in 8 lesbian women and 1 in 2 bisexual women have been raped in their lifetime.

- CDC, 2010 statistics

Sexual Abuse

Sexual abuse is when something sexual is done to a person without their consent. A person cannot legally consent to sexual activity when they are drunk or high on other drugs. Sexual abuse can also happen when a person doesn't want to do something sexual but consents to do it anyway because of pressure, manipulation, threats or out of fear.

Sexual abuse happens to people of all ages, from babies to older adults. It can range from touching the genitals to other forms of sexual activity. It can include rape, incest, or sexual harassment. All forms of sexual abuse can deeply hurt a person.

Patients are not always willing to tell you that they have been sexually abused at some time in their lives. This is especially true if they were abused by someone close to them, such as a father or mother.

This is where taking a good sexual history can help. Asking questions about sex carefully and respectfully can sometimes help patients tell you about current or past sexual abuse.

If a patient tells you that they have been forced to have sex or have been abused in some way, listen carefully and caringly. You will need to talk with a supervisor before the patient leaves. Some abuse cases must be reported outside the clinic. Follow your health site's guidelines for reporting and responding to patient disclosures of sexual abuse. You may also be able to refer the patient to an expert for help.

Helping patients with sexual concerns

There are some things that only a specially trained counselor can do to help patients with sexual concerns. And there are some things that you can do as a health worker. It will be easier for you to help your patients if you understand what those things are.

The **P-LI-SS-IT** model can help. This model for treating sexual problems has four levels:

P Permission-giving

LI Limited Information

SS Specific Suggestions

IT Intensive Therapy

The first two levels (P and LI) are things that a health worker with some training in sex education can do.

The third and fourth levels (SS and IT) are things that only a specially trained counselor can do.

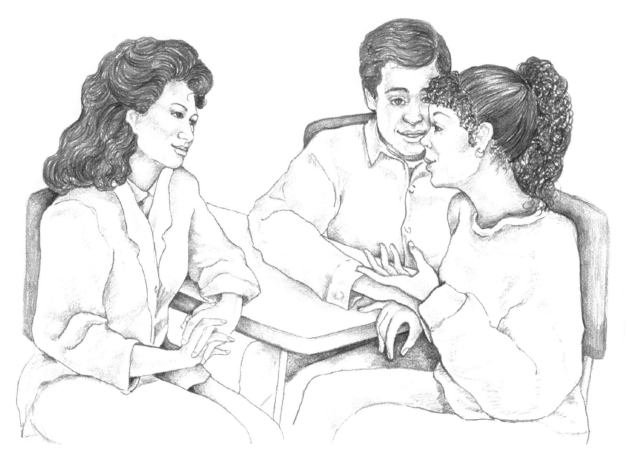

The P-LI-SS-IT Model for Treating Sexual Problems

This model describes four levels of treatment for sexual problems.

What health workers can do

Level 1: Permission-giving (P)

You can tell your patients that it is okay to talk about sexual matters. Make sure patients know you understand and respect their concerns and feelings. Use good listening skills and encourage your patients.

Level 2: Limited Information (LI)

This means that you can give correct information to patients who have a sexual question or concern. Many sexual problems are caused by a lack of information. You can help when you give the patient needed information.

What only specially trained counselors can do

If you have patients with serious problems or concerns, always refer them to a specially trained counselor or provider for the next two levels of treatment.

Level 3: Specific Suggestions (SS)

This involves giving detailed advice to help treat a problem. Only a trained sex counselor should do this.

Level 4: Intensive Therapy (IT)

To solve sexual problems, patients sometimes need to work with a person trained in sex therapy and other forms of therapy for short or long periods of time.

How *you* can help

Start by helping your patients feel safe. Build trust.

Here are some of the things you can do.

Give patients permission to talk about sex.

Let patients know sex is a safe topic to discuss.

> ▸ Ask your patients if they have any questions or concerns about sex. Patients may be embarrassed to bring up concerns on their own. But they may share their sexual concerns if you ask them.

> ▸ Let them know that it is okay to talk about these concerns.

> ▸ Be open and accepting. It is important not to judge the patient's thoughts or ideas.

Educator Tip

Give permission to your patients to talk about sex. You can say, "I want you to know that if you have any questions or concerns about sex, you can ask me. I am here to help you get answers."

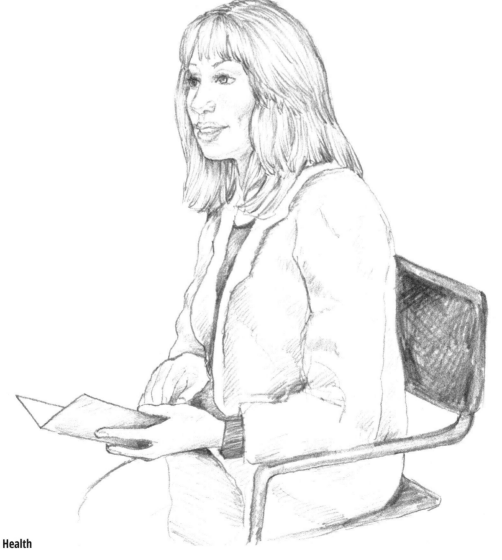

Give your patients the correct information they need.

Knowing the facts can help your patients feel more confident and less confused.

- ► Answer questions and give basic information about sexuality.

- ► Find out what they already know.

- ► Explain things clearly.

For example, your patient may be worried that their vagina gets moist during sex. You can explain that getting wet during sex is normal and helps sex feel good. Just knowing it is normal can often help.

If you don't know the answer to your patient's questions, find the answer or refer the patient to someone else. When in doubt, always check with a supervisor.

Validate your patient's feelings, concerns, and choices.

- ► You can often do this just by letting patients know that any thoughts, feelings, or actions that cause pleasure are "normal" as long as they don't cause any harm. Often, just listening and being accepting can help the patient feel better.

- ► Respect and accept your patient's feelings and choices even if they differ from your own. Set aside your own reactions.

- ► Practice active listening.

- ► Focus on what is best for this patient's life.

Talk about communication.

Remind patients that communication between partners is very important. It helps build the closeness that leads to fulfilling sex.

- ► Kind words, open discussion, and being thoughtful of each other can all help a relationship.

- ► Creating a warm and caring relationship can lead to sexual satisfaction for your patient.

Help patients think about their barriers to enjoying sex.

There can be many barriers to enjoying sex.

- ▸ It could be something temporary, like stress or worry. For example, someone could be worried about pregnancy or STIs during unprotected sex. That worry can keep them from relaxing enough to enjoy having sex.

- ▸ Sometimes it can be something deeper, like hurt or resentment in the relationship. For example, if someone is angry with their partner, they may have a hard time getting an erection or reaching orgasm.

Help patients learn about orgasms.

Some patients may worry about their own sexual ability if their partner does not have an orgasm at the same time they do. The truth is that it is common for partners not to have orgasms at the same time. The person with a penis and testicles often has an orgasm before their sex partner with a vagina and clitoris does.

Those who understand this are more likely to be comfortable helping their partners reach orgasm. During sex, the person with a vagina and clitoris may want to tell their partner if they have not climaxed so the partner can help them reach orgasm.

Referrals

It is important to know resources in your community to refer patients to for sex-related counseling. *AASECT.org* can help you locate a certified sex educator, counselor or therapist in your community.

Also, remember that there is a lot of information patients can learn on their own — if they know where to look. It is a good idea to have a list of books or websites patients can look at to learn more about sexuality.

Refer your patient for help.

You may have a patient who needs more help than you are trained to give. Or you may not have enough time to talk about the problem. In those cases, you can refer the patient to a trained counselor or health care provider. It is always best to give a referral if a patient has:

- ▸ Questions that you cannot answer

- ▸ A major sexual problem, such as not having orgasms, or an inability to get an erection, or pain with sex

- ▸ Multiple sexual conflicts and problems

- ▸ A difficult conflict with a partner

Check your health site's policies about referring patients for help with sexual problems. Perhaps there is someone in your facility who is trained to provide help with sexual issues.

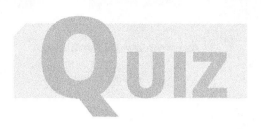

COMMON SEXUAL PROBLEMS

Directions: Circle the best answer.

1. If a patient tells you that they have been forced to have sex or has been abused in some way, you should:

    a. Change the subject to something easier to talk about.

    b. Listen carefully and caringly.

    c. Talk with a provider or your supervisor before the patient leaves the clinic.

    d. Both B and C

2. Based on the P-LI-SS-IT model, what two levels of help can a health worker with some training in sex education give?

    a. Permission-giving and Specific Suggestions

    b. Permission-giving and Limited Information

    c. Permission-giving and Intensive Therapy

    d. Specific Suggestions and Intensive Therapy

3. Before patients will speak openly about their sexual problems and concerns, they need to know it is okay to talk about these things. You can help them to do this by:

    a. Telling them that it is okay to talk about sex with you.

    b. Making sure they bring a friend along to listen.

    c. Asking only close-ended questions from the patient's history form.

    d. Acting uncomfortable when you talk about sex.

4. What should you do if you don't know the answer to a patient's questions?

    a. Guess at the correct answer.

    b. Find the correct answer or refer the patient to somebody else.

    c. Give them a brochure to read.

    d. All of the above

Go on to the next page.

Directions: Read each of the following statements. Is it true or false? Circle the best answer.

5. You need specialized training before you can give patients specific suggestions or intensive therapy for a sexual problem.   **True**   **False**

6. You don't need to tell patients that they can talk with you about their sexual problems and concerns. They will assume it is okay to because you are talking to them about birth control.   **True**   **False**

7. You should respect and accept your patient's feelings and choices even if they differ from your own.   **True**   **False**

8. You can help patients think about what barriers may be keeping them from enjoying sex.   **True**   **False**

Check your answers on the next page.

ANSWERS

COMMON SEXUAL PROBLEMS

Check your answers.

1. **D** Both B and C. If a patient tells you that they have been forced to have sex or have been abused in some way, you should listen carefully and caringly and talk with a provider or your supervisor before the patient leaves.

2. **B** Based on the P-LI-SS-IT model, the two levels of help that a health worker with some training in sex education can give are "Permission-giving and Limited Information."

3. **A** You can help patients to speak openly about their sexual problems and concerns by telling them that it is okay to talk about sex with you.

4. **B** If you don't know the answer to your patient's questions, you should find the correct answer or refer the patient to somebody else.

5. **True** You *do* need specialized training before you can give patients specific suggestions or intensive therapy for a sexual problem.

6. **False** You *do* need to tell patients that they can talk with you about their sexual problems and concerns. They *will not* assume it is okay to just because you are talking to them about birth control. Patients may be embarrassed to bring up concerns on their own. But they may share their sexual concerns if you tell them it is okay. You can say, "I want you to know that you can talk with me about any questions or concerns you have about sex. I am here to help you get answers."

7. **True** You should respect and accept your patient's feelings and choices even if they differ from your own.

8. **True** You can help patients think about what barriers may be keeping them from enjoying sex.

CHAPTER QUIZ

HUMAN SEXUALITY

Directions: Circle all that apply.

1. Which of the following are part of your sexuality?
   a. Gender roles
   b. Human growth and development
   c. Body image
   d. Sexual orientation
   e. Sexual expression
   f. Family and relationships

Directions: Read each of the following statements and write your best answer in the spaces below.

2. List five things that influence your sexuality.
   One is done for you.

   - The media _____

   - _____

   - _____

   - _____

   - _____

Go on to the next page.

3. List five ways that people express their sexuality.
   One is done for you.

   - _Fantasy_____

   - _____

   - _____

   - _____

   - _____

Draw a line from the description on the left to the sexual response phase on the right.

Description

4. Muscles throughout the body quickly tense and relax, but mostly those around the vagina, uterus, and anus.

5. Blood flows away from the penis.

6. The labia majora flatten and open and the labia minora swell.

7. The testicles rise to a point where they press against the body and get larger.

Sexual Response Phase

a. **Plateau Phase**

b. **Orgasm Phase**

c. **Excitement Phase**

d. **Resolution Phase**

Directions: Circle the best answer.

8. Which of the following are common sexual problems that your patients might tell you about?

   a. Vagina may not have enough lubrication.

   b. Feel pain during sex.

   c. Penis may not be able to become erect.

   d. All of the above

Directions: Circle the best answer.

9. Which of the following statements is true?

    a. About 1 out of every 5 women will be a victim of rape or attempted rape in her lifetime.

    b. About 1 in 3 girls under the age of 18 has been a victim of sexual abuse.

    c. About 1 in 5 boys under the age of 18 has been a victim of sexual abuse.

    d. All of the above

10. Which of the following can you do to help patients who have a sexual concern?

    a. Help patients think about barriers to enjoying sex.

    b. Tell them not to worry about it, it's probably normal.

    c. Start giggling to lighten the mood.

    d. None of the above

11. When should you refer a patient to someone else?

    a. When they have questions you can't find the answer to.

    b. When it's a major problem, such as not having orgasms.

    c. When they have multiple sexual problems.

    d. All of the above

Check your answers on the next page.

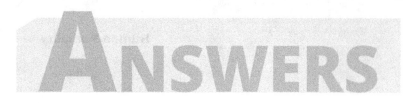

HUMAN SEXUALITY

Directions: Check your answers.

1. **A, B,** Gender roles, human growth and development,
   C, D, body image, sexual orientation, sexual expression,
   E, F and family and relationships are all part of your
            sexuality.

2. Some things that can influence your sexuality include:
   - Gender roles
   - Family
   - Body image
   - Media
   - Peers
   - Past sexual experiences
   - Knowledge about sexuality
   - Values and attitudes
   - Culture and religion
   - Sexual orientation

3. People express their sexuality in many ways. Some
   of those ways include abstinence, fantasies, touching,
   masturbation, oral sex, anal sex, and vaginal sex.

4. **B** **Orgasm Phase.** In people with a vagina and
         clitoris, the muscles throughout the body quickly
         tense and relax during this phase, but mostly
         those around the vagina, uterus, and anus.

5. **D** **Resolution Phase.** In people with a penis and
         testicles, blood flows away from the penis during
         this phase.

6. **C** **Excitement Phase.** In people with a vagina and
         clitoris, the labia majora flatten and open and the
         labia minora swells during this phase.

7. **A** **Plateau Phase.** In people with a penis and
         testicles, the testicles rise to a point where they
         press against the body. They also start to get
         much larger as they fill with blood.

8. **D**   All of the above. Some common sexual problems your patients might tell you about include:
- Their vagina may not have enough or any lubrication.
- They may feel pain during sex.
- Their penis may not be able to become erect or fully erect.

Some other problems a patient might tell you about include:
- A person with a penis may ejaculate sooner than they would like.
- They may have low desire for sex.
- They may not be able to have an orgasm.

9. **D**   All of the above. All of these statements are true:
- About 1 out of every 5 women will be a victim of rape or attempted rape in her lifetime.
- About 1 in 3 girls under the age of 18 has been a victim of sexual abuse.
- About 1 in 5 boys under the age of 18 has been sexually abused.

10. **A**   To help patients who have a sexual concern, you could help patients think about barriers to enjoying sex. You could also:
- Give patients permission to talk about sex.
- Give your patients the correct information they need.
- Validate your patient's feelings, concerns, and choices.
- Talk about communication.
- Refer your patient to someone specially trained to help them.

11. **D**   All of the above. You should refer patients to someone else if:

- They have questions you can't answer.
- They have a major sexual problem, such as not having orgasms.
- They have many sexual conflicts and problems.

You should also refer a patient to someone specially trained to help if they are having a difficult conflict with a partner.

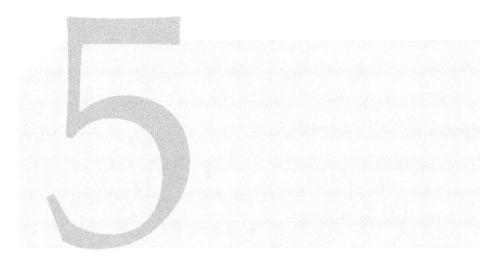

Sexually Transmitted Infections (STIs)

Sexually Transmitted Infections (STIs) are infections that people can get by having sex with someone who has an STI. As a health worker, you can play a key role in helping your patients keep from getting an STI.

This chapter gives you basic information about the STIs you are most likely to see in your health care site. As a health worker, you can talk to patients about these infections. But it is up to a health care provider to diagnose and treat them.

If you will be doing a lot of STI counseling, you will need to know more about each STI and how your health care site treats it. For more information, talk with a provider or take a class on STIs.

Note: We use the newer term "sexually transmitted infections" (STIs) in this manual because it is more accurate. You might also hear the term "sexually transmitted diseases" (STDs) to refer to these same infections. Talk to your supervisor about the term your health care site prefers.

Topics in this chapter

▸ What are sexually transmitted infections (STIs)?

▸ Preventing STIs

▸ Getting tested and treated

▸ Common STIs and vaginal infections:

Curable

- Chlamydia
- Gonorrhea
- PID (Pelvic Inflammatory Disease)
- Syphilis
- Trichomoniasis
- Vaginal infections

Not Curable

- Genital herpes
- HPV (types of viruses that can cause genital warts or cervical cancer)
- Hepatitis B
- HIV (the virus that causes AIDS)

Objectives

By the end of this chapter, you will be able to:

▸ Tell how most common STIs are spread.

▸ List three things that make patients more likely to get an STI.

▸ List steps patients can take to help prevent STIs.

▸ List five things you should tell a patient who needs treatment for an STI.

▸ Describe four common STIs.

What are STIs?

STIs are infections that people usually get by having sex with someone who has one. Make sure your patients understand the basic facts about STIs. This will help them avoid getting them. Some STIs can be treated and cured with antibiotic medicine. Others, like HIV, cannot be cured, but they can be treated to make them easier to live with. HIV can be prevented with PEP and PrEP. HPV may go away on its own with time and some strains can be prevented with a vaccine.

If patients do not get the treatment they need, STIs can:

- ▶ Be painful and make them very sick. A few can even cause death.
- ▶ Make it hard for someone to get pregnant or to cause a pregnancy
- ▶ Cause birth defects or other health problems for a newborn, and if left untreated can even cause death.

Millions of people have STIs. And most people who get them are under the age of 30. Be sure to tell your patients that:

- ▶ STIs are common.
- ▶ You can have more than one STI at a time.
- ▶ You can get the same STI more than once.

It is important to give your patients the knowledge they need to protect themselves and their partners. This section gives you a way to explain STIs to them.

STIs that can be treated and cured

- Chlamydia
- Gonorrhea
- PID
- Syphilis
- Trichomoniasis

These STIs are caused by bacteria or a parasite (kinds of germs).

STIs that can be treated but not cured, and some prevented by a vaccine* or medication**.

- Genital herpes
- HPV*
- Hepatitis B*
- HIV**

These STIs are caused by a virus (another kind of germ).

How are STIs spread?

Most often, STIs are spread by having sex with someone who has an STI. People can get them by having sex using a penis, vagina, mouth, or by skin to skin contact.

Germs that cause STIs live in warm, moist places like the mouth, vulva, vagina, anus, urethra (the tube that carries urine), penis, and testicles. You can get an STI from someone who has one if you:

> ▸ Share body fluids like blood, semen or vaginal fluids.

> ▸ Touch or rub infected parts of their body.

> ▸ Share needles or use needles that have not been cleaned with bleach.

What are body fluids?

Body fluids include:

- Blood
- Semen
- Vaginal fluids
- Pre-ejaculate
- Breast milk

How people talk about sex

Having sex:	When talking about birth control, "having sex" means any contact between a penis and a vagina or anus. When talking about STIs, "having sex" means any contact between the penis, vagina, mouth, or anus.
Vaginal sex:	When a penis enters a vagina. Sometimes vaginal sex is called "sex" or "making love."
Oral sex:	When a person's mouth is used to stimulate the vulva, vagina, anus, or penis of another. Some people call these blowjobs, BJs, tossing salad, eating out, going down on, or diving.
Anal sex:	When a penis, finger or sex toy enters an anus.

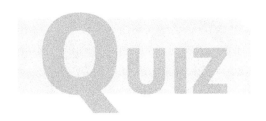

What are Sexually Transmitted Infections (STIs)?

Directions: Read each of the following and write your best answer in the space provided.

1. What are STIs?

_____

_____

2. List three things that can happen if people with STIs don't get the treatment they need.

   ▪ _____

   ▪ _____

   ▪ _____

Directions: Read each of the following statements.
Is it true or false? Circle the best answer.

3. STIs can be passed by blood, semen, vaginal fluids, and sometimes by touch.   True   False

4. All STIs can be cured.   True   False

5. Syphilis and chlamydia are examples of STIs that can be cured.   True   False

6. A person can get the same STI more than once.   True   False

7. A person can only get one STI at a time.   True   False

8. Some STIs can be spread by sharing needles.   True   False

Check your answers on the next page.

© Essential Access Health

181

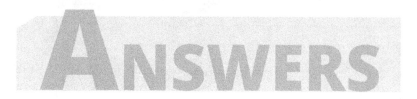

ANSWERS

What are Sexually Transmitted Infections (STIs)?

Check your answers.

1. STIs are infections that people usually get by having sex with someone who already has one. You can get them by having sex using a penis, vagina, mouth, or anus.

2. If people with STIs do not get the treatment they need, STIs can:

    - Be painful and make them very sick. A few can even kill them.
    - Make it hard for a person to get pregnant or to cause a pregnancy.
    - Cause birth defects or other health problems for a newborn.

3. **True**   Blood, semen, and vaginal fluids all may contain germs that cause STIs. Some STIs, like herpes or genital warts, can be spread if someone touches a sore or wart.

4. **False**   Not all STIs can be cured. *Some* STIs *can* be cured. Others can be treated but *not* cured.

5. **True**   Syphilis and chlamydia can be cured. Some STIs that cannot be cured include: genital herpes, genital warts, hepatitis B, and HIV.

6. **True**   A person *can* get the same STI more than once. Even though some STIs can be cured, a cured person can get the STI again. That is one reason it is important for patients who have an STI to tell their sex partners to get treated too.

7. **False**   People *can* have more than one STI at a time.

8. **True**   Some STIs *can* be spread by sharing needles.

Preventing STIs

You can help your patients learn how to protect themselves from STIs.

The surest way not to get an STI is to not have sex with a penis, vagina, mouth, or anus. But when patients do have sex, there are ways they can help protect themselves.

Some methods of birth control can help prevent STIs. The external or internal condom can be used along with nearly any other birth control method your patient uses. No matter which birth control method your patients choose, be supportive. But if their choice does not protect them from STIs, be sure to talk about that too.

Example:

If your patient chooses the Pill for birth control, you can say:

"The Pill is a great choice for birth control. Tell me what you're going to do to protect yourself from STIs." OR,

"The Pill is a great way to prevent pregnancy but you still need to use a condom every time you have sex to protect yourself from STIs."

What does "Risk" mean?

As a health worker, you may hear other staff use the words "risk" and "at risk" when they talk about STIs. It is good for you to know what these words mean even though it may be best not to use them when talking with patients.

▶ **Risks** are things that could harm or hurt someone.

▶ If someone is **at risk** for an STI, that person has a chance of getting an STI.

▶ If someone is **at high risk** for an STI, that person has a very high chance of getting an STI.

▶ If an activity **puts a patient at risk** for an STI, it gives that patient a chance of getting the STI.

Ways to prevent STIs

Share these tips on preventing STIs with your patients.

Do's

▶ **Use a condom every time you have sex.**

External condoms (worn on the penis or sex toys) are made from latex rubber or a soft plastic called polyurethane. Internal condoms (worn inside the vagina or anus) are made from nitrile, another type of plastic. All these types of condoms help protect you from many STIs. Be aware that condoms made from lambskin do not protect against STIs.

If you have oral sex, use condoms or dental dams. Dental dams are square pieces of latex rubber that are used to cover the area around the vulva or anus during oral sex.

Use a condom even if you use other types of birth control. The only birth control methods that helps protect you from STIs are the external or internal condom.

STI Vaccines

Hepatitis B and some types of HPV can be prevented by a vaccine.

Preventive Medicine

There are drugs that can prevent the transmission of HIV. They include: PEP (post-exposure prophylaxis) and PrEP (pre-exposure prophylaxis).

Learn more at CDC.gov

▶ **Talk with your partner about sex and STIs.**

Before you have sex with someone, ask them if they have other partners, or if they have an STI or any symptoms. Talk about what each of you can do to protect yourselves from getting an STI. For example, you can talk about using condoms. Or you both may want to get tested for STIs before you start having sex.

▶ **Have sex with only one person who has sex only with you.**

If you have sex with only one person and if that person has sex only with you, your chances of getting an STI are lower. If you have more than one partner, it is very important to use a condom every time you have sex.

▶ **Get checked and treated for STIs.**

If you have an STI, both you and your partner should get treated. You should wait to have sex until your health care provider says it is safe.

Don'ts

▶ **Don't have sex while you or your partner is using alcohol or other drugs.**

When people drink or use drugs, they may do things without thinking. For example, someone might forget to use a condom or may not use it the right way.

▶ **Don't share needles from injection drugs, body piercing, or tattoos. And don't have sex with someone who shares needles.**

Some STIs, like HIV (the virus that causes AIDS), can be spread by needles. These could be needles used for drugs, steroids, body piercing, vitamins, hormone shots and so on. If a person with HIV uses a needle and shares that needle with a friend, that friend can get HIV. You can also get HIV if you have sex with someone who got HIV sharing or reusing needles. Do not share needles. Find a needle exchange program to get clean needles.

▶ **Don't have sex with someone who has signs of an STI. And don't touch the sores of someone who has signs of an STI.**

If you or your partner has any signs of an STI, get checked. Signs to look for are sores, blisters, warts, or bumps. These could be in the area around the penis, vulva, anus, or on the mouth. People with an STI could also have a discharge from the penis or vagina. Talk to your health care provider to learn more about how to protect yourself.

Safe sex

Let patients know that they can be sexual without sharing body fluids such as semen, vaginal fluids, or blood. They can flirt, hug, kiss, talk dirty, or give each other a massage.

▶ **Don't have sex if it isn't right for you.**

Sex is your choice. It is your body. Decide ahead of time if sex is right for you, and talk about it with your partner. Even if you think you want to have sex at first and then later change your mind, that's OK. Be clear and tell your partner what you really want.

Protect yourself

It is a good idea to:

▶ Get a Hepatitis B vaccine. Ask about the HPV vaccine.

▶ Get tested for HIV and other infections people get from having sex. Get tested for STIs every year and with every new partner. Ask your provider if PrEP is right for you.

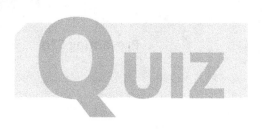

Quiz

Preventing STIs

Directions: Circle the best answer.

1. When patients choose a birth control method that does not protect them from STIs, you should:

    a. Tell them their birth control method is a bad choice.

    b. Tell them the method is a good way to prevent pregnancy. Then ask them what they will do to protect themselves from STIs.

    c. Not talk about STIs at all. It's not the reason for their visit to the health care site.

2. _____ is one STI that can be prevented by a vaccine.

    a. Herpes

    b. Chlamydia

    c. Syphilis

    d. Hepatitis B

3. External condoms made from _____ will help protect against some STIs.

    a. Latex or polyurethane

    b. Lambskin or polyurethane

    c. Latex or lambskin

Go on to the next page.

Directions: Read each of the following statements. If it is something a patient <u>should</u> do to help prevent STIs, circle "Do." If it is something a patient should <u>not</u> do, circle "Don't."

4. Have sex with only one person who has sex only with you.   *Do*   *Don't*

5. Have sex while you or your partner is drinking alcohol or using drugs.   *Do*   *Don't*

6. Have sex with someone who has signs of an STI.   *Do*   *Don't*

7. Use a condom every time you have sex.   *Do*   *Don't*

Check your answers on the next page.

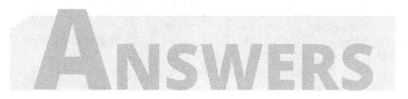

Preventing STIs

Check your answers.

1. **B**   Tell them the method is a good way to prevent pregnancy. Then ask them what they will do to protect themselves from STIs.

2. **D**   *Hepatitis B* is one STI that can be prevented by a vaccine. Some types of HPV can also be prevented by vaccines.

3. **A**   External condoms made from *latex* rubber or a plastic called *polyurethane* help protect against many STIs. Condoms made from lambskin do *not* protect against STIs.

4. **Do**   Do have sex with only one person who has sex only with you. If you have sex with only one person and if that person has sex only with you, your chances of getting an STI are lower.

5. **Don't**   Don't have sex while you or your partner is drinking alcohol or using drugs. When people drink or use drugs, they may do things without thinking. For example, someone might forget to use a condom or may not use it the right way.

6. **Don't**   Don't have sex with someone who has signs of an STI. If you or your partner have any signs of an STI, get checked. Signs to look for are sores, blisters, warts, bumps, or a discharge from the penis or vagina.

7. **Do**   Do use a condom every time you have sex. Use a condom even if you use other types of birth control.

The Fundamentals of Family Planning

Getting Tested and Treated

You play a role in helping patients know what to look for and when to get tested. You also can encourage them to get proper treatment and talk to their partners. Here is language you can use to talk to your patients about the importance of getting tested and treated.

How do you know if you or your partner has an STI?

Sometimes STIs have signs that people can see or feel. But sometimes they don't. That means that someone can have an STI without knowing it. And they can still pass the STI to another person.

The best way to know for sure if you have an STI is to have a physical exam and tests. Each STI has its own test.

Common symptoms of STIs

Patients who tell you that they have any of the following signs should be checked. They should also be checked if they tell you that a partner has any of these signs.

Here are some common signs of STIs that people may get.

- Burning or pain while urinating (peeing)
- Any discharge from the opening of the penis
- A change in vaginal discharge or smell
- Sores, blisters, rashes, bumps, swelling, or growths around the penis, vulva, anus, or mouth
- Itching, burning, or pain around the penis, vulva, anus, or mouth
- Pain during sex
- Pain in the lower abdomen (stomach/tummy)

Getting tested

Patients should come to the health care site to get checked any time they think they might have an STI.

The sooner an STI is found, the better. You should get checked if:

▶ You have any signs.

▶ A sex partner has any signs.

▶ You had sex with a new partner and didn't use a condom.

▶ You think your partner is having sex with another person.

Getting treated

You may be asked to go over treatment plans with your patients to be sure they can understand and follow it.

Some STIs are caused by bacteria. Most of these STIs can be cured if they are treated early with the right medicine.

Other STIs are caused by viruses. Most of these STIs can be treated but not cured. There are medicines and treatments to help get rid of the symptoms. But the virus that causes the infection can stay in the person's body.

If a test finds an STI or if enough signs of an STI are seen during the exam, the health care provider may give you medicine or other kinds of treatment. There are many forms of medicine. Some of them are:

▶ Pills that you take by mouth

▶ A cream to rub on the genitals or to put in the vagina with a special applicator

▶ Shots

Helping patients understand their treatment plan

To help patients understand their treatment plan, start with the basics. You may need to tell them:

▸ The name of the medicine. Has it given them any problems before?

▸ How to take it. Is it by mouth? With meals? Rubbed on the skin? Put into or on the genitals?

▸ When to take it. Once a day? Two times a day? What time?

▸ How to fit the treatment into their lives. What times may make them less likely to forget to take their medicine.

▸ When and where to go for follow-up care. How often?

Also be sure to talk to them about:

▸ Any side effects of the medicine. Will the patient have an upset stomach? Will there be redness where a cream is rubbed in?

▸ What to do if they have side effects. Should they keep taking the medicine? Should they call the health care site?

▸ Why it is important to complete their treatment. Explain that the STI may not be cured or improved.

If patients understand the following, they are more likely to complete their treatment successfully:

▸ What this medicine will do. Will it cure the infection? Will it just reduce the signs?

▸ What they should do about sex. Should they stop having sex for a while? How long should they wait?

▸ The reasons their partner needs to be treated. Explain that the partner could become very sick. Or the partner could give the STI back to the person, or give it to someone else.

▸ How to keep from getting an STI again. Let them know that a person can get the same STI over and over.

Supporting your patients

Patients with an STI should tell their partners so they can also be treated. This can be hard to do. You can help your patients choose the best way to talk to their partners. You can ask your patients these questions to help get started:

- Have you thought about what you will say to your partner?

- Have you thought about how your partner might react?

- Would it help to think about it out loud with me?

- Would it help to practice with me?

- Do you think it would help to bring your partner to the health care site with you?

- Would you like me to give you a website that will send an anonymous email to your partner so you don't have to say anything yourself?

You can also be a great support for patients who have an STI that can't be cured. They may be scared, angry, or sad. They may feel that they can never have sex again or that no one will ever love them. They may need help figuring out how to live with the infection and how to keep from giving it to someone else. They may also need to discuss how to talk to future partners about the infection.

To learn more, ask your supervisor about taking classes on STI counseling.

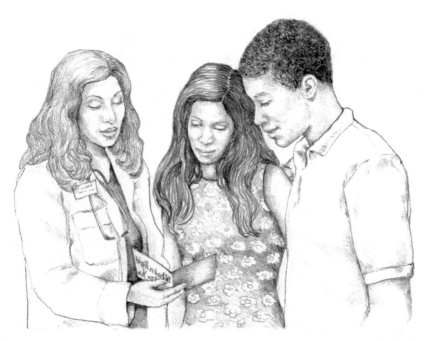

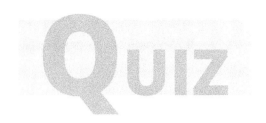

Getting Tested and Treated

Directions: Read each of the following, and write your best answer in the space below.

1. The best way for patients to know if they have an STI is:

_____

_____

_____

2. List three common signs of STIs:

   ▪ _____

   ▪ _____

   ▪ _____

Directions: Circle the best answer.

3. When should people be tested for an STI?
   a. Only if they have two or more symptoms of an STI.
   b. If they shake hands with a person who has been sneezing hard.
   c. If they have signs of an STI, think they may have been exposed to an STI, or it is recommended per STI screening guidelines.

4. STIs can be caused by:
   a. Viruses
   b. Bacteria
   c. Both a and b
   d. None of the above

Go on to the next page.

5. Which of the following are things you can tell your patients to help them understand their STI treatment plan?

   a. The name of their medicine

   b. How to take it

   c. When to take it

   d. When to come back for follow-up care

   e. All of the above

Directions: Write your best answer in the space below.

6. Your patient just learned they have an STI. What might you ask them about how to talk to their partner about it?

   _____

   _____

   _____

   _____

   _____

Check your answers on the next page.

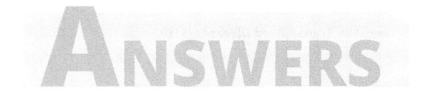

Getting Tested and Treated

Check your answers.

1. The best way for patients to know if they have an STI is to have a physical exam and tests. Each STI has its own test.

2. Sometimes STIs have no signs that people can see or feel. But sometimes they do. Some signs a patient might have are:

   - Burning or pain while urinating (peeing)
   - Any discharge from the opening of the penis
   - A change in normal vaginal discharge or smell
   - Sores, blisters, rashes, bumps, swelling, or growths around the penis, vulva, anus, or mouth
   - Itching, burning, or pain around the penis, vulva, anus, or mouth
   - Pain during sex
   - Pain in the lower abdomen

3. **C** People should be tested for STIs if they have signs of an STI, think they may have been exposed to an STI or per the STI Screening Guidelines. Some reasons for patients to think they have been exposed to an STI include:

   - A sex partner has any signs of an STI.
   - They had sex with a new partner and didn't use a condom.
   - They think their partner is having sex with another person.

   A patient should also be tested for STIs before having an IUD placed in their uterus.

4. **C** Both A and B. STIs can be caused by both viruses and bacteria.

Go on to the next page.

5. **E** All of the above. To help patients understand their STI treatment plan, you can tell your patients:
   - The name of their medicine
   - How to take it
   - When to take it
   - When to come back for follow-up care

   You might also tell patients any of the following:
   - How to fit the treatment into their lives
   - Any side effects of the medicine
   - What to do if they have side effects
   - Why it is important to complete their treatment

   Other information patients may need includes:
   - What the treatment will do
   - What they should do about sex
   - Why their partner needs to be treated
   - How to keep from getting an STI again

6. You could help your patient think through talking to their partner by asking any of the following questions:
   - What do you think you might say to your partner?
   - How do you think your partner might react?
   - Would it help to think about it out loud with me?
   - Would it help to practice with me?
   - Would it help to bring your partner to the health care site with you?

Common STIs and Vaginal Infections

Your patients may need to know about a number of STIs and vaginal infections, like yeast infections. This section gives you the basic information you can share with patients who have an STI. It is written as though you are talking to a patient with that infection.

It is important for patients to know that even STIs that cannot be cured can be treated. Treatment can often make the symptoms less severe, cut down on outbreaks, or slow the progress of the infection.

This section is divided into two parts:

Curable (STIs and other infections of the reproductive tract that can be treated and cured)

▶ Chlamydia

▶ Gonorrhea

▶ PID (Pelvic Inflammatory Disease)

▶ Syphilis

▶ Trichomoniasis

▶ Vaginal infections (bacterial vaginosis and yeast infections — these are not sexually transmitted)

Not Curable (STIs that can be treated but *not* cured)

▶ Genital herpes

▶ HPV (the viruses that cause genital warts or cervical cancer)

▶ Hepatitis B

▶ HIV (the virus that causes AIDS)

Curable

Chlamydia

What is it?

Chlamydia is an infection of the penis, vagina, cervix, throat, anus, or urethra (the tube that carries urine).

- ▸ It is caused by bacteria (a kind of germ).
- ▸ You get it by having sex with someone who has chlamydia.
- ▸ It can be spread by the vagina, penis, mouth, or anus.

Symptoms

Most people do not have any signs of chlamydia. That's why most people don't know they have it. The best way to find out if you have it is to have a test done.

Signs of PID

Your patient should tell the health care provider right away, if they have:

- Pain or cramping in the lower abdomen. The pain can be mild, such as a dull ache or it can hurt a lot
- Abnormal discharge from the vagina that may smell
- Bleeding between periods
- Pain during sex
- Fever or chills
- Pain when urinating

A few people may have these signs:

- ▸ Abnormal discharge from the penis or vagina
- ▸ Pain or burning when they urinate (pee)
- ▸ Pain during sex
- ▸ Vaginal bleeding between periods and during or after sex

Long-term effects

Chlamydia can be cured. But if you don't get treated, these things could happen:

- ▸ You could pass it on to others.
- ▸ You increase your chances of getting HIV.

A person with untreated chlamydia could get an infection that causes scars in their uterus or in the tubes that carry their eggs. If this happens:

- ▸ They could have a pregnancy in their tubes (ectopic pregnancy).

- They could have pelvic pain and an infection called pelvic inflammatory disease (PID).
- They might become sterile (unable to get pregnant).

If someone has chlamydia while they are pregnant, chlamydia could harm the baby's eyes or lungs during birth.

Treatment

To cure chlamydia:

- You may take antibiotic medicine. You may take it in one dose. Or you may take pills for a week.
- You and your partner(s) must get treated.
- Take all of your pills, even if you feel better.
- Do not have sex for at least one week after you start your treatment. Do not have sex with your partner(s) until one week after they have completed their treatment.

If you think you might be pregnant, be sure to tell your health care provider *before* you get treated.

Keep from getting it again

To help keep from getting chlamydia again:

- Take all of your medicine.
- Tell your partner(s) to get checked for chlamydia. You *and* all of your partners must be treated. This protects you. It also helps keep chlamydia from spreading to other people.
- Do not have sex until you and all of your partners have finished treatment.
- Use condoms every time you have sex.

It is also a good idea to:

- Get re-tested in 3 months.
- Ask about the HPV vaccine.
- Get a hepatitis B vaccine.
- Get tested for HIV and other STI's.
- Ask to get checked for these infections every year or if you have a new partner(s).
- Ask if PrEP is right for you.

Gonorrhea

What is it?

Gonorrhea is an infection of the penis, vagina, anus, or throat.

- ▸ It is caused by bacteria (a kind of germ).
- ▸ You get gonorrhea by having sex with someone who has it.
- ▸ It can be spread by having sex with the penis, vagina, anus, or mouth.

Symptoms

You can have gonorrhea without knowing it. Many people have no signs at all. The best way to find out if you have it is to get tested.

Some people may have these signs:

- ▸ Pain when they urinate (pee) or have a bowel movement.
- ▸ Abnormal or increased discharge from the penis or vagina
- ▸ Pain in the testicles
- ▸ Pain or tenderness in the abdomen, or bleeding between periods or right after sex.
- ▸ A sore throat

Long-term effects

Gonorrhea can be cured. But if you don't get it treated, the following could happen:

- ▸ You can pass it on to others.
- ▸ You have a higher chance of getting other STI's including HIV.

If you have gonorrhea too long before being treated, it can cause these problems:

- ▸ Your joints may swell and hurt.
- ▸ The vagina or penis may swell and hurt.

A person with untreated gonorrhea could get an infection that causes scars in their uterus or in the tubes that carry their eggs. If this happens:

▶ They could have a pregnancy inside their tubes (ectopic pregnancy).

▶ They could have pelvic pain and infection (PID).

▶ They might become sterile (unable to get pregnant).

If someone has gonorrhea while they are pregnant, gonorrhea could harm the baby's eyes during birth or cause other health problems.

Treatment

To cure gonorrhea:

▶ You must get a shot and take pills.

▶ You and your partner(s) must be treated.

▶ Take all of your pills, even if you feel better.

▶ Do not have sex until you and your partner(s) have been treated.

If you think you may be pregnant, be sure to tell your health care provider *before* you get treated.

Keep from getting it again

To help keep from getting gonorrhea again:

▶ Tell your partner or partners to get checked for gonorrhea. You *and* all of your partners must be treated. This protects you. It also helps keep gonorrhea from spreading to other people.

▶ Don't have sex until you and all of your partners have finished treatment.

▶ Use condoms every time you have sex.

It is also a good idea to:

▶ Get re-tested in 3 months. Ask about the HPV vaccine.

▶ Get tested for HIV and other STI's.

▶ Ask to get checked for these infections every year or if you have a new partner.

▶ Ask if PrEP is right for you.

PID (Pelvic Inflammatory Disease)

What is it?

PID is caused by an infection in the ovaries, tubes, or uterus.

▶ You can get PID when another STI, like gonorrhea or chlamydia, goes untreated. Without treatment, the STI gets worse and can spread to your ovaries, tubes, or uterus. You can also get PID from other normal types of bacteria that are in your vagina.

Symptoms

The main sign of a PID is:

▶ Pain or cramping in your lower abdomen. The pain can be mild, such as a dull ache. Or it can hurt a lot.

Other signs include:

▶ Abnormal discharge from your vagina

▶ Bleeding between periods

▶ Bleeding or pain when you have sex

▶ A fever or chills

▶ Pain when you urinate

Long-term effects

PID can be cured. But if you don't get it treated, you could have:

▶ Severe pain in your abdomen

▶ A higher chance of getting HIV (the virus that causes AIDS)

PID can also cause serious health problems:

▶ You may become sterile (unable to get pregnant).

▶ You could have a pregnancy in your tubes.

▶ You may have to have surgery.

▶ You could die.

If someone has PID while they are pregnant, it can cause these problems for their baby:

- The baby can be born too soon.
- The baby's eyes and lungs can be infected during birth.

Treatment

To treat PID:

- You must take antibiotic pills and get a shot.
- Take all of your pills even if you feel better.
- Your health care provider may want to see you again in about 3 days to make sure the medication is working.
- Do not have sex for 2 weeks and until you and all of your partners have finished treatment.
- Get another checkup after you have been treated. You need to make sure you are cured.

If you think you may be pregnant, tell your health care provider *before* you get treated.

Keep from getting it again

To keep from getting PID again:

- Tell your partner or partners to get checked for STIs. You *and* all of your partners must be treated.
- Take all of your pills or get all of your shots.
- Do not have sex until you and your partner or partners are cured.
- Use condoms every time you have sex.

It is also a good idea to:

- Ask about HPV vaccine.
- Get tested for HIV and other STIs.
- Ask to get checked for these infections every year or if you have another partner.
- Ask if PrEP is right for you.

Syphilis

What is it?

Syphilis is a dangerous infection that can affect the whole body.

▸ It is caused by bacteria (a kind of germ).

▸ You get syphilis by having sex with someone who has it.

▸ It can be spread during sex with the penis, vagina, mouth, or anus and sometimes by touching a syphilis sore or rash.

Symptoms

The signs of syphilis can be so mild that you may never notice them. The first sign is a painless sore, called a chancre (pronounced "shank-er").

▸ This sore can be on or near the vagina, penis, mouth, or anus.

▸ You may not even see or feel the sore.

▸ It heals by itself even if it is not treated. But you still have syphilis.

After a few weeks or months, you may have some of these signs:

▸ Rash	▸ Joint pain
▸ Fever	▸ Hair loss
▸ Sore throat	▸ Headaches
▸ Weight loss	▸ Fatigue

These signs may also go away without treatment. But you still have the infection.

Long-term effects

Syphilis can be cured with medicine. But if you don't get treated, you could:

▸ Pass it on to others.

▸ Have a higher chance of getting HIV.

If not treated, over time syphilis can cause serious health problems, such as:

▸ Blindness

▸ Heart disease

▸ Brain damage or damage to other nerves

▸ Death

If someone has syphilis while they are pregnant:

▸ The baby could have birth defects.

▸ The baby may be born dead or die soon after birth.

Treatment

To cure syphilis:

▸ You must get one or more shots.

▸ You and your partner(s) must be treated.

▸ Get all of the shots you need, even if you feel better.

▸ Do not have sex until you and all of your partners have finished treatment.

▸ You may need another checkup and re-test to be sure the infection is fully treated. Ask your health care provider when you need to return to be sure you are cured.

If you think you may be pregnant, be sure to tell your health care provider *before* you get treated.

Keep from getting it again

To help keep from getting syphilis again:

- ▶ Tell your partner or partners to get checked for syphilis. You *and* all of your partners must be treated. This protects you. It also helps keep syphilis from spreading to other people.

- ▶ Do not have sex until one week after you and all of your partners have finished treatment.

- ▶ Use condoms every time you have sex.

It is also a good idea to:

- ▶ Ask about the HPV vaccine.

- ▶ Get tested for HIV and other STIs.

- ▶ Ask to get checked for STIs every year or if you have a new partner.

- ▶ Ask if PrEP is right for you.

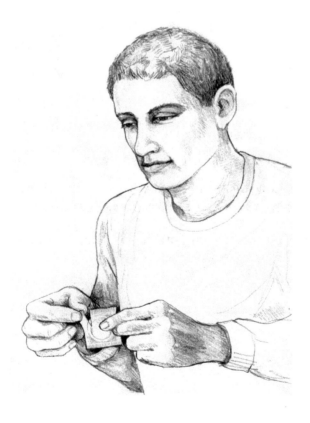

Trichomoniasis (Trich)
(also called "trich"; pronounced "trick")

What is it?

Trichomoniasis is an infection of the vagina or penis.

▶ It is caused by a parasite. In this case, the parasite is a tiny one-celled protozoa that lives, grows, and feeds off a person's body.

▶ You get it by having sex with someone who has it.

▶ It is spread by fluids from the vagina or penis.

Symptoms

Most often, people with a penis don't have signs. Sometimes, they may have an itching in the urethra (the tube that carries urine) or a burning feeling when they urinate (pee).

Some people with vaginas don't have signs. But many do. These signs include:

▶ A discharge from the vagina that can be, smelly, yellow, green, or gray

▶ Itching or burning of the vagina

▶ A burning pain when they urinate

Long-term effects

Trich can be cured. But if you don't get treated, the following can happen:

▶ You can pass it to others.

▶ You may have a higher chance of getting HIV or another STI.

If someone has trich while they are pregnant, the baby may be born too small or too early.

Treatment

Trich can be cured with antibiotics. To cure trich:

▸ You must take antibiotic pills.

▸ You and all of your partners must be treated.

▸ Take all of your pills, even if you feel better.

▸ Don't have sex until you and all of your partners have finished treatment.

If you think you may be pregnant, be sure to tell your health care provider *before* you get treated.

Keep from getting it again

To help keep from getting trich again:

▸ Tell your partner or partners to get checked for trich. You *and* all of your partners must be treated. This protects you. It also helps keep trich from spreading to other people.

▸ Take all of your medicine.

▸ Do not have sex until you and all of your partners have finished treatment.

▸ Always use condoms when you have sex. This can help protect you from infections.

It is also a good idea to:

▸ Ask about the HPV vaccine.

▸ Get tested for HIV and other STIs.

▸ Ask to get checked for these infections every year or if you have a new partner.

▸ Ask if PrEP is right for you.

Vaginal Infections

There are several kinds of vaginal infections (vaginitis). They can be passed during sex, when genitals touch other genitals. But people with vaginas can also get these without having sex. The most common vaginal infections are:

► Bacterial vaginosis (BV)

► Yeast infections

A health care provider can find each of these by looking at a drop of vaginal discharge under the microscope or sending a test to the lab.

Tips for keeping the vagina healthy

Always wipe yourself from front to back when you go to the bathroom. This can keep germs from your anus away from your vagina.

Don't douche. You don't need to clean inside your vagina. It keeps clean by itself. When you douche, you may be washing away what the vagina needs to keep healthy.

Wear cotton underwear and don't wear tight pantyhose. This will keep you cool and dry so bacteria won't grow as easily.

Bacterial Vaginosis (BV)

What is it?

BV is an infection of the vagina.

► It is caused by bacteria (a kind of germ). BV happens when some normal bacteria in the vagina grows too much.

► It can be passed by sex. But some people with vaginas can also get this without having sex.

People with vaginas get BV more often when they:

► Have a new sex partner.

► Have more than one sex partner.

► Rinse out the inside of the vagina with a douche.

Symptoms

You may have these signs:

▸ A fishy-smelling discharge from your vagina

▸ Abnormal discharge from your vagina

▸ Itching or burning in or around the vagina

Long-term effects

BV can be cured with medicine. But if you don't get treated, the following could happen:

▸ Your tubes and uterus can get infected.

▸ You may have a higher chance of getting or spreading HIV or other STIs.

If someone has BV while they are pregnant, the baby could be born too soon or too small.

Treatment

To cure BV:

▸ You must take pills or use a gel or cream that you put in your vagina.

If you think you may be pregnant, tell your health care provider *before* you get treated.

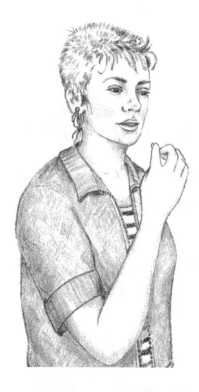

Yeast Infection

What is it?

A yeast infection is a common infection of the vagina. It is caused by yeast (candida). Every person with a vagina has some yeast in their vagina. But if you have too much yeast, this is called a yeast infection. This may happen for many reasons. It could happen because you:

- Are pregnant.
- Wear tight underwear or panty hose.
- Take certain kinds of medicines, like antibiotics.
- Rinse out the inside of your vagina with a douche or soap.
- Have diabetes or HIV.

Symptoms

You may have these signs:

- Abnormal thin or thick, white discharge, like cottage cheese
- Itching in or around the vagina and vulva
- A burning pain when you urinate (pee)

Long-term effects

There are no long-term effects of yeast infection.

Treatment

To cure a yeast infection, you must:

- Take a pill or put a gel or cream in your vagina. Use the medicine even if you get your period.

Not Curable

Genital Herpes

What is it?

Genital herpes is an infection caused by a virus (a kind of germ).

- ▸ You get the herpes virus by having sex with someone who has it.
- ▸ It can be spread by the penis, vagina, mouth, or anus. It can also be spread by touching the infected area of someone who has it.
- ▸ It causes small, painful sores or blisters. The sores can come and go. But once you get herpes, the virus stays in your body.

Symptoms

Some people with herpes don't get signs of infection. But other people do.

The people that do get signs and symptoms get blisters and sores. They can show up in any of these places:

- ▸ The vulva, vagina, penis, scrotum or anus
- ▸ The thighs or buttocks
- ▸ The mouth

These blisters or sores are different for everyone:

- ▸ Some people get a painful rash of blisters or sores.
- ▸ Some get only a blister or two that just itch.
- ▸ Some people feel like they have the flu along with the blisters. This usually only happens the first time you get an outbreak.

Cold sores

Cold sores on the lips are a kind of herpes. The virus can be spread by mouth to the penis, vagina, or anus.

The sores and blisters will heal.

- ▸ Some people get the sores only once.
- ▸ Some people get them many times.

Even when you have no sores or blisters, the herpes virus is in your body, sometimes without knowing it you can pass herpes to others.

Long-term effects

Herpes cannot be cured. It can cause these problems:

- You can pass it on to others.
- You have a higher chance of getting HIV (the virus that causes AIDS).

If you have herpes and get pregnant:

- Tell your doctor you have herpes.
- Get prenatal care.

Treatment

Genital herpes can't be cured, but there are medicines that may help the sores heal more quickly. Some medicines may also make the blisters come less often, stay a shorter time, and be less painful.

To treat genital herpes:

- Take the medicine your provider gives you.
- Your partner or partners should get checked for herpes if they have signs.

If you think you may be pregnant, be sure to tell your health care provider *before* you get treated.

To take care of the sores:

- Keep the area clean and dry. Wash gently and dry with a clean, soft towel. Or use a hair dryer set on cool.
- Wear cotton underwear and loose clothes.
- Don't put any cream or ointment on the sores unless your health care provider tells you to.
- Wash hands with soap after touching the sores.

Protect yourself and others

If you have genital herpes:

- **Don't touch the sores.** If you or anyone else touches the sores, you could get new sores or give herpes to your partner or partners.
- **Don't have sex when you have sores.** There is a higher chance of spreading herpes when you have sores. And you have a much higher chance of getting HIV when you have sores.

- **Wash your hands with soap and water right away** if you touch the sores. You can spread herpes to your eyes and other parts of your body. You can also give it to other people you touch.

- **Always use condoms when you have sex.** You can give herpes to a partner even when you don't have blisters or sores. Condoms can help protect them.

- **Don't let anyone else use your towel or washcloth.** Don't ever share underwear or bathing suits.

- **Pay attention to your body.** Many people can learn to tell when they are about to get blisters ("have an outbreak").

It is also a good idea to:

▸ Ask about the HPV vaccine.

▸ Get tested for HIV and other STI's.

▸ Ask to get checked for these infections every year or if you have a new partner.

▸ Ask if PrEP is right for you.

Human Papilloma Virus (HPV)

What is it?

HPV is the most common virus that people get from having sex with someone who had it. There are many types of this virus spread by sex.

▸ Almost everyone who has sex, has had HPV at some time in their life. Most HPV infections go away on their own and cause no health problems.

▸ Some types of HPV can lead to cancer of the cervix. These same types of HPV, which are called "high risk strains," can cause cancer of the anus, penis, vagina, or throat. These strains have no symptoms.

▸ Other types of HPV cause genital warts. We call these types of HPV "low risk" strains. They often have symptoms (warts) that the patient sees and feels.

Symptoms

HPV is spread when the skin around the penis, scrotum, vulva, vagina, cervix or anus touches during sex. A person can have HPV and not know it. You can't tell when you look at a person if they have it. Some people have no signs of HPV. Others do have signs.

▸ You may see small bumps (warts) in or around the vagina, penis, or anus.

▸ The bumps may grow in bunches or clusters.

▸ They may itch.

You can spread the virus to others even when you have no signs.

Long-term effects

HPV can be treated but not cured. The treatment can help make you feel better. Some treatments can help take away the genital warts if you have them. But remember that with time most HPV infections go away on their own. Having HPV can cause these problems:

▸ You can pass it to others.

▸ You have a higher chance of getting HIV (the virus that causes AIDS).

▸ You may have one of the types of HPV that can lead to cancer.

If a pregnant person has genital warts, the baby could get the virus.

Genital Warts and Cervical Cancer

- Just having genital warts does not lead to cancer.

- However, if a person with a vagina has the kind of HPV that causes genital warts, they may also have another kind of HPV that causes cancer of the cervix.

Treatment

Genital warts (which is a low risk strain of the HPV virus) may be treated by your health care provider.

▸ You may need an exam of the cervix or penis called a colposcopy. Your health care provider uses a magnifying glass with a bright light to see the warts.

▸ The warts can be removed by freezing or burning. Most people need to have more than one visit to remove all the warts.

▸ There are also some medicines (cream or lotion) that you can use at home.

Talk to your provider about what treatment is right for you.

If you think you may be pregnant, tell your health care provider *before* you get treated.

If you have a high-risk strain of HPV, there are no symptoms.

- The only way you would know that you have a high-risk strain of HPV is if it were to show up on your screening test for cervical cancer. This might be an abnormal pap test or a "positive" HPV test. If either test is "positive," it means that you are at risk for cervical cancer or precancer.
- The provider will decide on what would be best to do, based on the results of your test(s).
- You may need an exam of the cervix called a colposcopy.
- The provider uses a magnifying lens and a bright light to carefully check your cervix.
- If your Pap test is abnormal, talk with your provider about what to do next.
- If you think you may be pregnant, tell the medical provider.

Learn more about the HPV vaccine.

Tell your patients that HPV vaccines prevent cancer of the cervix, penis, anus and throat as well as preventing genital warts. You can also tell them:

- The HPV vaccine is for pre-teens (age 11-12) and some young adults up to 26 years of age.
- It works best when you get the series of two or three shots before you ever start having sex.
- You can still get the vaccine even if you have already had sex before.
- If you are 27 to 45 years-old, you can get the vaccine but you will have to talk to your provider first.

Protect yourself and others

If you have HPV:

- Come back for all the treatments you need.
- Use condoms every time you have sex.

You can also help lower your chances of getting cancer of the cervix:

- Get a Pap test as often as your health care provider says.
- Don't smoke.
- Use condoms every time you have sex
- Ask about the HPV vaccine.

It is also a good idea to:

- ▶ Get tested for HIV and other STIs.
- ▶ Ask to get checked for STIs every year or if you have a new partner.
- ▶ Ask if PrEP is right for you.

Hepatitis

Hepatitis is an infection of the liver caused by the hepatitis virus. The most common three strains of this virus are hepatitis A, B and C. There are similarities and differences with these three infections. The symptoms of liver disease are similar across all three strains. There are ways that both hepatitis A and hepatitis B can be transmitted sexually. Here is more information about the most common strains of hepatitis.

Hepatitis A

The hepatitis A virus is mainly transmitted by the fecal-oral route, either by consumption of fecal-contaminated food and/or water, or through person-to-person contact. If hepatitis A is transmitted sexually, it is through direct fecal-oral contact such as mouth to anus sex, but this is not common. Transmitting hepatitis A through blood is also rare. Vaccination is the most effective means of preventing hepatitis A transmission.

Hepatitis C

Unlike hepatitis A, hepatitis C is mainly transmitted through blood, such as sharing needles for drugs or tattoos, or less commonly, by sharing household items that may contain blood like razors, toothbrushes and nail clippers. Hepatitis C is very rarely transmitted sexually, but an infected pregnant person can infect their unborn baby. Hepatitis C causes chronic infection in most people who get the virus. Many of those with chronic hepatitis C infection develop evidence of active liver disease, which can progress to liver cancer. Most people with hepatitis C do not know they have it because they don't feel ill, but they can still pass it to others. There is no vaccine for hepatitis C. Prevention includes not sharing needles of any sort, and using a condom if you are unsure of your partner's status.

Let's take a closer look at hepatitis B.

Hepatitis B

What is it?

Hepatitis B is a virus which causes severe infections of the liver. It cannot be cured, but in some people the infection can clear on its own, which can sometimes create lasting immunity. In other persons infected with hepatitis B, the virus can stay with them the rest of their lives and cause serious liver disease, even death. When this happens, it is called "chronic hepatitis."

Hepatitis B is caused by a virus (a kind of germ).

Get vaccinated

Hepatitis B can be prevented by getting the hepatitis B vaccine. It is a series of three shots.

Everyone should be vaccinated — even children.

You could get hepatitis B if you:

▶ Have unprotected sex with someone who has the virus.

▶ Share needles or drug "works."

▶ Share earrings, razors, nail clippers or toothbrushes.

▶ Pierce your body or get a tattoo with a dirty needle.

▶ Expose an open wound to infected blood or bodily fluids that contain blood.

▶ Were exposed during childbirth.

Symptoms

You can have hepatitis B without knowing it. You may feel fine or you may feel like you have the flu. The only way to know for sure that you have it is to have a blood test. Even if you have no symptoms, you can spread hepatitis B to others.

Some people get these signs:

▶ Yellow skin or eyes

▶ No appetite (they don't want to eat)

▶ Feeling tired

▶ Brown or dark urine (pee)

▶ Light or gray stools

▶ Pain in their stomach or abdomen, muscles or joints

Long-term effects

There is no cure for hepatitis B. But in some people, it goes away on its own. There is medicine that can help the liver of people who have chronic hepatitis.

Hepatitis B can cause these problems:

- ▶ You can give it to others.
- ▶ You have a higher chance of getting other STIs and infections.
- ▶ Chronic hepatitis can badly damage your liver. It can lead to cancer and even death.

If someone has hepatitis B while they are pregnant, they should tell their health care provider right away. The baby could be born with it. The baby will need special shots right after birth.

Treatment

Your provider will make a treatment plan just for you.

- ▶ You may need special medicines to help your liver.
- ▶ Tell your partner(s) and anyone you live with that you have hepatitis B. They will need to get the vaccine.
- ▶ If you think you may be pregnant, be sure to tell your health care provider *before* you get treated. You cannot take some kinds of medicines while you are pregnant.

Protect yourself and others

If you have hepatitis B:

- ▶ Get the treatment you need. Go back to your health care provider as often as you need to.
- ▶ Use condoms every time you have sex.
- ▶ Tell your partner(s) and family members to get the series of three shots (the vaccine) over six months. These shots help prevent them from getting hepatitis B.
- ▶ Don't share needles or drugs.
- ▶ Don't share earrings, razors, nail clippers, piercing jewelry, toothbrushes, or sex toys.
- ▶ Cover cuts or skin lesions to reduce contact with blood or body fluids.

It is also a good idea to:

- ▶ Get tested for HIV and other infections people get from having sex.
- ▶ Ask to get checked for STIs every year or if you have a new partner or partners.
- ▶ Ask if PrEP is right for you.

HIV (Human Immunodeficiency Virus)

What is it?

How HIV spreads
HIV is passed through:
■ Blood
■ Pre-ejaculate/pre-come
■ Semen
■ Vaginal fluids
■ Breast milk

HIV is the virus that causes AIDS. You can get HIV if you:

▶ Have sex with someone who has HIV. It can be spread by the vagina, penis, mouth, or anus. Your partner could have HIV and not know it.

▶ Share needles with someone who has HIV. They could have it and not know it.

Be aware that:

▶ A pregnant person who has HIV can pass it on to the baby, during childbirth or through their breast milk.

▶ If you are exposed to HIV and have any other STI, it could be easier for you to get infected with HIV.

Symptoms

HIV positive
People with HIV are HIV positive (HIV+).

You or your partner can have HIV and not know it. It can be months or years before you feel sick or have any serious signs. But you can still pass HIV to others. Though some people have no symptoms, some signs of HIV may include:

▶ Rapid weight loss

▶ Diarrhea

▶ Feeling very tired

▶ Fever

▶ Night sweats

▶ Pain in joints

Note: People with HIV who regularly take medication can become undetectable. This means there is not enough of the virus present in their body to be transmitted to someone else. Someone who is undetectable cannot spread HIV to another person.

Long-term effects

If you get HIV, it can affect every part of your body. Treatment can help with this, but the virus is still in your body and you can pass it to others.

HIV can cause these problems:

- You can give it to others.
- You have a higher chance of getting other STIs and infections.
- Over time, HIV can stop your body from fighting off other diseases.

When your body can't fight off diseases, you could get infections often. You might also have:

- Dangerous weight loss
- Cancer
- Mental problems
- Blindness

You could also die.

If a pregnant person has HIV, they should tell their health care provider. Their baby will need special care all through the pregnancy. Treatment can prevent the baby from getting HIV.

Treatment

HIV can't be cured. There are some medicines that can slow down the growth of HIV for a long time. Unless you are taking medication that has made your viral load undetectable, the virus is still in the body and can be passed to others.

- Your provider will make a treatment plan just for you.
- You may need special medicines.
- Tell your partner(s) that you have HIV. Tell them about PEP and PrEP. Use condoms every time you have sex.

If you think you may be pregnant, be sure to tell your health care provider *before* you get treated. If you are planning to get pregnant it is important to discuss it with your medical provider first. That way you can prepare for the pregnancy.

PEP (post-exposure prophylaxis)

This is medicine you can take if you've been exposed to HIV. It can reduce your chances of getting HIV. It is used in case of an emergency.

PrEP (pre-exposure prophylaxis)

This is medicine you can take before and during exposure to HIV. It can lower your chances of getting HIV.

Learn more at:

www.greaterthan.org

Protect yourself and others

If you have HIV:

▶ Tell your partner(s) to get checked for HIV.

▶ Get the treatment you need.

▶ Use a condom every time you have anal, oral, or vaginal sex.

▶ Use a latex barrier, like a dental dam, if you have oral sex on a vulva or anus.

▶ Don't share needles.

▶ Hugging, kissing, and touching are safe.

It is also a good idea to:

▶ Get a pap test once a year.

▶ Ask about the HPV vaccine.

▶ Get tested for other STIs.

▶ Ask to get checked for STIs every year or if you have a new partner or partners.

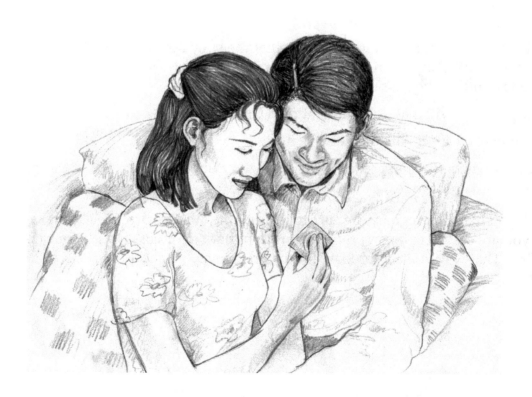

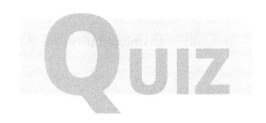

Common STIs

Directions: Draw a line from the description on the left to the STI on the right that it describes.

Description	**STI**
1. This is one of the most common STIs. Most people don't know they have it. Most people have no signs. It can be cured with antibiotics.	**a.** HPV
2. This STI causes fever blisters or cold sores. People get these on or near their genitals or mouth. Symptoms go away in a week or two. The virus stays in the body and can cause sores to break out again.	**b.** HIV
3. This STI causes bumps to appear around the genitals or inside the vagina, anus, or penis. Even if you don't have these bumps, the virus can be spread to others. Many people don't know they have this because they haven't noticed the bumps.	**c.** Chlamydia
4. Some people have no symptoms of this infection for many years. Others get sick and quickly die. It may keep your body from being able to fight off other diseases. There is no cure for this infection.	**d.** Herpes

Go on to the next page.

Directions: Circle the best answer.

5. Which of the following STIs can be cured?
    a. Trichomoniasis, HIV, and chlamydia
    b. Syphilis, HPV, and genital herpes
    c. Syphilis, trichomoniasis, and chlamydia

6. Which of the following STIs cannot be cured?
    a. Syphilis, gonorrhea, and HIV
    b. Genital herpes, HPV, and HIV
    c. Chlamydia, trichomoniasis, and syphilis

Check your answers on the next page.

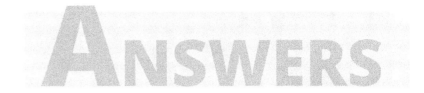

Common STIs

Check your answers.

1. **C**   **Chlamydia** is one of the most common STIs. Most people don't know they have it. Most people have no signs. It can be cured with antibiotics.

2. **D**   **Herpes** causes fever blisters or cold sores. People get them on or near their genitals or mouth. Symptoms go away in a week or two. The virus stays in the body and can cause sores to break out again.

3. **A**   **HPV** causes bumps that appear around the genitals or inside the vagina, anus or penis. Even if you don't have these bumps, the virus can be spread to others. Many people don't know they have this because they haven't noticed the bumps.

4. **B**   **HIV** Some people have no symptoms of HIV for many years. Others get sick and quickly die. It keeps your body from being able to fight off other diseases. There is no cure for this infection.

5. **C**   Syphilis, trichomoniasis, and chlamydia *can* be cured.

6. **B**   Genital herpes, HPV and HIV *cannot* be cured.

Sexually Transmitted Infections

Directions: Circle the best answer.

1. STIs are infections that people can get when they:

    a. Have sex with someone who has an STI.

    b. Shake the hand of someone who sneezes a lot.

    c. Swim in a pool with someone who has an STI.

2. People might get an STI if they do which of the following things with a person who has an STI?

    a. Have anal sex.

    b. Have oral sex.

    c. Have vaginal sex.

    d. Touch the genitals of that person.

    e. All of the above

3. These STIs can be cured:

    a. Chlamydia, gonorrhea, and genital herpes

    b. HIV, syphilis, and HPV

    c. Hepatitis B, chlamydia, and gonorrhea

    d. Chlamydia, trichomoniasis, and syphilis

Directions: Read each of the following and write your best answer in the space below.

4. Your patient has chosen a birth control method that doesn't protect them from STIs. What can you ask to find out what they will do to protect themselves from STIs?

    _____

    _____

    _____

Go on to the next page.

5. List three things you can tell your patients to do to protect themselves from STIs:

   - _____

   - _____

   - _____

6. List three things that make a patient more likely to get an STI:

   - _____

   - _____

   - _____

7. List five things you can tell patients about their STI treatment plan:

   - _____

   - _____

   - _____

   - _____

   - _____

Go on to the next page.

Directions: Fill in the blanks.

8. Although _____ is one of the most common STIs, many people don't know they have it.

9. The first sign of _____ is a painless sore called a chancre. It will go away on its own. A few weeks later, a person with this STI might have a rash, a fever, and headaches.

10. _____ is a group of viruses that can cause genital warts or cervical cancer.

11. Over time, _____ keeps your body from fighting off other infections.

Check your answers on the next page.

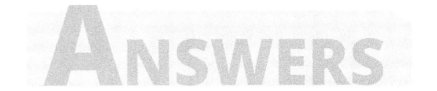

Sexually Transmitted Infections

Check your answers.

1. **A**   STIs are infections that people usually get by having sex with someone who already has one.

2. **E**   All of the above. People can get an STI if they have anal sex, oral sex, or vaginal sex with a person who has an STI. They can also get some STIs if they touch the genitals of another person who has the STI. If they use condoms, they lower their chances of getting an STI.

3. **D**   Chlamydia, trichomoniasis, and syphilis are STIs that *can* be cured.

4. To find out what patients will do to protect themselves from STIs, you can say:

   "Tell me what you're going to do to protect yourself from STIs."

5. These are things you can tell your patients to do to protect themselves from STIs:

   - Use a condom every time you have sex.
   - Use a condom even if you use other types of birth control.
   - Talk with your partner about sex and STIs.
   - Have sex with only one person who has sex only with you.
   - Get checked and treated for STIs.

Go on to the next page.

© Essential Access Health

6. Patients are more likely to get an STI if they:

   - Have sex while they or their partners are drinking alcohol or using drugs.

   - Share needles from injection drugs or tattoos, or if they have sex with someone who shares needles.

   - Have sex with someone who has signs of an STI, or if they touch the sores of someone who has signs of an STI.

   - Have sex without using a condom.

7. Some things you can tell patients about their STI treatment plan are:

   - The name of the medicine

   - How to take it

   - When to take it

   - How to fit the treatment into their lives

   - When to come back for follow-up care

   You can also talk about:

   - Any side effects of the medicine

   - What to do if they have side effects

   - Why it is important to complete their treatment.

   - What this treatment will do

   Patients may also need to know:

   - What they should do about sex while they are being treated

   - Why their partners need to be treated

   - How to keep from getting an STI again

   Go on to the next page.

8. **Chlamydia**	Although chlamydia is one of the most common STIs, many people don't know they have it.
9. **Syphilis**	The first sign of syphilis is a painless sore called a chancre. It will go away on its own. A few weeks later, an infected person might have a rash, fever, and headaches.
10. **HPV**	HPV (human papilloma virus) is a group of viruses that can cause genital warts or cervical cancer.
11. **HIV**	Over time, HIV keeps your body from fighting off other infections.

Birth Control Methods

As a health worker, one of your main goals is to teach patients about birth control methods — especially about the birth control method they have chosen. This chapter gives you the correct, up-to-date information you will need when talking with your patients. It also gives you an idea of how to present that information.

An easy way to present birth control information is to use a tiered-effectiveness approach. That means you introduce the most effective methods first and then talk about the other birth control methods in order of effectiveness. Using a chart that shows the methods arranged in three rows or tiers, with the most effective methods in the top tier, makes it easy for your patients to see how well a method works compared to other methods.

To help you learn about the many birth control methods, this chapter groups them into
five types:

> **Tier One — Long-Term Methods:** These methods prevent pregnancy for 3 or more years.

> **Tier Two — Hormonal Methods:** These methods use hormones made in a lab to keep the hormones in the body at a level that will prevent pregnancy.

Other words for Birth Control

Other words you may hear that mean the same thing as 'birth control' are:

- Contraception
- Prophylactic
- Family planning

▸ **Tier Two or Three — Information-Based Methods:** These methods use the patient's knowledge about their body and about how pregnancy happens.

▸ **Tier Three — Barrier Methods:** These methods keep sperm from traveling through the cervix and into the uterus.

▸ **Emergency Contraception:** This is the only kind of birth control that works to prevent pregnancy after having sex.

Topics

▸ Special Notes About This Chapter

▸ Tier One: Long-Term Methods

- Implants

- Intra-uterine Devices (IUDs)

- Sterilization Methods

▸ Tier Two: Hormonal Methods

- Birth Control Pill

- Birth Control Patch

- Birth Control Ring

- Progestin-Only Pills (POPs)

- Birth Control Shot (Depo-Provera)

▸ Tier Two or Three: Information-Based Methods

- Abstinence

- Fertility Awareness-Based (FAB) Methods

- Withdrawal

- Lactation Amenorrhea Method (LAM)

- Tier Three: Barrier Methods
  - External Condom
  - Internal Condom
  - Diaphragm
  - Birth Control Cap
  - Birth Control Sponge
  - Spermicides
- Emergency Contraception (EC)

Objectives

After reading this chapter you will be able to:

- Explain how each birth control method works.
- Tell how well each method works to prevent pregnancy.
- Describe how to use each method correctly.

You will also be able to:

- Tell what side effects each method may have.
- Tell what complications or warning signs each method may have.
- Discuss the advantages of each method.
- Describe problems some people may have with each method and how they can deal with these problems.

A note about transgender patients and birth control

Transgender patients also need information about birth control. A transgender patient who is on hormone replacement therapy (HRT) and still has their reproductive organs can cause a pregnancy or get pregnant.

It is important to note that testosterone or estrogen replacement therapy is NOT birth control.

Patients taking testosterone can choose any birth control method, but should speak to their provider about possible side effects and interactions.

Methods with progestin **do not** counteract the effects of testosterone. Patients using methods with progestin may experience similar side effects to those seen in cisgender (non-transgender) women. Methods like the Implant, hormonal IUD, shot and Progestin-only pills may be used to control, lessen or stop bleeding during the menstrual cycle in combination with testosterone therapy.

Methods with estrogen (pill/patch/ring) **can** counteract the effects of testosterone. This may result in a reversal of the desired effects of testosterone by patients who may become pregnant (e.g. further breast development, fat redistribution, menstruation).

Patients taking estrogen who still have a penis can choose any birth control method approved for persons who can cause pregnancy (sterilization, condoms and/or withdrawal).

Educator Note: To learn more about birth control and transgender patients:

Reproductive Health Access Project
www.reproductiveaccess.org/
(Birth Control Across the Gender Spectrum)

American College of Obstetrics and Gynecologists
www.acog.org (Contraception for Transmasculine Patients)

Special Notes About This Chapter

Suggestions for where to start

This chapter has a lot of information. You don't need to learn everything all at once. You may want to focus first on the methods your patients use most. Once you are comfortable with those, you can read about the other methods.

It is a good idea to look for things that methods have in common. For example, all of the hormonal methods that use both estrogen and progestin work the same way. So, once you learn how the Birth Control Pill works, you will also know how the Birth Control Patch and Birth Control Ring work.

Ways to talk to your patients

This chapter is set up in a slightly different way than others. Like Chapter 5, it is written mostly as though you are talking to your patient. Things are explained using plain, easy-to-understand language. You do not have to use this language word for word. Use it as a model for how to talk with your patients. You should use words and phrases that you are comfortable with and that work for your individual patients.

Here are a few points to keep in mind when talking with your patients:

- Use words and phrases that your patient understands.
- If you must use a word that is hard to understand, such as a medical term, be sure to explain it.
- Be sure to ask patients to tell you what they have learned in their own words. This will help you know what was and was not understood.

Notes to you

Of course, this chapter also includes notes written directly to you, the health worker, not to the patient. You will find some of those notes in boxes in the margins. You will find others in text-boxes that look like this:

> Information written in boxes that look like this are notes to you, the health worker.

Information for Informed Consent

In Chapter 1, you learned about the importance of patients giving informed consent for the birth control method they have chosen. In this chapter you will find the information a patient needs to have so that she or he can give their informed consent.

Remember that patients only need this detailed information for the method they have decided to use. Before they make that decision, they should be given basic information about each of the methods available. You don't need to cover all of that information personally. Many health care providers introduce patients to their many choices through DVD's, booklets or pamphlets, or online resources before they meet with you. When they do meet with you, you can answer any questions they may have.

Once patients decide on a birth control method, you must give them details on that method. As you learned in Chapter 2, before patients can give informed consent for a method, they need to know:

- ▶ What it is
- ▶ How it works
- ▶ How well it works
- ▶ How to use it
- ▶ Possible side effects (minor reactions or body changes the method can cause)

Patients also need to know about:

- ▶ Complications (rare, but serious, health problems that could happen because a method is used)
- ▶ Warning signs (physical signs that warn of a possible complication)
- ▶ Advantages and disadvantages to using the method
- ▶ What to do if they want to stop using the method

To make it easier to remember, the information for each method in this chapter is set up in that same order.

Sometimes there are reasons that a patient should not use a certain method. Those reasons are called *precautions*. For example, a patient might have high blood pressure. That is a precaution against using a hormonal method. It is the health care provider who must discuss precautions with each patient and decide if the patient should choose a different method for medical reasons. This chapter includes the basic information on such precautions to help you answer questions your patients may have.

A special word about how well methods work

This chapter tells you how well each method works (how effective it is). This information is based on the most recent research.

For most methods, this chapter gives you a number for *perfect use* and for *typical use*.

The number for "perfect use" tells you how many users out of 100 may get pregnant in a year if the method is used exactly the right way *every* time.

The number for "typical use" tells you what happens to a typical patient in real life. Even though patients may plan to and try to use their method exactly the right way every time, sometimes they might make a mistake -- especially during the first year they use the method. So, the number for "typical use" tells you how many users out of 100 may get pregnant during the first year that they use a method.

Even though these numbers are based on research, they rarely apply directly to any one patient. Let your patients know that:

▶ If they use their method correctly every time, their chances of getting pregnant would be closer to the number under "perfect use."

▶ If they don't always use their method correctly, their chances of pregnancy could be much higher than the number under "typical use."

You can help your patients compare choices by telling them:

▶ If 100 users have sex using no birth control method at all, 85 of them may get pregnant in a year.

Also talk to your patients about:

▶ Any reasons a method might fail

▶ Things they can do to prevent or solve that problem

▶ What to do if the method fails or if they forget to use it

NOTE: Perfect and typical use effectiveness percentage rates for all birth control methods covered in this manual have been updated using *Contraceptive Technology*, 21st Edition, 2018 (Table 26-1 on page 844).

Tips you can give your patients

There are many ways you can help your patients use their method successfully. But sometimes they will need a back-up method to use along with their regular birth control method. Sometimes they may need help *after* they have had unprotected sex.

Back-up method

A back-up method of birth control is another method the patient can use if their first choice is not available or not working.

Example: A patient wants to start using the birth control patch. They want to start using the patch that day. For the first week that they use the patch, they must use an additional method (a back-up method) or not have reproductive sex to protect themselves from pregnancy that first week.

Example: A patient is using the pill. They forget to take two pills in a row. When that happens, they may not be protected from pregnancy. To protect themselves, they should use a back-up method along with the pill for 7 days. They can use condoms, withdrawal, spermicides, or abstain from reproductive sex as their back-up method.

Ask your patients what methods they will use as a back-up when they need it.

Emergency Contraception (EC)

All patients should be told that they have a second chance to prevent pregnancy even if they realize *after* sex that their method may have failed. EC is a special type of birth control that can be used in such a situation. They can take an EC pill or pills up to 5 days after having unprotected sex to help prevent a pregnancy. Or, an IUD can be placed into their uterus up to 5 days after unprotected sex to prevent pregnancy.

EC pills *should not* be used as a regular birth control method because they are much less effective than other methods.

If placing an IUD for emergency contraception, the user will continue to have very effective birth control if they decide to keep their IUD.

Tier One: Long-Term Methods

Long-term methods of birth control include long acting reversible contraceptives (LARCs) such as birth control implants and intra-uterine devices, and permanent methods of birth control like sterilization procedures.

Terms for IUDs

Intra-uterine devices (IUDs) have many names: intra-uterine contraceptives (IUCs), and intra-uterine system (IUS)

- Birth control implants work for up to 3 to 5 years.
- IUDs work for between 3 and 12 years. How long yours works depends on which IUD you choose.
- Sterilization for patients who make sperm (vasectomy) or for patients who ovulate (tubal sterilization) should be thought of as permanent methods of birth control. Sterilization is only for those who **know** they do not want to have any or any more children.

Long-term methods work very well to prevent pregnancy. But, they do **not** help protect against HIV or other STIs. Use condoms every time you have sex to help protect yourself from these infections.

Words you may need to know

Here are some words you may need to know when you talk with your patients about long-term methods.

Words	Description
Implant	A small flexible plastic rod about the size of a match. It is placed right beneath the surface of the skin in the inner part of the patient's upper arm. It has a hormone (progestin) in it that helps prevent pregnancy.
Intra-uterine devices (IUDs)	A small piece of plastic that has either copper on it or the hormone progestin in it that is placed in a patient's uterus by a health care provider to prevent pregnancy.
Sterilization	A permanent method of birth control that is done when people no longer want to have children.
Tubal sterilization	The tubes that carry the eggs are cut, blocked or removed.
Vasectomy	The tubes that carry the sperm are cut.

Birth Control Methods

Topics in this section

▸ Birth Control Implant

▸ IUDs

▸ Sterilization

Objectives

After reading this section, you will be able to:

▸ Tell how well each method works to prevent pregnancy.

▸ Explain how the long-term methods work.

▸ Describe how to use the methods correctly.

You will also be able to:

▸ List a side effect of each method.

▸ List a complication and warning sign for each method.

▸ Describe the advantages of each method.

▸ Describe problems some people may have with each method and how they can deal with these problems.

Birth Control Implant

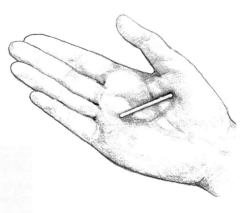

This section is mostly written as though you were talking to your patients. It gives you an idea of how to explain the birth control implant in a way your patients can understand. This section also has notes written directly to you, the health worker. Those "health worker notes" will look like this one.

What is it?

The birth control implant is a small plastic rod the size of a matchstick that is placed under the skin in the inner, upper part of your arm. It can prevent pregnancy for up to 3 to 5 years. It has one hormone in it to make it work. That hormone is progestin. The implant has no estrogen in it. That means that those who cannot take estrogen for some reason can use this method.

The implant must be placed and taken out by a health care provider. Once it is placed in your arm, you will hardly notice it and most can barely see it. You will be able to feel it with your fingertips.

The implant works well to prevent pregnancy. But it does not protect against HIV or other STIs. Use condoms every time you have sex to help protect against these infections.

How does it work?

The implant works mostly by keeping the egg from leaving the ovaries. If there is no egg to meet with sperm, you can't get pregnant. The implant may also:

▶ Keep the mucus of the cervix thick. This helps keep sperm from getting into the uterus and meeting with an egg.

How well does the Implant work?

There is no difference between perfect and typical users of the implant. Once the implant is placed in the arm by the health care provider, there is nothing you can do to make it less effective. If your health care provider puts it in the right way, the implant is one of the most effective methods of birth control.

For perfect and typical users, the implant is over 99.9% effective.

That means that if 100 patients use the implant, only 1 (and probably none) of them may get pregnant in a year.

How do you use the Implant?

Teach your patients these steps so they can use the implant the right way. Your provider's advice may differ from the advice given here. Be sure to give your patients the advice used at your health care site.

1. **Talk to the health care provider about whether the implant is right for you.**

   The health care provider will ask you some questions. Talk to the provider about:

   ▸ Any health problems you may have

   ▸ Any medicine you may be taking

   ▸ Any questions you may have

   You may also need to have an exam. Your health care provider will help you decide if the implant is right for you.

2. **The provider will place the implant in your arm.**

   If the implant is right for you, the health care provider can place it in your arm that day. Or you may need to come in to have the implant put in during the first 5 days of your next period.

   If you are left-handed, the implant will be placed in your right arm. If you are right-handed, the implant will be placed in your left arm.

   You will lie on your back with your arm up. Your health care provider will numb the area on your inner arm where the implant will be put in. It will look like you are getting a shot. The health care provider will put the implant just under the skin of your inner upper arm. It will not be in your muscle.

   The health care provider will put a small bandage over the implant. They will have you rub the area so that you can see what it feels like. Then they will put a second, larger bandage over the first.

Get FREE Reminder Notifications

Sign-up for free email and/or phone notifications via the bedsider.org website or via an app for your smartphone that will help you keep track.

3. **Ask about using a back-up method.**

   Depending on when during your cycle your implant is placed, you may need to use a second method for the first 7 days. Ask your medical provider whether it is needed.

4. **Keep the area around your bandages dry and clean.**

   This will help prevent infection. After 24 hours, take off the larger, outside bandage. After 3-5 days, take off the smaller, inside bandage. You may have a little bruising. But there should be little or no scarring.

5. **Keep track of when you will need to have your implant removed.**

    A health care provider will need to remove the implant within 3-5 years of when it was placed. The date when you need to have it taken out is called your 'removal date.' Your health care site will keep track of this date. If you can't remember you can call your provider and ask when you need to have it removed. Your health care site can remind you when it's time to have a new implant placed.

    Think about different ways to help you remember to schedule an appointment in 3-5 years:

    ▶ Enter it on your paper, phone, or email calendar.

    ▶ Write the date on a card that you keep in your purse or wallet.

    ▶ Have your partner help you remember.

    Make sure to come in to have it taken out on or before your removal date.

6. **Get the implant removed or replaced.**

    Make an appointment to have the implant taken out. Call 2 or 3 weeks before your removal date. To prevent pregnancy, you must either have a new implant placed or switch to another birth control method by your removal date. If you want to keep using the implant as your birth control method, your provider can place a new one on the same day, in the same place in your arm where you have your current implant. If you don't want a new implant, you should know that once the implant is taken out, you could get pregnant right away — even the very day that the implant is removed.

    To remove the implant, the provider will ask you to lie back with your arm up. They will touch your arm to find it. Then they will numb the area and make a small cut to take out the implant. If you don't want a new implant, the provider will put a small bandage over the cut. To prevent infection, keep the area dry and clean. If you want a new implant, the provider can place one in the same place in your arm.

7. **If you see a doctor for any reason, tell the doctor that you are using the implant.** Add it to your list of daily medications you take.

What if you are late getting a new Implant after the three years is up?

If you forget to get your implant replaced on time, you could get pregnant. Follow these steps:

> ▶ Call the health care site right away to make an appointment to have the new implant put in and the old one taken out.

Talk to your patients about Emergency Contraception.

Emergency Contraception (EC), in the form of EC pills or an IUD, can prevent pregnancy *after* sex. Patients can use EC up to 5 days after unprotected sex. Read more about it in the section on EC.

> ▸ If you had sex since the date you should have had a new implant put in, ask about Emergency Contraception (EC).

> ▸ Use a second method of birth control, like condoms, until you can get the new implant put in.

Are there any side effects?

All patients using the implant have one or more side effects.
A very common side effect is for the patient to notice changes in their menstrual bleeding. Patients can talk to the medical provider if their side effects bother them.

Counsel your patient about changes in their period.

The main reason patients stop using the implant is because of irregular bleeding. Talk with your patient about how they will deal with any changes in their bleeding pattern. This may help them to know what to expect.

Ask your clients:

- How do you think you might feel if you had no periods at all?
- How do you think you might deal with it if you had frequent or continuous or unpredictable spotting for awhile?
- Let them know if they are not happy with their bleeding pattern once they are using the implant, they can talk with the provider about ways to make it better.

Changes in periods

While you use the implant, it is normal to have bleeding you can't predict. No one knows exactly what your bleeding pattern will be like. This is normal and it is caused by the progestin in the implant. After 3-6 months the bleeding may become more regular and usually becomes lighter and less crampy.

Patients who use the implant will have changes in their periods:

> ▸ You may not bleed while you are using the implant or may go long stretches of time without bleeding.

> ▸ You may not know when you will have your period.

> ▸ You may have spotting between periods.

> ▸ You may have longer or shorter periods.

Other possible side effects

These are the most likely side effects you could have:

- Headaches
- Acne
- Depression

These are less common, but other side effects some patients get include:

- Breast pain
- Stomach pain
- Painful periods
- Nervousness

- Nausea
- There can be temporary pain, swelling or bruising where the implant was put in.

Some of these side effects may not go away until the implant is taken out. If you have any problems, talk to a health care provider. There may be something that can be done to help. But you may have to wait until the implant is removed.

What about complications and warning signs?

Serious problems are **rare** with the implant. But here are some possible problems you should know about:

- **The implant may not be placed correctly or it may come out of your arm.**
  Right after your implant is placed in your arm, check to see if you can feel it. If you can feel the implant under your skin it is in a perfect position! If you can't, it may not have been put in the right way. Tell your health care provider right away. You may not be protected from pregnancy.

- **Rarely patients get an infection** where the implant was put in. Signs of infection include redness, swelling, heat, and tenderness. If you get any of these warning signs, call the provider right away.

- **There's a small chance the implant could break.**

The Implant and Weight Concerns

Q: Does the implant cause weight gain?

A: No.

Q: If a patient is overweight, will the implant still work well?

A: Yes!

Q: Would a patient who is overweight have a higher chance of health problems while using the implant?

A: No.

Research shows that the implant does not cause weight gain. Most people gain weight over time whether they use the implant or not. This is especially true for teens and young adults who may still be growing.

The implant has not been shown to increase the risk of cancer, blood clots, stroke, or heart attack. Even so, some drug company inserts for the implant may list these estrogen-related risks. Check with your supervisor about how to discuss this with patients.

Are there any precautions to using the Implant?

A health care provider may advise you to use a different method if any of the following is true:

- ▸ You have had breast cancer.

- ▸ You have liver disease.

- ▸ You have irregular bleeding from the vagina for no known reason.

The health care provider will talk with you about your health to make sure that there is no reason for you not to use the implant.

Breastfeeding

Patients who breastfeed can use the implant, but they may have to wait for awhile after childbirth. The health care provider can tell the patient how long they have to wait.

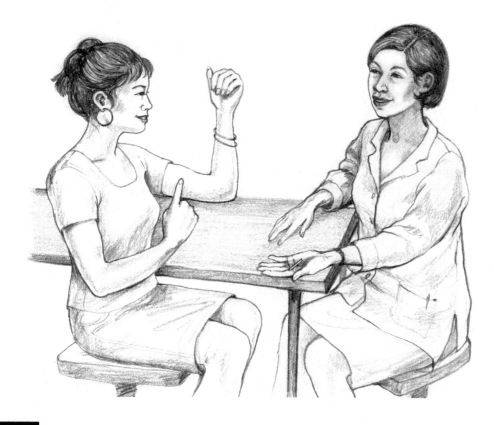

What are the advantages and disadvantages of using the Implant?

There are many things patients like about using the implant. And there are things some patients don't like. Find out what your patient likes. Encourage them to focus on those things.

What some people like about the implant:

▸ It is excellent at preventing pregnancy.

▸ Using it doesn't interrupt sex.

▸ It is simple to have it placed.

▸ Once in place you don't have to do anything to make it work and you don't have to worry about it.

▸ It is very safe to use.

▸ It can be used by those who can't take estrogen.

▸ It can be used by those who don't like the side effects of estrogen.

▸ It may help prevent cancer of the ovary and cancer of the lining of the uterus.

▸ It usually prevents menstrual cramps.

▸ Many patients don't get a period at all or bleed rarely.

▸ For those who still have periods, they are usually light.

Ask your patients if they have any concerns about using the implant. Then talk to them about their concerns. Help them think through how to solve any problems they might have while using the implant. Try to get them to come up with their own solutions first. Read the chart that follows for some ideas on how to deal with concerns.

Keep in mind that the implant isn't the best method for everyone. It is the patient's choice.

The Implant: Some Problems and Ways to Solve Them

Problem	Ways to Solve the Problem
I don't like having it put in and taken out.	It only takes a few minutes to put it in and to take it out. And the health care provider will numb the area where it will be put in so you won't feel any pain. Ask your patient what troubles them the most about this. Perhaps they don't know what to expect. It may help to explain it to them. For example, if they have a piercing, you may want to say that placing the implant feels a lot like getting a piercing.
I don't like being able to feel the implant in my arm.	Most patients don't notice the implant unless they touch it with their fingertips.
I have to remember to come in to the health care site in 3-5 years.	Make sure to come to your annual exams. Your provider will tell you when it's time for a new implant. You also can: • Enter it on your phone or a calendar. • You can use a free app that sends notifications like Bedsider. • Write the date on a card that you keep in your purse or wallet. • Have your partner help you remember.
I may get some side effects.	Some side effects go away after 3-6 months. But some don't. If your side effects bother you, talk to your health care provider to see if they can do anything to help.

The Implant: Some Problems and Ways to Solve Them

Problem	Ways to Solve the Problem
It would really bother me if the spotting kept going on and on.	In most, there will be less spotting over time. There are medications that a provider can give you to help stop or control the spotting. But there is no way to know how long the spotting might go on for you. If on-going spotting would bother you, the implant may not be the best method for you. **Most users spot for many days in a row when they are using the implant. Patients should think about whether they would be comfortable with this. For some patients, the added expense of panty liners may be a problem.**
I want to have a period every month.	If having a period every month is important to you, the implant may not be the best method for you. There are other methods you can choose from that will let you bleed every month or will not stop you from getting a period every month.
I could get a serious complication.	Serious problems are very rare with the implant. If you are ever worried about something you think is not normal, call the provider for advice.
What if I forget to get my implant taken out on time and a new one put in?	Call the provider for advice. You may still prevent pregnancy after sex by using emergency contraception.
The implant does not protect me from HIV and other STIs.	Use condoms every time you have sex to help protect against these infections.

What if you want to stop using the Implant?

If you want to stop using this method, a health care provider must take the implant out. Do not take it out yourself. This could harm you.

Once the implant is removed, you can become pregnant right away. Start using another birth control method the same day the implant is removed if you don't want to be pregnant.

There are no health problems to watch for when you stop using this method.

Make sure your patient understands.

Before your patients leave, make sure they understand how to use the implant successfully. Here are some things you can ask to make sure they understand.

- ▸ Tell me what you know about the implant.
- ▸ How does the implant work?
- ▸ How will you take care of your arm to avoid infection after the implant is placed?
- ▸ How will you remember to have the implant taken out in 3 to 5 years?
- ▸ What might be the most difficult problem for you when using the implant?
- ▸ How would you solve that problem?
- ▸ What warning signs will you look for while you are using the implant?
- ▸ How will you deal with the spotting you might get from using the implant?

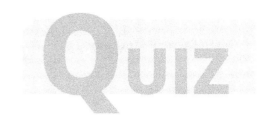

Birth Control Implant

Directions: Circle the best answer.

1. The Birth Control Implant:
    a. Works for 3 to 5 years.
    b. Has only one rod.
    c. Has one hormone in it named progestin.
    d. All of the above

2. The Implant works because:
    a. It keeps eggs from leaving the ovaries.
    b. It keeps the cervical mucus thick.
    c. Once it is placed, it releases progestin every moment of the day without the user having to do anything.
    d. All of the above

3. To have the Implant placed, a patient should:
    a. Go to a health care provider.
    b. Read the instructions and carefully put it in their arm themselves.
    c. Have a friend read the instructions and carefully put it into their arm.
    d. None of the above

4. Which of the following is true about the Implant?
    a. It can get lost in the arm.
    b. It has the highest effectiveness rate of all birth control methods.
    c. A patient needs to check their arm once a month to make sure the implant is still in.
    d. None of the above

Go on to the next page.

Directions: *Read each of the following and write your best answer in the spaces below.*

5. List one concern that a patient may have about using the Implant and what you might say to help them deal with that concern.

- **Patient's concern:**
  _____

  _____

- **What you can say:**
  _____

  _____

Check your answers on the next page.

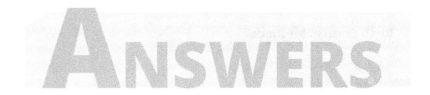

Birth Control Implant

Check your answers.

1. **D** All of the above. The Implant works for 3 to 5 years. It has only one rod, and it has one hormone in it to make it work. That hormone is called progestin.

2. **D** All of the above. The Implant works because:
   - It keeps eggs from leaving the ovaries.
   - It makes the mucus from the cervix thick.
   - Once it is placed, it releases progestin every moment of the day without the user having to do anything.

3. **A** To have the Implant placed, a patient should go to a health care provider. The health care provider will place it in their arm.

4. **B** The Implant has the highest effectiveness rate of any method of birth control. It is 99.95% effective for both perfect and typical users.

5. Here are two concerns a patient might have about using the Implant and what you might say to help them. For other possible concerns and responses, please see "The Implant: Some Problems and Ways to Solve Them" chart near the end of the Birth Control Implant section.

   - *Patient's concern:* "It would really bother me if the spotting kept going on and on."

     What you could say: "In most patients, there will be less spotting in 3-6 months. But there is no way to know how long it might go on for you. If that would bother you, the implant may not be the best method for you."

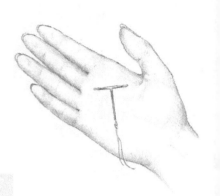

Intra-uterine Devices (IUDs)

This section is mostly written as though you were talking to your patients. It gives you an idea of how to explain IUDs in a way your patients can understand. This section also has notes written directly to you, the health worker. Those "health worker notes" will look like this one.

What are IUDs?

An IUD (intra-uterine device) is a small piece of plastic. A health care provider places it inside the uterus to prevent pregnancy. It stays there and works for up to 3 to 12 years, depending on which kind of IUD is used.

A health care provider can take the IUD out any time you wish to get pregnant or to change your birth control method.

There are five IUDs being used in the United States:

> ▸ The **Paragard** IUD (also called the **Copper T**) is partly wrapped in a fine copper wire. It works for up to 12 years.

> ▸ There are four IUDs with the hormone progestin in it. **Skyla** works up to 3 years, **Kyleena** works up to 5 years, **Mirena** works up to 5 or 6 years and, **Liletta** is currently approved for up to 6 years. Ongoing studies show that **Liletta** may work even longer so the recommendations may change again.

IUDs work very well to prevent pregnancy. But they do not help protect against HIV and other STIs. Use condoms every time you have sex to help protect against these infections.

Other Names for an IUD

People use different names for IUDs. Use whatever term your patients are comfortable with. Other names for IUDs are:

- IUS Intra-uterine System
- IUC Intra-uterine Contraceptive

How does it work?

IUDs keep sperm from meeting an egg. They do this in several ways:

▶ All IUDs change the environment in your uterus. This causes your uterus to make chemicals that make sperm unable to move. It doesn't cause any health problems while you are using it or later in life. Once placed, you cannot feel the IUD at all.

▶ The **Paragard** IUD has copper wrapped around the plastic T. The copper limits sperm function or survival and prevents the sperm and egg from meeting.

▶ The **Mirena**, **Skyla**, **Liletta** and **Kyleena** IUDs release small amounts of the hormone progestin into the uterus. This thins the lining of the uterus, slows sperm movement and reduces sperm survival. This also keeps the mucus of your cervix thick and sticky. The thick mucus keeps sperm from getting into the uterus. If sperm can't get into the uterus, they cannot meet with an egg. The progestin may sometimes keep the egg from leaving the ovary but this is not the main way that IUDs work to prevent pregnancy.

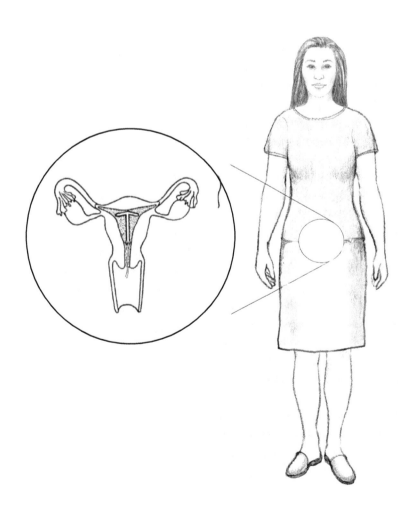

How well do IUDs work?

When you talk to your patients, discuss how well the IUD works (how effective it is). There is little or no difference between "typical" and "perfect" use for IUDs. Here's how well each IUD works.

ParaGard is 99.2% effective.

That means that if 100 patients use ParaGard, only 1 (and probably none) of them may get pregnant in a year.

Hormonal IUDs are 99.6 to 99.9% effective.

That means that if 100 patients use a hormonal IUD, only 1 (and probably none) of them may get pregnant in a year.

Talk to your patients about Emergency Contraception.

Emergency Contraception (EC), in the form of EC pills or an IUD, can prevent pregnancy after sex. Patients can use EC up to 5 days after unprotected sex. Read more about it in the section on EC.

How do you use an IUD?

Teach your patients these steps so they can use the IUD successfully.

1. **Talk to a health care provider about whether the IUD is right for you.**

   The health care provider will give you an exam. You will be checked to make sure your uterus and cervix are suitable for the IUD. You may be tested for certain STIs at the same time.

2. **A provider must place the IUD into your uterus.**

   The IUD can be placed any time that you are not pregnant.

   ▸ The provider uses a special applicator to place the IUD through the vagina and cervix and into your uterus.

   ▸ Some patients feel a mild or sharp cramp during placement but this is usually just for a few seconds.

   ▸ The provider will cut the two IUD strings short so they hang just outside your cervix in the back of the vagina.

   ▸ Placing the IUD takes just a few minutes.

Checking strings

Let your patients know that the IUDs work well even if patients aren't able to check their strings every month.

Signs that the IUD is coming out

- Cramps
- Spotting
- Change in the length of the strings
- Feeling the hard plastic at the cervix

Talk to your patients about Emergency Contraception.

Emergency Contraception (EC) can prevent pregnancy after sex. If a patient thinks that the IUD might have come out, or have partly come out, they might need EC. Patients can take EC up to 5 days after unprotected sex. Read more about it in the section on EC.

3. **Checking the strings about once a month.**

Once you have had your IUD placed, the provider may suggest that you feel for the IUD strings in the back of your vagina about once a month. This is to check that it is still in place. If you are getting your period once a month, then after your period is a perfect time to check. If you aren't getting your period regularly (as may happen if you use a hormonal IUD), then simply choose a time about once a month to "check your strings."

- ▶ Put one or two fingers inside of your vagina and reach towards the back until you feel the soft plastic strings (also called threads). You can feel them coming out of the little opening to the cervix.
- ▶ If the strings feel the same as always, the IUD is probably in place.
- ▶ The IUD may be out of place if:
  - The strings feel longer or shorter than usual.
  - You can't find the strings.
  - You feel a hard bump of plastic at the opening of your cervix.
  - It's a good idea to feel for your strings if you have abnormal cramping at any time.

If you think the IUD may be out of place, call your health care provider right away.

If the IUD is out of place:

Be aware that if the IUD is out of place, **you could get pregnant.**

- ▶ It is best not to have sex until a health care provider checks the IUD.
- ▶ If you do have sex, use a back-up method, like condoms or spermicides or abstain from vaginal sex, to keep from getting pregnant.

4. **A health care provider must take the IUD out when it is time.**

The following are reasons you may need to have the IUD removed:

- ▶ It stops working.
- ▶ With any of the IUDs you can ask to have a new one placed the same day the old one is removed if you still want to prevent pregnancy with an IUD.
- ▶ You want to get pregnant.
- ▶ You want to change your method.
- ▶ You think you might be pregnant.

The IUD and Weight Concerns

Q: Does the IUD cause weight gain?

A: No.

Q: If a patient is overweight, does the IUD still work?

A: Yes.

Q: Are there health risks for using the IUD if a patient is overweight?

A: No.

Research shows IUDs do not cause weight gain. Most people gain weight over time whether they use an IUD or not. This is especially true for teens and young adults who may still be growing.

Are there any side effects?

All IUD's can have these possible side effects:

▸ Cramping when the IUD is placed or removed.

▸ Spotting between periods, especially right after it is placed.

ParaGard may also have these side effects:

▸ Heavier or longer periods each month.

▸ More cramps with your period.

Mirena, **Liletta** and **Kyleena** may have these side effects:

▸ For first 3-6 months, irregular periods, frequent spotting or light bleeding.

▸ Headaches, dizziness, abdominal or pelvic pain, sore breasts, or acne. All symptoms usually get better after the first 3-6 months.

Skyla may have these side effects:

▸ Irregular bleeding or no periods.

▸ Lighter or heavier periods.

▸ These side effects usually get better after the first 3-6 months.

What about complications and warning signs?

Serious health problems from an IUD are rare, but some patients do get them. Here are some of the possible complications you should tell your patients about.

▸ **Infection or Pelvic Inflammatory Disease (PID)**

This is RARE and if it happens, it would be during the first few weeks after the IUD is placed. If you get symptoms of foul discharge, a fever, pelvic pain, abdominal pain, or pain with sex tell your provider right away.

▸ **A tear or hole in the uterus or cervix**

This is RARE but can happen when the IUD is placed into the uterus. In most cases, the uterus repairs itself with no long-term problems and the IUD placement can be tried again.

▸ **The IUD comes out**

This is RARE but if the IUD comes out part way or all the way, you could get pregnant.

▸ **Pregnancy**

Rarely, patients using the IUD get pregnant. Even more rarely, a patient could have a pregnancy in the tubes instead of in the uterus (an **ectopic pregnancy**). If you get pregnant, the IUD must be taken out as soon as possible. If it stays in, it could cause an infection or a miscarriage. If you have symptoms of pregnancy either get a pregnancy test from a drug store or go to a health care setting for a pregnancy test.

Are there any precautions?

IUD Warning Signs

P = **P**eriod late (only w/ copper IUD), abnormal bleeding. These could mean pregnancy or infection.

A = **A**bdominal or pelvic pain, pain with intercourse. These could mean pregnancy or infection.

I = **I**nfection, abnormal discharge.

N = **N**ot feeling well, fever, chills. These could be signs of an infection.

S = **S**tring missing or changed. The IUD may be out of place.

**If you have any of these warning signs,
call a health care provider right away.**

A health care provider may advise you to choose a different method if any of the following is true:

▸ You have a current infection of the uterus and tubes (PID).

▸ You have vaginal bleeding for no known reason.

▸ You are pregnant.

▸ You have cancer of the cervix or uterus..

You will also be advised not to use hormonal IUDs if you have ever had breast cancer.

Breastfeeding

Those who breastfeed can use either type of IUD. They may be able to have the IUD placed right after childbirth.

A health care provider will talk with you about your health to make sure an IUD is a good choice for you.

What are the advantages and disadvantages of using IUDs?

There are many things patients like about using an IUD. And there are some things they don't like. Find out what your patient likes about using an IUD.

What some patients like about IUDs:

- ▸ It doesn't interrupt sex.
- ▸ It works very well to prevent pregnancy.
- ▸ It is easy to use.
- ▸ It lasts a long time.
- ▸ You may eventually have lighter periods or no periods at all with hormonal IUDs.

Hormonal IUDs may help prevent Pelvic Inflammatory Disease (PID).

- ➤ The progestin in hormonal IUDs makes the mucus of the cervix thick and sticky. This helps keep an STI from getting into the uterus and causing a PID.
- ➤ The hormone may also help protect against cancer of the lining of the uterus.

Find out what your patient might not like about using an IUD.

Ask your patients if they have any concerns about using an IUD. Then talk to them about their concerns. Help them think through how to solve any problems they might have while using an IUD. Try to get them to come up with their own solutions first. Read the chart that follows for some ideas on how to deal with possible concerns.

Keep in mind that the IUD isn't the best method for everyone. It is up to the patient and their health care provider to decide.

IUDs: Some Problems and Ways to Solve Them

Problem	Ways to Solve the Problem
I don't want to get an exam. And I'm worried about having the IUD put in.	We will explain just how it is done and what you can expect. It doesn't take very long at all. You can take some pain medication ahead of time to help with any cramping you may have. We are glad to talk about any worries and questions you may have.
I don't like having something stay inside my body that I can't take out myself.	Some people do have that concern. This is a method that a health care provider will have to place and remove. **Talk with the patient about their concerns. If they don't think they can get used to the idea, they might want to choose another method.**
I don't like having to put my fingers inside my vagina to check the strings.	Checking the strings can be helpful, but you don't have to do it every month for the IUD to work well. It feels odd to some when they first start checking the strings. But after they have done it for a few months, many get used to it. **Talk to your patient about their concerns. And ask if they think they can get used to it. If they say "no," they might want to choose a different method.**
I have to remember to make an appointment to have it taken out when it is time.	Your medical records will always be on file here. If you forget how long the IUD has been in, you can ask your health care provider or call the health care site any time.
I could get side effects.	With hormonal IUDs, most side effects go away after the first few months. But you will continue to have light or no bleeding. With ParaGard, the heavier menstrual bleeding and cramping, may go away or get much better after 3-6 months. It also could go on as long as you have it. You can ask your medical provider about using a medication to help. **Ask the patient what they think they could do to deal with the cramps and heavier bleeding.**

IUDs: Some Problems and Ways to Solve Them

Problem	Ways to Solve the Problem
I could get a serious complication.	**These are very rare**. But you need to remember to watch for the warning signs. If you have any warning signs, come to the health care site right away.
What if I have sex and then find out the IUD was out of place?	Call the health care site for advice. You may still prevent pregnancy after sex by taking emergency contraceptiive pills.
The IUD does not protect me from STIs.	Use condoms every time you have sex to help protect against these infections.

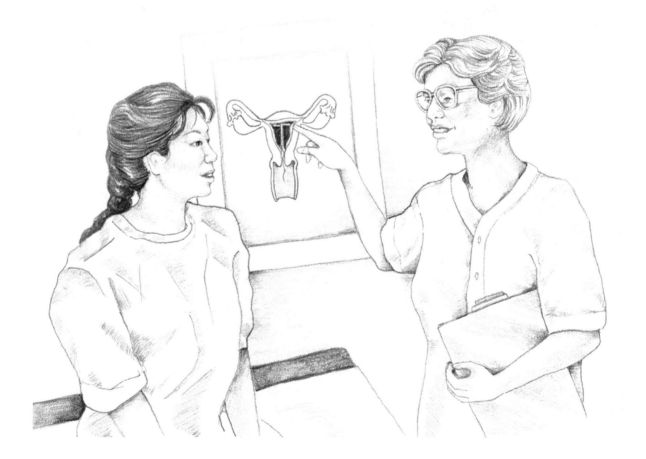

What if you want to stop using this method?

If you want to stop using this method, a health care provider must take the IUD out. Do not take it out yourself. This could harm you.

Once the IUD is taken out, you could become pregnant right away. Use another birth control method if you don't want to be pregnant.

There are no health problems to watch for when you stop this method.

Make sure your patient understands.

Before your patients leave, make sure they understand how to use the IUD successfully. Here are some things you can ask to make sure they understand.

- ▸ Tell me what you know about the IUD.
- ▸ How does the IUD work?
- ▸ When will you check your strings?
- ▸ How will you protect yourself from STIs?
- ▸ When do you have to get the IUD taken out?
- ▸ How will you remember to have it removed?
- ▸ What might be the most difficult problem for you when using the IUD?
- ▸ How would you get around that problem?
- ▸ What warning signs will you watch for while using the IUD?

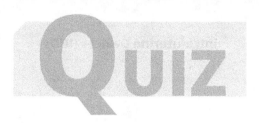

INTRA-UTERINE DEVICES (IUDS)

Directions: Read each of the following statements.
Is it true or false? Circle the best answer.

1. A health care provider places the IUD into the fallopian tubes.　　True　　False

2. Paragard has copper wrapped around it; Mirena, Skyla, Liletta and Kyleena release a hormone.　　True　　False

3. All IUDs change the environment in the uterus.　　True　　False

4. Those using the IUD need to check the strings every day.　　True　　False

5. A patient should never take out the IUD themselves.　　True　　False

Directions: Each of the following statements is true for either ParaGard or hormonal IUDs.

- **If it is true for Hormonal IUDs, circle "Hormonal"**
- **If it is true for ParaGard, circle "ParaGard."**

6. The hormone in this IUD makes the cervical mucus thick and sticky.　　Hormonal　　ParaGard

7. This IUD will work for up to 12 years.　　Hormonal　　ParaGard

8. This IUD may cause heavier or longer periods.　　Hormonal　　ParaGard

9. Those using this IUD may have very light or no periods.　　Hormonal　　ParaGard

Check your answers on the next page.

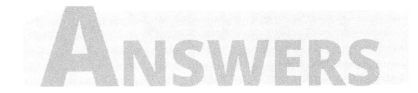

INTRA-UTERINE
DEVICES (IUDS)

Check your answers.

1. **False**   The health care provider places the IUD into the uterus.

2. **True**   ParaGard does have copper. And hormonal IUDs release a hormone.

3. **True**   All IUDs change the environment in the uterus and make sperm unable to move.

4. **False**   Those using the IUD do not need to check the strings every day. A provider may recommend that a patient check their strings about once a month. If they are having a monthly period, then the time after the period is over is a good time to check the strings. They should also check the strings any time they have abnormal cramping or bleeding.

5. **True**   An IUD must be removed by a health care provider, NOT by the patient.

6. **Hormonal**   The progestin in hormonal IUDs makes the cervical mucus thick and sticky. Paragard does not have hormones and does not change the cervical mucus.

7. **ParaGard**   ParaGard works for up to 12 years.

8. **ParaGard**   ParaGard may cause heavier or longer periods.

9. **Hormonal**   Patients using a hormonal IUD may have very light or no periods after the first 3 – 6 months.

Sterilization Methods

Sterilization is a surgery or other procedure done on those who decide not to have any children or any more children in the future. It works by keeping the sperm away from the egg.

Sterilization is considered a permanent method of family planning. This means that once a person is sterilized, they cannot change their mind and have children later on.

- Sterilization for a body that ovulates is called *tubal sterilization.*
- Sterilization for a body that produces sperm is called a *vasectomy.*

Patients must make their own decisions about being sterilized. Before making an appointment, they should talk with a trained counselor. The counselor asks questions to help them decide whether they truly want this permanent method of birth control. The counselor also explains the procedures and follow-up.

As a health worker, you can present permanent contraception as an option to your patients. You can also answer basic questions about it. The information in this section will help you do that.

Then, if your patient is seriously thinking about sterilization, refer them to a trained sterilization counselor.

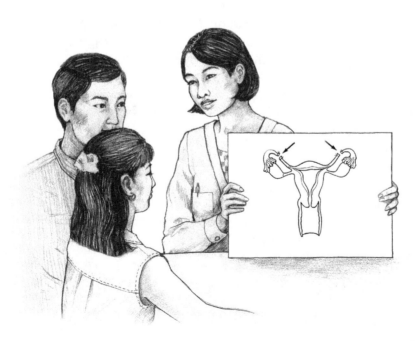

Topics in this section

▸ Tubal Sterilization

▸ Vasectomy

Objectives

After reading this section you will be able to:

▸ Explain how permanent contraceptive methods work to prevent pregnancy.

▸ Discuss the advantages and disadvantages of sterilization.

▸ Tell how well sterilization works to prevent pregnancy.

Precaution

Tell your patient:

"If you are not sure about whether or not you want children in the future, sterilization is not the method for you."

Sterilization Counselor Training

Sterilization is a permanent method. This method is not like other methods. Choosing this method means carefully thinking through difficult questions. These include:

- "What if one of my children dies? What if all of my children die? How will I feel if I am not able to have more children?"

- "What if, for any reason, I'm not with the same partner in the future? What if my current partner dies? How will I feel if I want to have a child with a new partner?"

A sterilization counselor must be specially trained to help patients think through these issues and to make sure they have been given all the information they need to make an informed decision.

Without special training, you should not try to counsel patients on sterilization. If you would like to do sterilization counseling, you can talk to your supervisor about getting the training you will need.

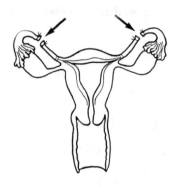

Tubal Sterilization

What is it?

Tubal sterilization is a permanent method of birth control. Patients can choose tubal sterilization if they know they don't want to have children in the future.

Tubal sterilization works very well to prevent pregnancy. But it does not help protect against HIV and other STIs. Use a condom every time you have sex to help protect against these infections.

How does it work?

Educator Tip

You can tell your patients the basics about sterilization. But patients who are thinking about sterilization need special counseling. If you have not been specially trained to give this counseling, refer the patient to someone who has.

With tubal sterilization, the tubes that carry the eggs (the **fallopian tubes**) are permanently blocked or removed. Afterwards, the patient still releases an egg each menstrual cycle as always. They will also still have a period. But because the tubes are blocked or gone, sperm cannot reach an egg. And that means they cannot get pregnant.

Tubal sterilization is usually done with surgery. Another name for this is **tubal ligation**. The tubes can be cut and the ends tied off or burned to close them. Or a surgical clip can be placed on each tube to close them.

No matter how it is done, tubal sterilization keeps sperm from getting to eggs. And it is permanent. The tubes cannot be reopened without an expensive and difficult surgery that most often doesn't work.

How well does Tubal Sterilization work?

When you talk to your patients about tubal sterilization, discuss how well it works (how effective it is).

Tubal sterilization is 99.5% effective.

That means that if 100 patients are sterilized, only 1 (and probably none) of them may get pregnant in a year.

How do you get it done?

Explain these steps to your patients so they will know what to expect.

You will first need to get special counseling from a trained sterilization counselor.

If you then decide you want to use sterilization as a birth control method, you will most likely need a physical exam. At that time, if everything is okay, you can schedule an appointment. You will be told what to expect, how to prepare for the procedure, and what to do afterwards.

A patient can get a tubal sterilization done in a hospital or outpatient health care setting. It does not take long to do it and most of the time the patient can go home that same day. They are usually put to sleep with general anesthesia. For a few days afterwards, the patient needs to rest.

Be sure to remind patients that they can change their minds about getting this permanent method of birth control even at the last minute.

Talk to your patients about Emergency Contraception.

Emergency Contraception (EC), in the form of EC pills or an IUD, can prevent pregnancy *after* sex. Patients can use EC up to 5 days after unprotected sex. Read more about it in the section on EC.

Tubal Sterilization and Weight Concerns

Q: Does tubal sterilization cause weight gain?

A: No.

Q: If a patient is overweight, does tubal sterilization still work?

A: Yes.

Q: Are there health risks having a tubal sterilization if a patient is overweight?

A: Many surgical procedures have higher risks for patients who are very overweight. Tubal ligation may not be the best choice for them.

Research shows tubal sterilization does not cause weight gain. Most people gain weight over time whether they have had a tubal sterilization or not.

What about complications and precautions?

Rare complications after tubal ligation include wound infection, possible prolonged pelvic or abdominal pain or ectopic pregnancy.

What are the advantages and disadvantages of Tubal Sterilization?

What some patients like about having tubal sterilization:

- No other method of birth control is ever needed.
- It is safe. It does not take long to heal.
- It does not interrupt sex.

What some patients don't like:

- Once it is done, it cannot not usually be undone. If you change your mind later on, the tubes can often not be repaired, even with costly surgery. And most insurance does not cover the cost.
- There may be a small chance of infection.
- You may need to rest for a few days afterwards.
- There may be some pain or discomfort for a little while.
- It doesn't protect against HIV and other STIs.

If your patient is interested in permanent contraception, refer them to a trained sterilization counselor.

Vasectomy

What is it?

Vasectomy is a surgery patients can choose to have if they know they don't want to have children in the future. It is safe and simple. This is a permanent method of birth control.

A vasectomy works very well to prevent pregnancy. But it does not help protect against HIV and other STIs. Use a condom every time you have sex to help protect against these infections.

How does it work?

The tubes inside the scrotum that carry sperm (the **vas deferens**) are blocked. This keeps sperm out of the fluid the penis ejaculates. The look of the semen and the quantity stay the same even if there is no sperm in it. Since there is no sperm in the semen, they cannot cause a pregnancy.

To do a vasectomy, the health care provider makes a small cut in the scrotum to get to the sperm-carrying tubes. The tubes can then be cut or blocked with a clip. If the tubes are cut, the ends of the cut tubes are sealed either by being tied off or burned.

After a vasectomy, there are still sperm in the semen for a while. It can take about 20 ejaculations or 3 months to get rid of all the sperm. To be sure there are no sperm left, the patient should have their semen checked by a health care provider. Until they are told there are no more sperm, they need to use another method of birth control, like condoms, to prevent pregnancy.

This surgery does not change the patient's sexual feelings or their ability to have sex.

Educator Tip

You can tell your patients the basics about sterilization. But patients who are thinking about sterilization need special counseling. If you have not been specially trained to give this counseling, refer the patient to someone who has.

How well does a Vasectomy work?

When you talk to your patients about vasectomy, be sure to tell them how well it works (how effective it is).

Vasectomy is about 99.85% effective.

This means that if 100 patients have vasectomies, 1 or none of them, may cause a pregnancy in a year, especially if they follow the health care provider's directions.

Note: After a vasectomy, patients should use condoms or some other birth control method for the first 3 months. They should get a check-up to be sure that the surgery worked before they have sex without another method.

How do you get it done?

Explain these steps to your patients so they will know a little about what to expect.

Before you can get a vasectomy, you will need to get special counseling from a trained sterilization counselor.

If you then decide you want one, you will most likely need a physical exam. At that time, if everything is okay, you can schedule an appointment. You will be told what to expect, how to prepare for surgery, and what to do afterwards.

Remember

Be sure to remind patients they can change their mind about vasectomy even at the last minute.

A patient can get a vasectomy done at an outpatient health care site. It takes less than 30 minutes to do and they can usually go home in an hour or two afterwards. They stay awake for the procedure and the area is made numb. For a few days afterwards, they need to take it easy and do no heavy lifting. Most of the time, the patient is able to go back to their normal activities after a few days.

What are the advantages and disadvantages of a Vasectomy?

What some patients like about vasectomies:

- ▸ No other method of birth control is ever needed.

- ▸ It does not change your feelings, your sex drive, or your ability to have sex.

- ▸ It does not interrupt sex.

- ▸ It's done in a local clinic (no general anesthesia needed) and you go home the same day.

- ▸ The procedure is safe. It does not take long to heal. It is safer, easier, faster and cheaper than tubal ligation.

What some patients don't like:

- ▸ Once it is done, you usually cannot change your mind and have it undone.

- ▸ There can be some soreness, swelling, and bruising of the scrotum for a little while after the surgery.

- ▸ It doesn't protect against HIV and other STIs.

Before referring patients to a trained sterilization counselor, you can ask them if they have any concerns about using sterilization. The chart that follows can help you talk to them about some of their concerns. If they are interested in using this method, you can refer them to the trained sterilization counselor to get more information.

Vasectomy and Weight Concerns

Q: Does vasectomy cause weight gain?

A: No.

Q: If a patient is overweight, does vasectomy still work?

A: Yes.

Q: Are there health risks having a vasectomy if the patient is overweight?

A: No.

Research shows that vasectomy does not cause weight gain. Most people gain weight over time whether they have had a vasectomy or not.

Sterilization: Some Problems and Ways to Solve Them

Problem	Ways to Solve the Problem
What if I change my mind and want to have children later on?	If you are not *sure* about wanting any children in the future, *sterilization is not the method for you.* Sterilization is a permanent method. A trained sterilization counselor will help guide you through this important decision.
If I did change my mind, couldn't I get it reversed?	In some cases, people can get their sterilization reversed. But it is hard to do, can be costly, and most often doesn't work. Before you get a sterilization done, you must think of it as a permanent method. Your sterilization counselor can give you more information about this.
I'm worried about having the sterilization done. Is it safe?	Both vasectomy and tubal sterilization are safe. The counselor will be glad to talk about any worries and questions you may have.
I may have a hard time remembering when to come back to make sure the sterilization worked.	Your medical records will be on file. It is important to follow your health care provider's instructions carefully. Call the health care site anytime, if you wonder: ■ When you can start having sex without worrying about pregnancy. ■ When you should could come for a follow-up visit.
I could get side effects.	Most side effects are minor. Your sterilization counselor will tell you just what you should do.
I could get a serious complication.	These are very rare. Your sterilization counselor will tell you the warning signs to watch for. If you have any warning signs, come to the health care site right away.
What if I have sex before my health care provider tells me it is safe?	Call the provider for advice. You can still prevent pregnancy after sex. Find out about EC.
Sterilization does not protect me from STIs.	Use a condom every time you have sex to help protect against these infections.

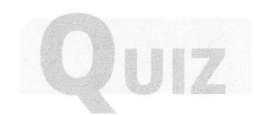

STERILIZATION METHODS

Directions: Circle the best answer.

1. Which of the following is true about sterilization?

    a. It is permanent birth control.

    b. People should only think about having sterilization if they are sure they do not want any more children in the future.

    c. It is easy to reverse.

    d. Both A and B

2. Patients who are thinking about sterilization should:

    a. First get sterilization counseling from a trained sterilization counselor.

    b. Get it done quickly before they change their minds.

    c. Not worry about getting counseling. They are grown adults who don't need any help.

    d. All of the above

3. Tubal ligation works by:

    a. Keeping the eggs from leaving the ovaries

    b. Blocking the fallopian tubes so that an egg and a sperm cannot meet

    c. Thinning the lining of the uterus

    d. All of the above

4. Which of the following sterilization choices does a patient who ovulates have?:

    a. A health care provider cuts or blocks the tubes by surgery.

    b. A health care provider removes both fallopian tubes.

    c. The patient takes a pill.

    d. Both A and B

Go on to the next page.

Directions: Read each of the following and write your best answer in the spaces below.

5. List two things that some people like about sterilization.

- _____

_____

- _____

_____

Directions: Read each of the following statements. Is it true or false? Circle the best answer.

6. Sterilization is a permanent form of birth control.   True   False

7. During a vasectomy, the vas deferens are cut or blocked to keep sperm from being released during ejaculation.   True   False

8. A patient can still cause a pregnancy up to 3 months after having a vasectomy.   True   False

9. The scrotum may be swollen, sore, and bruised for a little while after the vasectomy.   True   False

10. Vasectomy is easier, safer and cheaper than tubal ligation surgery.   True   False

Directions: Read the following and write your best answer in the space below.

11. List one concern that a patient may have about sterilization and what you might say to help deal with that concern.

- **Patient's concern:**
_____

_____

- **What you could say:**
_____

_____

Check your answers on the next page.

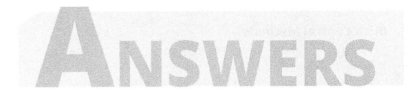

STERILIZATION METHODS

Check your answers.

1. **D**   Both A and B. Sterilization is permanent birth control. And people should only think about having a sterilization if they are sure they do not want any more children in the future. Trying to reverse a sterilization procedure is hard to do, can be costly, and most often doesn't work.

2. **A**   People who are thinking about sterilization should first get sterilization counseling from a trained sterilization counselor.

3. **B**   Tubal sterilization works by blocking the fallopian tubes so that an egg and sperm cannot meet.

4. **D**   Both A and B. Patients who ovulate have these sterilization choices:
   - A health care provider cuts or blocks block the tubes by surgery.
   - A health care provider removes both fallopian tubes.

5. Here are things that some people like about sterilization:
   - No other method of birth control is ever needed once your provider has made sure it really worked.
   - It is safe. It does not take long to heal.
   - It has no long-term side effects.
   - It does not change your feelings, your sex drive, or your ability to have sex.
   - It does not interrupt sex.

6. **True**   Sterilization is a permanent form of birth control.

7. **True**   During a vasectomy, the vas deferens are cut or blocked to keep sperm from being released during ejaculation.

8. **True**   A patient can still cause a pregnancy up to 3 months after having a vasectomy. After a vasectomy, sperm are still in the tubes for a while. It can take about 20 ejaculations or 3 months to get rid of all the sperm in the tubes.

9. **True**   The scrotum can be swollen, sore, and bruised for a little while after the vasectomy.

10. **True**   Vasectomy is easier, safer and cheaper than tubal ligation surgery.

11. Here are two concerns a patient might have about sterilization and what you might say to help. For other possible concerns and responses, please see the chart "Sterilization: Some Problems and Ways to Solve Them" near the end of the Sterilization section.

   - *Patient's concern:* "What if I change my mind and want to have children later on?"

     What you could say: "Sterilization is a permanent method. A trained counselor will help guide you through this important decision. If you're not sure, there are other methods you can use."

   - *Patient's concern:* "Is it safe?"

     What you could say: "Both vasectomy and tubal sterilization are safe. Talk to your counselor about any worries you may have."

Tier Two: Hormonal Methods

Hormones are chemicals made naturally by the body. They act as signals. The ovaries make two hormones: progesterone and estrogen. These hormones tell the body what to do during the monthly menstrual cycle.

Hormonal methods of birth control use hormones like the ones made by the ovaries. But the hormones in hormonal methods are made in a lab. When the methods are used correctly, they keep the hormones in a body that ovulates at a level that prevents pregnancy.

Some hormonal methods use only one hormone, called progestin. This hormone works like the progesterone made by the ovaries. Other hormonal methods use two hormones: progestin and estrogen.

All hormonal methods do one or more of the following things to keep someone from getting pregnant:

- They help keep the egg from leaving an ovary each month. If there is no egg, the sperm can't meet with it. That means there can be no pregnancy.

- They keep the mucus made by the cervix thick. This mucus is called **cervical mucus.** When it is thick, the sperm can't swim through the cervix to reach the egg. If sperm can't reach the egg, there can be no pregnancy.

- They keep the lining of the uterus thin (this happens more with methods that contain estrogen). When the lining is thin, a fertilized egg will not attach to the uterus. That means there can be no pregnancy.

Hormonal methods do **not** help protect against HIV or other STIs. To help prevent these STIs, people should use condoms every time they have sex.

Topics in this section

▸ Birth Control Pill (the combined pill)

▸ Birth Control Patch (the Patch)

▸ Birth Control Ring (the Ring)

▸ Progestin-Only Pills (POPs)

▸ Birth Control Shot (the Shot, Depo-Provera)

Objectives

After reading this section, you will be able to:

▸ Explain how hormonal methods work.

▸ Tell how well each method works to prevent pregnancy.

▸ Describe how to use each method correctly.

You will also be able to:

▸ List a side effect of each method.

▸ List a complication and warning sign for each method.

▸ Discuss the advantages of each method.

▸ Describe problems some people may have with each method and how they can deal with these problems.

Words you may need to know

Here are some words you may need to know when you talk with your patients about hormonal methods.

Words	Description
Hormones	Chemicals made naturally by the body. They can also be made in a lab.
Estrogen (ES-stro-juhn)	A hormone made by the ovaries. Estrogen can also be made in a lab. It is put in some hormonal methods of birth control to help prevent pregnancy.
Progesterone (pro-JES-tur-own)	A hormone made by the ovaries.
Progestin (pro-JES-tin)	A hormone made in a lab that works like progesterone. It is used in hormonal birth control methods to help prevent pregnancy.
Cervical mucus (SUR-vuh-kuhl MYU-kuhs)	The mucus made by the cervix (the opening to the uterus). When it is thin and stretchy, it helps sperm live and reach an egg. When it is thick and sticky, it helps keep sperm and germs out of the uterus.
Back-up methods	These are other methods of birth control (including abstaining from vaginal sex) you can use at the same time as or instead of your main method. They can help make sure you don't get pregnant.

Choosing a hormonal method

Patients who would like to use a hormonal method have many to choose from. These facts might help them narrow down the choices to methods that might work best for them.

Methods you need to take every day:

▸ Combined Pill
▸ Progestin-Only Pills (POPs)

Methods that usually give you a regular "period" or scheduled bleeding:

▸ Combined Pill
▸ Birth Control Patch
▸ Birth Control Ring

Methods that you have to do something with only once a month or less:

▸ Birth Control Ring
▸ Birth Control Shot
▸ Hormonal IUDs

Methods that often cause irregular periods or spotting - especially the first few months:

▸ Progestin-Only Pills (POPs)
▸ Birth Control Shot
▸ Birth Control Implant
▸ Hormonal IUDs

These methods have no estrogen in them — only progestin.

Scheduled Bleeding

When we talk about having a "regular period" with some of these hormonal methods, we can also call this scheduled bleeding. The pill, the patch, and the ring all regulate periods so that bleeding only happens on certain days. This scheduled bleeding is like a "regular period" but because of the hormones they are getting through these birth control methods, they are not having a real period. Users can control how often they have their period by working with their provider to use these methods for a long period of time without a break. This is also know as "continuous use". They use the method without a break to control how often they have a scheduled bleed.

Birth Control Pill

What is it?

The birth control pill is what most people think of as "the pill." It is a pill made with both estrogen and progestin. That is why it is sometimes called "the combined pill." You will take one pill at the same time each day.

There are many types and brands of birth control pills. They come in different colors and in different kinds of packs. Packs often come with enough pills for 21 or 28 days but some packs come with many more pills. The amount of hormones in the pills depends on the type and brand of pill. A health care provider decides which type and brand is best for you.

The pill works well to prevent pregnancy. But it does not help protect you against HIV and other STIs. Use condoms every time you have sex to help protect against these infections.

How does it work?

The pill works mostly by keeping the egg from leaving the ovaries. If there is no egg to meet with sperm, you can't get pregnant. The pill also:

- Keeps the mucus from the cervix thick. This helps keep sperm from getting into the uterus and meeting with an egg.
- Keeps the lining of the uterus thin so that the egg cannot attach to the uterus.

How well does the Pill work?

With perfect use, the pill is 99.7% effective.

This means that if 100 patients use the pill exactly the right way, only 1 (and probably none) of them may get pregnant in a year.

With typical use, the pill is 93% effective.

For those who don't always take their pill exactly the right way, 7 out of 100 may get pregnant in a year.

Talk to your patients about Emergency Contraception.

Emergency Contraception (EC), in the form of EC pills or an IUD, can prevent pregnancy after sex. Patients can use EC up to 5 days after unprotected sex. Read more about it in the section on EC.

How do you use the Pill?

Teach your patients these steps so they can use the pill the right way. Your health care site's advice may differ from the advice given here. Be sure to give your patients the advice used at your health site.

1. **Talk to a health care provider about whether the pill is right for you.**

   The health care provider will ask you some questions. Talk to the health care provider about:

   ▶ Any health problems you may have

   ▶ Any medicine you may be taking

   ▶ Any questions you may have

Your health care provider will help you decide if the pill is right for you. Always be sure to take your own pills. Don't borrow from others. And don't give someone else your pills. All birth control pills are not the same.

Be sure to explain to your patient:
▶ How and where they will pick up the pills
▶ How much they can expect to pay (if anything)

2. **Choose another birth control method to use as a back-up method along with the pill when you first start using it.**

   When you start taking the pill, it is a good idea to use a second method of birth control for a while. Your provider can tell you how long you should use this back-up method. You can choose the condom, the diaphragm, the cap, the sponge, spermicides, withdrawal or abstaining from reproductive sex.

   Tip: Keep this second method around in case you need it later.

3. **Talk to your health care provider about how to start taking the pill.**

There are a few different ways to start the first pack of pills. Each way has something good about it. Your health care site may use one way for all of your patients. Or the health care provider may decide which way will work best for each patient. Here are three ways for starting the pill. Talk to your patient only about the way or ways you do it at your health site.

Taking the Pill

Be sure your patient knows that:

- They must *swallow* the pill.

- They must take one pill *every* day, even if not having sex on that day.

▸ **You can start on the first day of your period.** The pill starts working right away to prevent pregnancy.

▸ **You can start on the first Sunday after your period starts.** For the first week or two you will also need to use a second method to keep from getting pregnant. When you start on a Sunday, your periods will always come during the week and not on weekends.

▸ **If you know you are not pregnant, you can start the day of your appointment.** You will also need to use a second method or abstain from vaginal sex for the first week.

Tip: It is a good idea to use a second method when you first start using the pill. It is not always easy to remember to take your pill each day at the same time. It takes practice.

4. **Take 1 pill each day at about the same time until the pack is finished.**

▸ **With a 28-day pack,** finish the whole pack. Start a new pack the next day. Don't skip any days between packs. Always start with the first pill in a new pack.

▸ **With a 21-day pack,** finish the pack and stop taking pills for 7 days. On the eighth day, start a new pack.

▸ **With a 24-day pack,** finish the whole pack and stop taking the pills for 4 days. On the fifth day, start a new pack.

A regular package of the birth control pill has 21 or 24 pills with hormones and 7 or 4 pills with no hormones. You have your scheduled bleeding during the 7 or 4 days of taking pills without hormones.

The *extended regimen* pill packs are different. Each package contains 84 pills with hormones and 7 pills with no hormones. You will take one hormone pill a day for 84 days in a row. Then take 7 pills with no hormones and get your scheduled bleeding at that time. This means that when you use the extended regimen pill pack, you will have scheduled bleeding once every 3 months instead of once a month. This is safe and causes no health problems.

The pills in the extended regimen packs are the same as the pills in regular pill packs. The side effects, complications, and warning signs are the same for both packs of pills. The main difference is that you

Educator Tip

Ask your patients:

- What time are you going to take the pill each day?

- What will you do to help you remember?

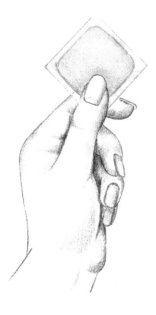

Birth Control Patch

This section is mostly written as though you were talking to your patients. It gives you an idea of how to explain the birth control patch in a way your patients can understand. This section also has notes written directly to you, the health worker. Those "health worker notes" look like this one.

What is it?

The birth control patch is a small patch you wear on your skin to keep you from getting pregnant. It sticks to the skin like a bandage. The patch has the same two hormones in it as the birth control pill: estrogen and progestin. The hormones go slowly into your body through the skin.

Each patch works for only 1 week. You wear 1 new patch each week for 3 weeks. During the fourth week, you wear no patch at all. This is when you will get your scheduled bleed.

The patch works well to prevent pregnancy. But it does not help protect you against HIV and other STIs. Use a condom every time you have sex to protect yourself from these infections.

How does it work?

The patch works mostly by keeping the egg from leaving the ovaries. If there is no egg to meet with sperm, you can't get pregnant. The patch also:

▸ Keeps the mucus from the cervix thick. This helps keep sperm from getting into the uterus and meeting with an egg.

▸ Keeps the lining of the uterus thin so that an egg cannot attach to the uterus.

How well does the Patch work?

When you talk to your patients, you will need to explain how well the patch works (how effective it is). Be sure to explain the difference between "perfect use" and "typical use." You can read more about this in the "Stage 3" section of Chapter 2.

With perfect use, the patch is 99.7% effective.

This means that if 100 patients use the patch exactly the right way, only 1 (and probably none) of them may get pregnant in a year.

With typical use, the patch is 93% effective.

For those who don't always use their patch exactly the right way, 7 out of 100 may get pregnant in a year.

How do you use the Patch?

Teach your patients these steps so they can use the patch the right way. Your health care site's advice may differ from the advice given here. Be sure to give your patients the advice used at your health care site.

Talk to your patients about Emergency Contraception.

Emergency Contraception (EC), in the form of EC pills or an IUD, can prevent pregnancy after sex. Patients can use EC up to 5 days after unprotected sex. Read more about it in the section on EC.

How do you get the patch?

First, you need to see a health care provider. The provider will ask you some questions. Talk to them about:

▸ Any health problems you may have

▸ Any medicine you may be taking

▸ Any questions you may have

Your provider will help you decide if the patch is right for you.

Learn how your health care site provides patches for patients. Be sure to explain to your patient:
- How and where they will pick up the patches
- How much they can expect to pay

How do you put the patch on?

When you explain this to your patient, remember to show them how to take the patch out of its packet and put it on their skin.

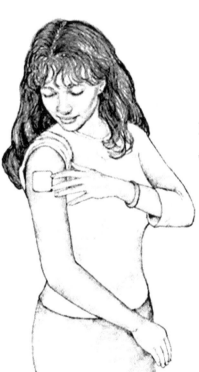

You can wear the patch on your:
- Upper arm
- Lower abdomen (stomach)
- Hip or buttock
- Upper torso (excluding breasts)

Never wear it on your breast or on the inside of your upper arm.

To put the patch on:

1. Wash and dry your hands and skin where you will put the patch.
2. The patch is covered with a plastic liner. Take the patch, with its liner, out of its foil package.
3. Peel off half of the patch's clear liner.
4. Press the sticky part of the patch onto your skin.
5. Peel off the rest of the liner.
6. Press the rest of the patch onto your skin. Be sure to press the edges of the patch down.
7. Press the palm of your hand over the patch for 10 seconds.

Tip: Try not to touch the sticky part of the patch with your fingers. That is where the hormones are.

When do you put the patch on?

There are different ways to start using the patch. Each way has something good about it. Your health care setting may use one way for all your patients. Or the health care provider may decide which way will work best for each patient. Here are two ways to start the patch. Talk to your patients only about the way or ways you do it at your health care setting.

Start using the patch on the day your health care provider suggests. There are two common ways to start.

▸ **You can start on the first day of your period.** The patch will start working right away to protect you from pregnancy.

▸ **You can start on the first Sunday after your period begins.** (If your period starts on Sunday, start the patch that day.) If Sunday is *not* the first day of your period, you will *not* be protected from pregnancy that first week. Use another birth control method (back-up method) along with the patch for 1 week.

Remember to:

▸ Put a new patch on once a week for 3 weeks in a row. Wear no patch at all during the fourth week.

▸ Change the patch on the same day each week. For example, if you start wearing the patch on a Sunday, always change it on Sunday.

Week 1:

▸ Put a new patch on clean, dry skin.

Weeks 2 and 3:

▸ Take off the used patch. Fold it in half, sticky side together, and throw it away.

▸ Put on the new patch. **Don't wear the patch in the exact same place 2 weeks in a row.**

Week 4:

▸ Take off the used patch. Fold it in half, sticky sides together, and throw it away.

▸ Go 7 days without wearing a patch. You are still protected from pregnancy for those 7 days. This is when you will get your period.

After 7 days without wearing a patch, start again with Week 1.

▸ Never go more than these 7 days without a patch. If you do, you could get pregnant.

▸ Put the new patch on — even if your period isn't over.

will bleed only 4 scheduled times a year when you use the extended regimen packs. Many pill users have spotting or unscheduled bleeding between their scheduled bleeding. This will most likely occur less after the first year.

If you don't have a scheduled bleed during your 7 days of non-hormone pills, you may be pregnant. Talk to your provider.

Be sure to start your new pack on the right day. If you are late starting your next pack, you could get pregnant.

Tip: You will always start your next pack of pills on the same day of the week that you started your first pack.

From one health worker to another

Q. My patient keeps forgetting to take the pill. They have a baby who is awake all hours of the day and night. Their life has no routine.

A. A patient of mine came up with a great idea. They set an alarm on their phone for 4 P.M. When it goes off, they take their pill.

Things to remember when you use the pill

▶ Take your pill every day at about the same time. It may help to think of something you do at the same time every day. For example, you could take it when you brush your teeth, when you eat a meal, or when you go to bed. You choose the time that is best for you.

▶ If you see a doctor for any reason, tell the doctor you are taking birth control pills. Doctors need to know if you are on the pill before they give you any medicine.

▶ If you are late taking your pills, follow the health care site's advice.

▶ Use a second method of birth control, like condoms, spermicides, withdrawal, along with the pill if you:

  ▪ Missed taking any pills.

  ▪ Had severe vomiting or diarrhea.

  ▪ Are taking medicines that keep the pill from working as well.

  Use the second method for as long as the provider advises. Also, ask about Emergency Contraception (EC).

What will your periods be like when you are on the pill?

Most patients are curious about what their periods will be like when they are on the pill. Here is what you could say: "Since your natural cycle stops when you are on the pill, you won't get a real "period." You can explain that the bleeding they will have when on the pill will be "scheduled bleeding" that is created by the use of the hormones. Below are some other things that you could say.

▶ **You may have light bleeding or just spotting during your scheduled bleeding or "periods".**

This is normal when you are on the pill. Your periods may be lighter and shorter than the ones you have when you are not on the pill. You may see no blood at all. Or you may see just a drop of blood. The color of the bleeding may change too. It may get darker, browner, and clumpy.

▶ **You may not bleed at all or you may bleed only once in a while.**

If you have taken all of your pills on time and don't bleed at the scheduled time, you are probably not pregnant. Start your next pack of pills as usual. If you don't bleed at the scheduled time again the next month, you should do a pregnancy test or, see your provider.

If you have missed a pill that month and don't bleed during the time that you are scheduled to bleed, you could be pregnant. Get a pregnancy test or contact your provider.

▶ **Keep track of your bleeding pattern.**

Once you have been on the pill for 2 or 3 months, your scheduled bleeding should become more regular. If you don't have your scheduled bleeding when you expect it, or if you have bleeding when you don't expect it, talk to your health care provider. A different type of pill might make your bleeding more regular. Some amount of unscheduled bleeding or spotting is not dangerous or bad for you. It does not mean you are more likely to get pregnant.

What if you forget to take your pills?

Teach your patients these steps so they will know what to do if they forget to take one or more pills. Your health care site's advice may differ from the advice given here. Be sure to give your patients the advice used at your health care site.

If you forget to take 1 pill at your usual time, follow these steps:

▶ Take your missed pill as soon as you remember.

▶ Take your next pill at your usual time. Do this even if it means taking 2 pills in 1 day.

If you miss taking 2 or more pills in a row, follow these steps:

▶ Take the last pill you missed as soon as you remember. Do not take any pills you missed earlier.

▶ Call your provider for advice. You may need Emergency Contraception.

▶ Use a back-up method, like condoms, spermicides, withdrawal, or abstaining from reproductive sex along with the pill for as long as your provider advises.

Educator Tip

- Be sure to tell your patients what to do if they forget to take any pills.

- Give them easy-to-read written materials about this to take home.

- Ask your patients which method they would use for a back-up if they needed one.

Important

If you miss any pills and have had sex within the past week:

- ▶ Call the provider right away to ask about Emergency Contraception (EC).

- ▶ It is especially important to ask about EC pills if you missed 2 or more of your birth control pills in a row.

- ▶ Follow the advice you are given about getting back on schedule with your birth control pills.

Get a pregnancy test if you don't get your period this month.

Calls about missed pills

At some point, a patient may call you for advice when they miss one or more pills. The advice you need to give them will depend on the following:

- ▶ The type of pill they are taking

- ▶ How many pills they have missed

- ▶ Where they are in their cycle when they missed the pills

- ▶ Whether they had sex near the time they missed the pills

Follow your health care site's guidelines for advising these patients.

Note: Remember that not all the pills in the pack have hormones in them. Some pill packs are set up with "placebo pills" which are sometimes called "sugar pills." If your patient forgets to take these "sugar pills," they will not have a greater chance of pregnancy.

Are there any side effects?

Some patients have one or more side effects with the pill. Most side effects go away after the first two or three months. Your patients can talk to a health care provider if the side effects last longer than that or really bother them. A different brand of pill may make some side effects go away. Here are some side effects to tell your patients about.

▸ **Changes in bleeding**

You may not bleed when you are scheduled to or you may spot or bleed "off schedule."

▸ **Nausea and vomiting**

This may happen during the first few months that you use the pill. Or it may happen during the first few pills of each pack. Taking your pill at night or after a meal may help. If this side effect bothers you, you may want to try a different brand of pill.

▸ **Tender or full breasts**

Your breasts may get bigger and be tender.

▸ **Mood changes**

The hormones in the pill can affect your emotions. However, some find that their PMS symptoms are improved on the pill.

▸ **Skin changes**

Mask of pregnancy (chloasma): The pill can cause the "mask of pregnancy" in a few users. The skin on the nose and cheeks get darker. Getting a tan can make it show up more. The darker skin should lighten some after you stop taking the pill.

Acne (pimples): Most acne gets better when you are on the pill. But for a few, it may get worse. Changing to a different brand of pills may help.

▸ **Headaches**

Some users get mild headaches when they start taking the pill. This is normal and they should go away with over-the-counter medication.

The Pill and Weight Concerns

Q. Does the pill cause weight gain?

A. No.

Q. If a user is overweight, will the pill still work well?

A. Most of the time, yes.

Q. Are there medical problems if a user is overweight and using the pill?

A. There could be. All users should talk to their provider about the risk of blood clots, heart attack, or stroke while using the pill.

Research shows that the pill does not cause weight gain. Most people gain weight over time whether they take the pill or not, especially teens and young adults who are still growing.

What about complications and warning signs?

Serious health problems from the pill are rare, but some users may get them. Here are some of the possible problems:

▸ **High blood pressure**

High blood pressure usually has no symptoms. Your health care provider will probably want to check your blood pressure a few months after you start the pill to make sure your blood pressure hasn't gone up. If your blood pressure does go up, you may be told to stop taking the pill. Your blood pressure will usually go back down once you stop the pill.

▸ **Blood clots**

Those taking the pill may have a slightly higher chance of developing a clot in their leg or belly. If a blood clot forms, it can travel to the heart or brain to cause a heart attack or stroke. Even with this slightly higher chance of developing a clot, a pill user still has a very, very low chance of having a heart attack or stroke. Your provider will talk through other things about your health which may add to your risk like smoking or older age.

▸ **Liver or gall bladder problems**

Rarely, a user may have problems with their liver or gall bladder.

Pill Warning Signs: A C H E S

Serious health problems are very **rare** with the pill. But it is important to know the warning signs.

A = **Abdominal pain** that is **severe**. This can be a sign of a liver tumor, gall bladder disease, blood clot, or pregnancy in your tubes.

C = **Chest pain** that is **severe**, or shortness of breath. These could be signs of a heart attack or blood clot.

H = **Headache** that is **severe** or that includes, dizziness, weakness, or numbness anywhere in the body.

E = **Eye problems** such as **severe** pressure behind the eyes or blurry vision. These could be signs of a stroke, blood clot, or high blood pressure.

S = **Severe leg pain** in the calf or thigh. This could be a sign of a blood clot.

**If you have any of these signs, call right away or
go to the emergency room.**

Are there any precautions?

A health care provider may advise you to use a different method if any of the following is true:

- You smoke and are over the age of 35.
- You have had blood clots, or a stroke or heart attack.
- You have high blood pressure, liver problems, or certain cancers.
- You have ever had breast cancer.

The health care provider will talk with you about your health to make sure that there is no reason for you not to use the pill.

Breastfeeding

Those who breastfeed should talk to their provider about when they can start using the pill. Using the combined pill may affect milk supply.

What are the advantages and disadvantages of using the Pill?

There are many things people like about using the pill. And there are some things they don't like. Find out what your patient likes and encourage them to focus on those things.

What some people like about the pill:

- It is easy to use.
- It is good at preventing pregnancy.
- The pill makes periods lighter and less crampy.
- The pill may make acne better.
- It does not interrupt having sex.
- The pill helps protect against cancer of the ovary and cancer of the uterus.

- It does not cause serious health problems in most users.
- The pill may prevent or improve PMS symptoms; particularly with "continuous use."
- Patients who use the pill can decide when they have their scheduled bleeding if they are taught how.

Find out what your patient might not like about taking the pill.

Ask your patients if they have any concerns about taking the pill. Then talk to them about their concerns. People hear a lot of myths about the pill that aren't true. This can make them afraid to take it. Give your patients the correct information.

Help them think through how to solve any problems they might have while using the pill. Have them come up with their own solutions first. Read the chart that follows for some ideas on how to deal with concerns.

Keep in mind that the pill isn't the best method for everyone.
It is the patient's choice.

The Pill: Some Problems and Ways to Solve Them

Problem	Ways to Solve the Problem
It is hard for me to get to my appointment.	Perhaps your partner could take you to the appointment. Talk to your provider about getting many months of pills at a time. That way you won't have to come as often.
I don't want to have an exam.	You will not need a full exam in order to get a prescription for the pill. But you may be due for an exam that is recommended for patients of your age. It may help to know that getting recommended health screenings is a key part of keeping healthy. Regular exams can help find things before they become a problem. Ask patients what troubles them about getting an exam. Perhaps they don't know what to expect. It may help if you explain what happens.
I have to remember to take it every day at the same time.	▶ Think of something you do at about the same time each day, like getting up or eating a meal. You could plan to take your pill at that same time. ▶ You could set a watch alarm or cell phone to remind you when to take your pill. ▶ You could use a website or a smartphone app that is designed to send you a daily reminder. If you do forget to take a pill, be sure to use a second method of birth control. Follow the provider's advice for getting back on schedule with your pills.
What if I have sex after forgetting to take 2 or more pills?	Call your provider for advice. You may still try to prevent pregnancy after sex by using emergency contraception.
I may get side effects.	Most side effects will go away after a few months of taking the pill. If your side effects bother you, talk to your health care provider. A different brand of pill may work better for you.

The Pill: Some Problems and Ways to Solve Them

Problem	Ways to Solve the Problem
I could get a serious complication.	Serious problems are **very rare** for those who are healthy when they start taking the pill. ▶ ***Before*** you start the pill, talk to your health care provider about any health problems you have. ▶ Call your health care provider right away if you have any of the warning signs.
I've heard the pill can cause cancer or make me sterile.	The pill doesn't cause cancer or infertility. Studies have shown that pill users do not have a higher risk of cancer or infertility. In fact, the pill helps protect against cancer of the ovary and cancer of the uterus. It also prevents ovarian cysts which can lead to fertility problems.
The pill does not protect me from HIV and other STIs.	Use condoms along with the pill every time you have sex to help protect you from STIs.

What if you want to stop using the Pill?

You can stop using the pill whenever you want to. But if you stop using it, you could become pregnant right away. Use another birth control method if you don't want to be pregnant.

There are no health problems to watch for when you stop this method.

Make sure your patient understands.

Before your patients leave, make sure they understand how to use the pill successfully. Some of these questions may help.

- ▸ Tell me what you know about the pill.
- ▸ What is one way the pill works to prevent pregnancy?
- ▸ When are you going to start your first pack?
- ▸ What time of day will you take the pill each day?
- ▸ What will help you remember?
- ▸ What will you do if you miss taking 1 pill? 2 pills? More than 2 pills?
- ▸ What might be the most difficult problem for you when using the pill?
- ▸ How would you solve that problem?
- ▸ What rare warning signs will you watch for while you are on the pill?

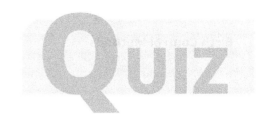

BIRTH CONTROL PILL

Directions. Circle the best answer.

1. What two hormones are in the Pill?
    a. Estrogen and testosterone.
    b. Estrogen and progestin.
    c. Testosterone and progestin.
    d. None of the above.

2. The Pill works because:
    a. It keeps eggs from leaving the ovaries.
    b. It keeps the mucus from the cervix thick.
    c. It keeps the sperm from entering the vagina.
    d. Both A and B.

3. To make the Pill work best, a user should:
    a. Take it only when they have sex.
    b. Take one pill at the same time every day.
    c. Use another person's pills if they are out, because birth control pills are all the same.
    d. None of the above.

4. If a user forgets to take two or more pills, they should:
    a. Take the last missed pill as soon as they remember.
    b. Call their provider for advice.
    c. Use a back-up birth control method, along with the pill for as long as the health care provider advises.
    d. All of the above.

Go on to the next page.

5. Which of the following is not a side effect of using the Pill:

   a. Bleeding changes

   b. Nausea and vomiting

   c. Weight gain

   d. Tender breasts

Directions. Read each of the following and write your best answer in the spaces below.

6. List two warning signs that you should tell a patient to watch for. Tell what health problem the sign may warn the patient of.

   ▪ _____

   _____

   ▪ _____

   _____

7. List one concern that a patient may have about using the Pill and what you might say to help them deal with that concern.

   Patient's concern:
   ▪ _____

   _____

   What you can say:
   ▪ _____

   _____

   _____

Check your answers on the next page.

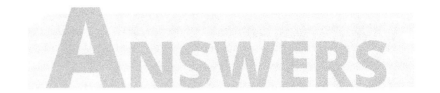

BIRTH CONTROL PILL

Check your answers.

1. **B**   Estrogen and progestin are the two hormones in the Pill.

2. **D**   Both A & B. The Pill works because:
   - It keeps the eggs from leaving the ovaries.
   - It keeps the mucus from the cervix thick.

3. **B**   To make the Pill work best, users should take one pill at the same time every day.

4. **D**   All of the above. If a user forgets to take one pill, they should:
   - Take the missed pill as soon as they remember.
   - Call the provider for advice.
   - Use a back-up birth control method along with the pill for as long as the provider advises.

5. **C**   Weight gain is not a side effect of using the Pill. Most people gain weight over time whether they take the Pill or not. Possible side effects of the Pill include:
   - Changes in bleeding
   - Nausea and vomiting
   - Tender or full breasts
   - Mood changes
   - Skin changes
   - Headaches

6. Warning signs that a patient should watch for include:

   A = **Abdominal pain** that is **severe**. This can be a sign of a liver tumor, gall bladder disease, blood clot, or pregnancy in your tubes.

   C = **Chest pain** that is **severe**, or shortness of breath. These could be signs of a heart attack or blood clot.

   H = **Headache** that is **severe** or that includes dizziness, weakness, or numbness anywhere in the body. These could be signs of high blood pressure or a stroke.

   E = **Eye problems** such as **severe** pressure behind the eyes or blurry vision. These could be signs of a stroke, blood clot, or high blood pressure.

   S = **Severe leg pain** in the calf or thigh. This could be a sign of a blood clot.

7. Here are two concerns a patient might have about using the Pill and what you might say to help. For other possible concerns and responses, please see the "The Pill: Some Problems and Ways to Solve Them" chart near the end of the Birth Control Pill section.

   - *Patient's concern:* "I have to remember to take it at the same time every day."

     What you could say: "Think of something you do at the same time each day, like brushing and flossing your teeth or eating a meal. You could plan to take your pill at that same time."

   - *Patient's concern:* "The pill does not protect me from HIV and other STIs."

     What you could say: "Use condoms along with the pill every time you have sex to help protect you from getting STIs."

Things to remember when you use the patch:

Educator Tip

Ask your patients, "What will you do to help you remember to change your patch on the same day each week?"

Do's

▶ Put on a new patch once a week for 3 weeks in a row. Then go 7 days without wearing a patch.

▶ Check your patch every day. Make sure it is not loose.

▶ Change your patch on the same day each week.

▶ Use a calendar or some other way to help you remember when to change your patch.

▶ Keep a second birth control method, like condoms, handy to use in case you have a problem with your patch.

▶ If you ever miss two periods in a row, take a pregnancy test.

▶ If you see a doctor for any reason, tell them you are using the patch.

Don'ts

▶ Don't use lotion, make-up, or powder on or near the skin where the patch will be. It is also a good idea not to use soaps with moisturizers in them. Any of these could make the patch come loose.

▶ Don't put the patch on your breast or on the inside of your upper arm.

▶ Don't put the patch in the exact same place two weeks in a row.

▶ Don't put the patch on skin that is red, irritated, or cut.

How do you clean the dark ring that the patch may leave on your skin?

This dark ring on your skin is like those you may get when you use a bandage. Don't try to clean the ring off while you are wearing the patch. When you change your patch, you can rub a little baby oil on the dark ring to remove it.

What if you forget to change your patch or it comes loose or falls off?

The instructions for what to do if something goes wrong while using the patch can be complicated. And if you tell your patients all the details at this first meeting, most patients won't remember them. Instead, teach patients the basic steps listed below.

This chapter also gives you, the health worker, more detailed advice. You may want to refer to those details if a patient calls for specific advice on what to do.

Note: Your provider's advice may differ from the advice given here. Be sure to give your patients the advice used at your health care site.

To keep from getting pregnant, try to use the patch the right way every time. Two basic things could go wrong when using the patch:

- The patch could come loose or fall off.
- You could forget to change your patch on the right day.

You should know what to do to keep from getting pregnant if either of these things happens. Here are the basics. Be sure to call the provider if you ever have any questions.

What if a patch comes loose or falls off?

What you do depends on how long the patch has been loose or off.

If it has been *less* than 24 hours:

- Try to stick the patch back on. If it won't stick smoothly, throw it away. Put on a new patch.
- Change this patch on your usual day.

You are still protected against pregnancy.

If it has been off or loose for 24 hours or *more*, call the provider for advice.

What if you forget to change your patch on the right day?

If you forget for 1 day or less, here is what you should do:

- Put the new patch on as soon as you remember.
- Change this patch on your usual day.

The patch should still protect you from getting pregnant.

If you forget for more than 1 day, here is what you should do:

- Change your patch right away and call the provider for advice. Find out what else you may need to do to protect yourself from getting pregnant.
- Be sure to use a back-up method, like condoms, until you find out exactly what to do.

Important

If you forgot to change your patch and have had sex within the past 7 days:

▶ Call the provider right away to ask about Emergency Contraception (EC).

▶ Follow the advice you are given about getting back on schedule with your patch.

Get a pregnancy test if you don't get your scheduled bleed this month.

Calls from patients

At some point, you may take a call from a patient whose patch has come loose or fallen off, or who has forgotten to change their patch on time. You may find that they need more information than "the basics" you give patients at their first patch visit. Here is some additional advice the patient may need.

Note: This advice may differ from the advice given at your health care site. Always follow your site's guidelines for advising these patients.

Calls about patches that have come loose or fallen off.

- If a patient calls for advice and says their patch has been off or loose for ***more than 24 hours,*** here is what you might tell them:

  Put a new patch on right away. This day will begin Week 1 of a ***new*** 4-week cycle. In other words, you will change your patch on ***this*** day each week. After wearing a new patch each week for 3 weeks, you will go 7 days without wearing a patch.

  Use a back-up method, like condoms, for the first week to keep from getting pregnant.

Follow your health care site's guidelines on talking to the patient about Emergency Contraception (EC).

Are there any side effects?

Some patients have side effects with the patch. Most side effects go away after using the patch for two or three months. Your patients can talk to a provider if the side effects last longer than that or really bother them. Below are some side effects to tell your patients about.

▸ **Changes in bleeding**

When first starting the patch, you may experience longer or crampier periods. You may experience spotting in the first two months.

▸ **Tender or full breasts**

Your breasts may get bigger and be tender. You can try wearing the patch on the lower part of your body, like your hips, instead of on your arms or upper torso.

▸ **Headaches**

These headaches are usually mild and go away with over-the-counter medication.

▸ **Nausea**

This may happen during the first few months you use the patch or during the first few days of wearing each "Week 1" patch.

▸ **Rash**

You may get a mild rash where you wear the patch. This is less likely to happen if you wear the patch in a different place each week.

The Patch and Weight Concerns

Q. Does the patch cause weight gain.

A. No.

Q. If a user is overweight, will the patch still work well?

A. Yes.

Q. Are there medical problems if a user is overweight and using the patch?

A. There could be. All users should talk to their provider about the risk of blood clots, heart attack, or stroke while using the patch.

Research shows that the patch does not cause weight gain. Most people gain weight over time whether they are using the patch or not, especially teens and young adults who are still growing.

Calls about forgotten patches	
If a patient calls because they have forgotten to change their patch, the advice you give them will depend on the following: ▶ Which week of their 4-week patch cycle they forgot to change it ▶ How many days they forgot to change it	
If it is the first week of their 4-week cycle:	*If it is week 2 or 3:*
If they have forgotten for more than 1 day, tell them: ▶ Put on your first patch right away. From now on, change your patch on *that* day each week. ▶ Use a second method of birth control, like condoms, for 1 week to help keep you from getting pregnant.	**If they have forgotten for only 1 or 2 days,** tell them: ▶ Change your patch right away. You are still protected from getting pregnant. ▶ Keep your usual day for changing your patch. **If they have forgotten for more than 2 days,** tell them: ▶ Change your patch right away. From now on, change your patch on *this* day each week. ▶ Use a second method of birth control, like condoms, for 1 week to help protect yourself from pregnancy.
If it is week 4 (their patch-free week):	
If they have forgotten to take their patch off during week 4, tell them: ▶ Take the patch off right away. You are still protected against pregnancy. ▶ You still put on your new patch on your usual day. (You don't have to wait 7 days to put it on.)	

What about complications and warning signs?

Serious health problems from the patch are rare, but some patients get them. Here are some of the possible complications:

▸ **High blood pressure**

   High blood pressure usually has no symptoms. This is why your health care provider will probably want to check your blood pressure a few months after you start the patch. If your blood pressure does go up, you may be told to stop using the patch. Your blood pressure will usually go back down once you stop.

▸ **Blood clots**

   In some users, clots can form in the legs or abdomen and travel to the heart, lungs, or brain. When blood clots travel, they can cause a *heart attack* or *stroke*. Patients who are *over 35 and smoke* are more likely than others to get clots when they are using the patch.

▸ **Liver or gall bladder problems**

   Rarely, a user may have problems with their liver or gall bladder.

Patch Warning Signs: A C H E S

Serious health problems are rare with the patch. But it is important to know the warning signs.

A = **Abdominal pain** that is **severe**. This can be a sign of a liver tumor, gall bladder disease, blood clot, or pregnancy in your tubes.

C = **Chest pain** that is **severe**, or shortness of breath. These could be signs of a heart attack or blood clot.

H = **Headache** that is **severe** or that includes, dizziness, weakness, or numbness anywhere in the body.

E = **Eye problems** such as **severe** pressure behind the eyes or blurry vision. These could be signs of a stroke, blood clot, or high blood pressure.

S = **Severe leg pain** in the calf or thigh. This could be a sign of a blood clot.

**If you have any of these signs, call right away
or go to the emergency room.**

Are there any precautions?

A health care provider may advise you to use a different method if any of the following is true:

- You have had blood clots, a stroke, or a heart attack.
- You have high blood pressure, liver problems, or certain cancers.
- You have ever had breast cancer.
- You smoke and are over the age of 35.

The health care provider will talk with you about your health to make sure that there is no reason for you not to use the patch.

Breastfeeding

Those who breastfeed should talk to their medical provider about when they can start using the patch.

What are the advantages and disadvantages of the Patch?

There are many things patients like about using the patch. And there are some things they don't like. Find out what your patient likes and encourage them to focus on those things.

What some people like about the patch:

- It is easy to use.
- It is very good at preventing pregnancy.
- They only have to change the patch once a week.
- Using the patch does not interrupt having sex.
- The patch stays on even when you exercise, shower, or take a bath.
- The patch may make menstrual periods lighter and less crampy.
- The patch may make acne better.
- The patch helps protect against cancer of the ovary and cancer of the uterus.
- The patch does not cause any serious problems in most users.

Find out what your patient might not like about using the patch.

Ask your patients if they have any concerns about using the patch. Then talk to them about their concerns. Help them think through how to solve any problems they might have while using the patch. Have them come up with their own solutions first. Read the following chart for some ideas on how to deal with concerns.

Keep in mind that the patch isn't the best method for everyone. It is the patient's choice.

The Patch: Some Problems and Ways to Solve Them

Problem	Ways to Solve the Problem
It's hard for me to get to the health care site to see a provider.	Perhaps your partner, family member, or friend could take you.
I don't want to have an exam.	You may not need an exam. But if you do, it may help to know that an exam is a key part of keeping you healthy. Regular exams can help find things before they become a problem. Ask your patient what troubles them about getting an exam. Perhaps they don't know what to expect. It may help if you explain it to them.
I have to remember to change it the same day each week.	<ul><li>You could mark it on your calendar or find some other way to help you remember.</li><li>You could sign-up for a weekly reminder through a website or an app for your smartphone.</li><li>Your partner could help remind you to change your patch.</li></ul>
The patch could show if my clothes don't cover it.	There are many places you can put the patch so it will be covered. Think about what you wear and place the patch where it won't show.
What if I have sex around the time I forget to change the patch?	Call the provider for advice. You can still try to prevent pregnancy after sex. Find out about EC.
I may get side effects.	Most side effects will go away after a few months of using the patch. If your side effects bother you, talk to your health care provider.

The Patch: Some Problems and Ways to Solve Them

Problem	Ways to Solve the Problem
I could get a serious complication.	Serious problems are very rare for patients who are healthy when they start using the patch. ▪ **Before** you start using the patch, talk to your health care provider about any health problems you have. ▪ Call your health care provider right away if you have any of the warning signs.
The patch does not protect me from HIV and other STIs.	Use a condom along with the patch every time you have sex to protect you from STIs.

What if you want to stop using the Patch?

You can stop using the patch whenever you want to. But if you stop using it, you could become pregnant right away. Use another birth control method if you don't want to be pregnant.

There are no health problems to watch for when you stop using the patch.

Make sure your patient understands.

Before your patients leave, make sure they understand how to use the patch successfully. Some of these questions may help.

▸ Tell me what you know about the patch.
▸ How does the patch work?
▸ When are you going to start using your first patch?
▸ What day of the week will you change your patch?
▸ What will help you remember?
▸ What will you do if you forget to change your patch?
▸ What might be the most difficult problem for you when using the patch?
▸ How would you solve that problem?
▸ What warning signs will you watch for while using the patch?

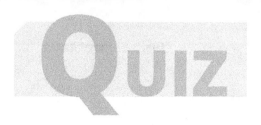

QUIZ

BIRTH CONTROL PATCH

Directions. Circle the best answer.

1. Which of the following hormones is in the Patch?
    a. Testosterone
    b. Estrogen
    c. Progestin
    d. Both B and C

2. How long does one patch work?
    a. 1 week
    b. 2 weeks
    c. 3 weeks
    d. 4 weeks

3. What is the main way that the Patch keeps a person from getting pregnant?
    a. It keeps them from wanting to have sex.
    b. It kills sperm.
    c. It keeps eggs from leaving the ovaries.
    d. All of the above

4. The Patch can be worn on the:
    a. Upper arm
    b. Hip
    c. Upper torso (excluding breasts)
    d. All of the above

Go on to the next page.

Directions. Read each of the following and write your best answer in the space below.

5. What should a person do if their Patch comes loose?

_____

_____

_____

6. List two side effects that could happen while using the Patch.

_____

_____

7. List two serious health problems (complications) that people who use the Patch could get.

_____

_____

Check your answers on the next page.

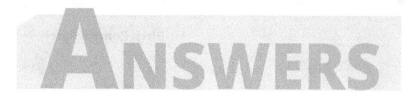

BIRTH CONTROL PATCH

Check your answers.

1. **D** The Patch, like the Pill, has two hormones in it: estrogen and progestin.

2. **A** Each patch works for 1 week.

3. **C** The Patch mostly prevents pregnancy by keeping the eggs from leaving the ovaries.

4. **D** All of the above. The Patch can be worn on the upper arm, hip, or upper torso. It can also be worn on the stomach or buttock.

5. If a Patch comes loose, they should do the following:
   - **If it has been loose for *less than* 24 hours:** Try to stick it back on. If it won't stick smoothly, throw it away and put on a new patch. Change this patch on the usual day.
   - **If it has been loose for 24 *hours or more.*** Call the provider for advice.

6. Possible side effects of using the Patch include:
   - Tender or full breasts
   - Changes in bleeding
   - Nausea
   - Headaches
   - Rash

7. Possible complications from using the Patch are rare, but they include:
   - High blood pressure
   - Blood clots
   - Liver or gall bladder problems

Birth Control Ring

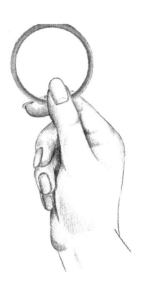

This section is mostly written as though you were talking to your patients. It gives you an idea of how to explain the birth control ring in a way your patients can understand. This section also has notes written directly to you, the health worker. Those "health worker notes" look like this one.

What is it?

The birth control ring (the ring) is a thin, flexible, plastic ring that is worn inside the vagina to keep you from getting pregnant. It comes in one size and has two hormones in it: estrogen and progestin. The hormones slowly go into your body through the skin in the vagina.

The ring works on a 4-week cycle. You will place a new ring in the vagina once a month.

- You can keep it in for 4 weeks so that there is no scheduled bleeding.
- Or, you can wear it for three weeks in a row. Then take it out and wear no ring for one week. During that week, you will have a scheduled bleed or period.

Most partners do not feel the ring during penile-vaginal sex.

The ring works well to prevent pregnancy but it does not help protect you against HIV and other STIs. Use a condom every time you have sex to help protect yourself from STIs.

How does it work?

The ring works mostly by keeping the egg from leaving the ovaries. If there is no egg to meet with sperm, you can't get pregnant. The ring also:

- Keeps your cervical mucus thick. This helps keep sperm from getting into the uterus and meeting with an egg.
- Makes the lining of the uterus thin so that the egg cannot attach to the uterus.

Talk to your patients about Emergency Contraception.

Emergency Contraception (EC), in the form of EC pills or an IUD, can prevent pregnancy after sex. Patients can use EC up to 5 days after unprotected sex. Read more about EC at the end of this chapter.

How well does the Ring work?

When you talk to your patients, you will need to explain how well the ring works (how effective it is). Be sure to explain the difference between "perfect use" and "typical use." You can read about this in the "Stage 3" section of Chapter 2.

With perfect use, the ring is 99.7% effective.

This means that if 100 patients use the ring exactly the right way, only 1 (and probably none) of them may get pregnant in a year.

With typical use, the ring is 93% effective.

For those who don't always use their ring exactly the right way, 7 out of 100 may get pregnant in a year.

How do you use the Ring?

Teach your patients these steps so they can use the ring the right way. Your provider's advice may differ from the advice given here. Be sure to give your patients the advice used at your health care site.

1. **Talk to a provider about whether the ring is right for you.**

    The health care provider will ask you some questions. Talk to the provider about:

    ▸ Any health problems you may have

    ▸ Any medicine you may be taking

    ▸ Any questions you may have

    Your health care provider will help you decide if the ring is right for you.

    Learn how your health care setting provides the ring for patients. Be sure to explain to your patient:

    ▸ How and where they will pick up the ring

    ▸ How much they can expect to pay

2. **Talk to your provider about when to start using the ring.**

> Here is basic advice for when to start using the ring. A medical provider may give different advice depending on the individual patient's birth control history. Give your patients whatever instructions your health care setting uses.

Start using the ring on the day your health care provider suggests.

Here is the basic advice for starting the ring:

- ▸ You can start the ring on any day.

- ▸ The very first time that you use the ring, use a second method of birth control, like condoms, until the ring has been in place for 7 days in a row.

Note: You will **not** need to use a second method if you put your first ring in on the *first day of your period.*

3. **Talk to the health care provider about how to use the ring for a scheduled bleed.**

Here are the steps to follow when you use the ring:

Step 1. Put a new ring in your vagina. Leave it in for 3 weeks in a row.

Step 2. At the end of 3 weeks:

- ▪ Take the ring out of your vagina on the same day of the week as you put it in.

- ▪ Throw the used ring away. (Do not flush it down the toilet.)

Step 3. Go 7 days (1 week) without wearing a ring. You should get your period during that week.

Step 4. After 1 week without wearing a ring, put in a new ring on the same day of the week as you did before. Put it in even if you are still on your period.

- ▪ Never go more than these 7 days without wearing a birth control ring. If you do, you could get pregnant.

No Scheduled Bleed

If you do not want a scheduled bleed, here are the steps you should follow.

Step 1. Put a new ring in your vagina. Leave it in for 4 weeks in a row.

Step 2. At the end of 4 weeks:

- ▪ Take the ring out of your vagina on the same day of the week as you put it in.

- ▪ Throw the used ring away. Do not flush it down the toilet.

Step 3: Put a new ring in right away. That way you will not have a scheduled bleed and you keep from getting pregnant. If you notice a small amount of bleeding, do not worry. This is not bad for your health and it does not mean you will get pregnant. If the bleeding bothers you, talk to your provider for advice.

How to put the ring in

1. Wash and dry your hands.

2. Take the ring out of its package. Squeeze the ring between your thumb and fingers until the sides come together.

Educator Tip

Ask your patients, "What will you do to help you remember to take out and put in your ring on time?"

3. To put the ring in, you can squat, lie down, or stand with one leg up.

4. Gently slide the ring into your vagina. When it is in right, you shouldn't notice it. If it feels uncomfortable, push it farther in. It can be anywhere in the vagina that is comfortable for you. There is no way to put the ring in "wrong." If it's inside of your vagina and it is comfortable, it is correct.

5. Wash your hands to wash off any hormones left on your fingers.

If they forget or the ring slips out . . .

- Be sure to tell your patients the basics about what to do if their ring slips out or if they forget to take it out or put it in on time.

- Give them easy-to-read written materials about this to take home.

- Ask your patients what method they would use for back-up if they needed one.

How to take the ring out

1. Wash your hands.

2. Put a finger into your vagina until you feel an edge of the ring. Curl your finger over the rim of the ring and pull gently. The ring will fold and slide out.

3. Wrap the ring in foil or plastic wrap and throw it away.

4. Wash your hands.

When you use the ring for a scheduled bleed, remember to:

▸ Leave the ring in the vagina for 3 weeks in a row. Then go just 7 days without wearing a ring.

▸ Put the ring in and take it out on the same day of the week, and at about the same time.

If you do not want a scheduled bleed, remember:

▸ Each ring works for exactly one month.

▸ A new ring must be put in every month.

- You can take out the ring for 4 days to have a scheduled bleed if you are having bleeding that bothers you.

- But do not not take the ring out unless you have had a ring in your vagina for at least 3 weeks in a row.

No matter how you use the ring, remember these important things:

- When you throw your used ring out, be sure it is out of the reach of children and pets. Some people put it back in its package before they throw it away.

- Find a way that helps you remember when to put the ring in and take it out. You may want to mark your calendar.

- Keep a second birth control method, like condoms, handy to use in case you have a problem with your ring. Never use the diaphragm or internal condom and the ring at the same time.

- If you ever miss two periods in a row or if you feel pregnancy symptoms, take a pregnancy test.

- If you see a health care provider for any reason, tell the provider you are using the ring.

What if you forget or the Ring slips out?

The instructions for what to do if something goes wrong while using the ring can be complicated. And if you tell your patients all the details at this first meeting, most patients won't remember them. Instead, teach your patients the basic steps listed below.

This chapter also gives you, the health worker, more detailed advice. You may want to refer to those details if a patient calls for specific advice on what to do.

Note: Your provider's advice may differ from the advice given here. Be sure to give your patients the advice used at your health care site.

To keep from getting pregnant, try to use the ring the right way every time. And be aware of the three basic things that could go wrong when using the ring:

- You could forget to put a new ring in on time.

- You could forget to take the ring out on time.

- Your ring could slip out.

You should know what to do to keep from getting pregnant if any of these things happens. Here are the basics. Be sure to call the provider if you ever have any questions.

What if you forget to put the ring in on time?

If you forget to put in a new ring on time (in other words, if you go *more than 7 days* without wearing a ring), you could get pregnant. You should do all of the following:

▸ Put the new ring in as soon as you remember. Keep that ring in for 3 weeks (21 days). Remember to take it out on the same day of the week as you put it in. Or keep the ring in for 4 weeks (the entire month). Remember to take it out on the same day of the week as you put it in.

▸ Use a second method of birth control, like condoms, withdrawal, spermicides or abstaining from reproductive sex, until the new ring has been in the vagina for 7 days in a row.

▸ *If you had sex within the past week,* call the provider right away for advice. Ask about EC.

What if you forget to take the ring out on time?

After wearing the ring for 3 weeks, you are supposed to take it out and go 7 days without wearing a ring. But what if you forget to take it out on time?

If you forget for 7 days or less (that means the ring has been in for a total of 4 weeks or less), you should still be protected from pregnancy. Here is what you should do:

▸ Take the ring out as soon as you remember.

▸ Then go 7 days without wearing a ring.

▸ After 7 days without wearing a ring, put in a new ring. Take that ring out 3 weeks later on the same day of the week as you put it in.

You could get pregnant if:

▸ You forget for more than 7 days (in other words, the ring has been in the vagina for more than 4 weeks in a row).

If that happens, do all of the following:

▸ Call the provider right away for advice.

▸ Be sure to use a back-up method, like condoms, until you find out exactly what you need to do.

▸ Ask about Emergency Contraception (EC).

What if the ring slips out?

Rarely, a ring can slip out. Or it could come out when you are taking out a tampon. The ring cannot get lost in your vagina.

If your ring slips out, here is what you should do:

> ▶ Rinse it with cool water, never hot. Then put it back in right away. If you can't find your ring, put a new ring in right away. Take this new ring out on the same day as you would have removed the lost ring.

> ▶ Some users like to take the ring out during sex. It is okay as long as it does not stay out longer than 3 hours in any *24 hour* period.

> ▶ *If the ring has been out for more than 3 hours,* you may *not* be protected from pregnancy. Be sure to use a second method of birth control, like condoms, until the ring has been in the vagina for 7 days in a row. *If you have had sex within the past week,* call the provider right away for advice.

Use this same advice if you ever take your ring out to have sex and forget to put it back in within 3 hours.

If they worry about the ring getting lost. . .

You can use a sock to demonstrate that a vagina is a "limited space" and that it can't can't get lost or travel deeper inside.

Important

You may not be protected from pregnancy if any of the following happens:

> ▶ After 7 days without wearing a ring, you forget to put a new ring in.

> ▶ You leave the ring in for *more than 4 weeks* in a row.

> ▶ The ring is out of the vagina for *more than 3 hours* when it should be in.

If any of those things happen *and you have had sex within the past 5 days:*

> ▶ Call the provider right away to ask about Emergency Contraception (EC). Or visit this website: cecinfo.org to learn more.

> ▶ Follow the advice the provider gives you for getting back on schedule with the ring and for using a second method of birth control as back-up to prevent pregnancy.

Get a pregnancy test if you don't get your period this month.

Calls from patients who have forgotten or whose ring has slipped out	
At some point, you may take a call from a patient who has forgotten to put their ring in or take it out on time, or whose ring has slipped out. You may find that they need more information than "the basics" you give patients at their first ring visit. Here is some additional advice the patient may need.	
If they have gone *more than 7 days* without wearing a ring	***If they have left their ring in for more than 4 weeks***
If they have had sex any time since they removed their last ring, they could get pregnant. This will depend on when they had sex. Follow your health care site's guidelines for talking to patients about: ▸ Emergency Contraception (EC) ▸ Getting back on schedule with their ring	Tell them to: ▸ Take that ring out and put in a new ring right away. ▸ Use a second method, like condoms, until the new ring has been in the vagina for 7 days in a row. If they have had sex within the past week, they could get pregnant. This will depend on when they had sex. Follow your health care site's guidelines for talking with patients about EC and pregnancy testing.
If their ring has slipped out and may have been out for *more than 3 hours*	**If they took their ring out to have sex and forgot to put it back in *within 3 hours***
Let them know that they may not be protected against pregnancy. Give them the usual advice for putting the ring back in. But tell them they also need to: ▸ Use a second method of birth control until the ring has been back in their vagina for 7 days in a row. If they have had sex within the past week, they could get pregnant. This will depend on when they had sex. Follow your health care site's guidelines for talking to patients about EC and pregnancy testing.	They may not be protected against pregnancy. Follow your health care site's guidelines for talking to patients about EC and pregnancy testing. Also, give them the usual advice for putting the ring back in. And tell them to: ▸ Use a second method of birth control, like condoms, withdrawal, spermicides or abstaining from reproductive sex until the ring has been back in their vagina for 7 days in a row.

Are there any side effects?

Some patients have side effects with the ring. Most side effects go away after they use the ring for two or three months. Your patients can talk to a provider if the side effects last longer than that or really bother them. Here are some possible side effects to tell your patients about.

▸ **Changes in bleeding**

You may miss periods or spot (bleed very lightly between periods). Spotting is most likely to happen during the first few months of using the ring. Some users get periods that are only spotting and last more than 7 days.

▸ **Headaches**

If you get headaches, they will probably be mild and go away with over-the-counter medication.

▸ **Increased vaginal discharge or irritation**

You may have more discharge from the vagina than is usual for you. Your vagina may be irritated. If this bothers you, talk to a health care provider.

What about complications and warning signs?

Serious health problems from the ring are rare, but some users do get them. Here are some of the possible complications:

▸ **High blood pressure**

There are usually no symptoms of high blood pressure. This is why your health care provider will probably want to check your blood pressure a few months after you start the ring. If your blood pressure does go up, you may be told to stop using the ring. This will usually make your blood pressure go down again.

▸ **Blood clots**

In some users, clots may form in the legs or abdomen and travel to the heart, lungs, or brain. When blood clots travel, they can cause a heart attack or stroke. Patients who are over 35 and smoke are more likely than others to get clots when they are using the ring.

▸ **Liver or gall bladder problems**

Rarely, a user may have problems with their liver or gall bladder.

The Ring and Weight Concerns

Q. Does the ring cause weight gain?

A. No.

Q. If someone is overweight, will the ring still work well?

A. Yes.

Q. Are there medical problems using the ring if a person is overweight?

A. There could be. A patient should talk to their provider about the risk of blood clots, heart attack, or stroke while using the ring.

Research shows that the ring does not cause weight gain. Most people gain weight over time whether they are using the ring or not, especially teens and young adults who are still growing.

Ring Warning Signs: A C H E S

Serious health problems are rare with the ring. But it is important to know the warning signs.

A = **Abdominal pain** that is **severe**. This can be a sign of a liver tumor, gall bladder disease, blood clot, or pregnancy in your tubes.

C = **Chest pain** that is **severe**, or shortness of breath. These could be signs of a heart attack or blood clot.

H = **Headache** that is **severe** or that includes, dizziness, weakness, or numbness anywhere in the body.

E = **Eye problems** such as **severe** pressure behind the eyes or blurry vision. These could be signs of a stroke, blood clot, or high blood pressure.

S = **Severe leg pain** in the calf or thigh. This could be a sign of a blood clot.

If you have any of these signs, call right away or go to the emergency room.

Breastfeeding

Those who breastfeed should talk to their provider about when they can start using the ring. Using the ring may affect milk supply.

Are there any precautions?

A health care provider may advise you to use a different method if any of the following is true:

- You have had blood clots, a stroke, or a heart attack.
- You have high blood pressure, liver problems, or certain cancers.
- You have ever had breast cancer.
- You smoke *and* are over the age of 35.

The health care provider will talk with you about your health to make sure that there is no reason for you not to use the ring.

What are the advantages and disadvantages of the Ring?

There are many things people like about using the ring. And there are some things they don't like. Find out what your patient likes and encourage them to focus on those things.

What some users like about the ring:

▶ It is easy to use.

▶ It is very good at preventing pregnancy.

▶ You only have to put the ring in once a month.

▶ Using the ring does not interrupt having sex.

▶ The ring may make periods lighter and less crampy.

▶ The ring may make acne better.

▶ The ring helps protect against cancer of the ovary and cancer of the uterus.

▶ The ring does not cause any serious health problems in most users.

▶ It can be removed before sex for up to three hours in a 24-hour time frame.

Ring Removal During Sex

Some people prefer or like to take the ring out when having vaginal sex.

Make sure patients know they can take the ring out for a total of three hours in a 24-hour window.

Find out what your patient might not like about using the ring.

Ask your patients if they have any concerns about using the ring. Then talk to them about their concerns. Help them think through how to solve any problems they might have while using the ring. Have them come up with their own solutions first. Read the chart that follows for some ideas on how to deal with concerns.

Keep in mind that the ring isn't the best method for everyone. It is the patient's choice.

The Ring: Some Problems and Ways to Solve Them

Problem	Ways to Solve the Problem
It's hard for me to get to my appointment	Perhaps your partner, family member, or friend could take you.
I don't want to have an exam.	You may not need an exam. But if you do, it may help to know that the exam is a key part of keeping you healthy. Regular exams can help find things before they become a problem. Ask your patient what troubles them about getting an exam. Perhaps they don't know what to expect. It may help if you explain it to them.
I don't like putting my fingers in my vagina.	This is something you may get used to with practice. If you don't think you can get used to it, the ring may not be the best method for you.
I have to remember to put it in and take it out at the right times each month.	You could mark it on your calendar or find some other way to help you remember. Your partner could help remind you to change your ring.
What if I have sex around the time the ring slips out or I forget to take it out or put it in?	Call the provider for advice. You can still try to prevent pregnancy after sex. Find out about EC pills.
I may get side effects.	Most side effects will go away after a few months of using the ring. If your side effects bother you, talk to your health care provider.

The Ring: Some Problems and Ways to Solve Them

Problem	Ways to Solve the Problem
I could get a serious complication.	Serious problems are very rare for patients who are healthy when they start using the ring. ■ *Before* you start using the ring, talk to your health care provider about any health problems you have. ■ Call your health care provider right away if you have any of the warning signs.
My partner is afraid of touching the ring during sex.	The ring will not be harmed if touched by a penis, fingers or sex toy. And if your partner touches the ring during sex, they will not be harmed either. If a partner is still concerned, you can take the ring out during sex. But you have to remember to put it back in within three hours. If you don't, you could get pregnant.
The ring does not protect me from HIV or other STIs.	Use a condom along with the ring every time you have sex to help protect you from STIs.

What if you want to stop using the Ring?

You can stop using the ring whenever you want to. If you stop using it, you could become pregnant right away. Use another birth control method if you don't want to become pregnant.

There are no health problems to watch for when you stop this method.

Make sure your patient understands.

Before your patients leave, make sure they understand how to use the ring successfully. Here are some things you can ask to make sure they understand.

- ▶ Tell me what you know about the ring.
- ▶ How does the ring work?
- ▶ When are you going to start using your first ring?
- ▶ What day of the week will you change your ring?
- ▶ What will help you remember?
- ▶ What will you do if you forget to take the ring out on time?
- ▶ What will you do if you forget to put a new ring in?
- ▶ What might be the most difficult problem for you when using the ring?
- ▶ How would you solve that problem?
- ▶ What warning signs will you watch for while using the ring?

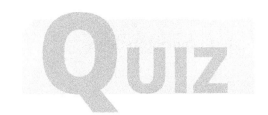

BIRTH CONTROL RING

*Directions. Read each of the following statements.
Is it true or false? Circle the best answer.*

1. A user wears a birth control ring inside   True   False
   their vagina for 3 weeks in a row.

2. The Ring helps protect against HIV   True   False
   and other STIs.

3. After wearing a ring in their vagina for 3   True   False
   weeks in a row, the user takes it out
   and goes 7 days without wearing a ring.

4. A user can go up to 15 days without   True   False
   wearing a ring and still be protected from
   pregnancy.

5. Headaches are one possible side effect   True   False
   of the Ring.

*Directions. Read each of the following statements and write your
best answer in the space below.*

6. List two warning signs to watch for when using the Ring.

   ▪ _____

   _____

   ▪ _____

   _____

Go on to the next page.

7. List two things some people like about using the Ring.

   ■ _____

   _____

   ■ _____

   _____

8. List one concern that a patient may have about using the Ring and what you might say to help them deal with that concern.

   ■ *Patient's concern:* _____

   _____

   ■ *What you can say:* _____

   _____

   Check your answers on the next page.

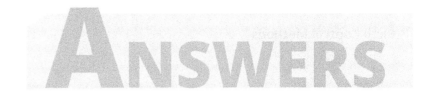

ANSWERS

BIRTH CONTROL RING

Check your answers.

1. **True** A user does wear 1 birth control ring inside their vagina for 3 weeks in a row.

2. **False** The Ring does *not* help protect against HIV or other STIs

3. **True** After wearing a ring in their vagina for 3 weeks in a row, the user does take the ring out and goes 7 days without wearing a ring.

4. **False** A user can *not* go up to 15 days without wearing a ring and still be protected from pregnancy. If they go more than the correct 1 week without wearing a ring, they could get pregnant.

5. **True** Headaches are one possible side effect of the Ring.

6. The warning signs to watch for when using the Ring are:

   A = **Abdominal pain** that is **severe**. This can be a sign of a liver tumor, gall bladder disease, blood clot or pregnancy in the tubes.

   C = **Chest pain** that is **severe** or shortness of breath. These could be signs of a heart attack or blood clot.

   H = **Headache** that is **severe** or that includes dizziness, weakness, or numbness anywhere in the body. These could be signs of high blood pressure or stroke.

   E = **Eye problems** such as **severe** pressure behind the eyes or blurry vision. These could be signs of a stroke, blood clot, or high blood pressure.

   S = **Severe leg pain** in the calf or thigh. This could be a sign of blood clots.

Go on to the next page.

© **Essential Access Health**

7. Here are things that some people like about the ring.
   - You only have to put the ring in once a month.
   - Using the ring does not interrupt having sex.
   - The ring can help protect the user from cancer of the ovaries and other diseases.
   - It's very good at preventing pregnancy.
   - Periods are less crampy, lighter.
   - The ring does not cause any serious problems in most users.

8. Here are two concerns a patient might have about using the Ring and what you might say to help them. For other possible concerns and responses, please see the "The Ring: Some Problems and Ways to Solve Them" chart near the end of the Birth Control Ring section.

   - *Patient's concern:* "I don't like putting my fingers in my vagina."

     What you could say: "This is something you may get used to with practice. If you don't think you can get used to it, the Ring may not be the best method for you."

   - *Patient's concern:* "I have to remember to put it in and take it out at the right times each month."

     What you could say: "You could find some way to help you remember. What do you think could help you remember?" (One suggestion you could make is marking it on a calendar.)

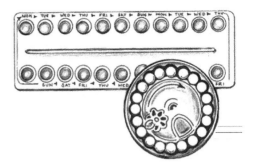

Progestin-Only Pills (POPs)

This section is mostly written as though you were talking to your patients. It gives you an idea of how to explain POPs in a way your patients can understand. This section also has notes written directly to you, the health worker. Those "health worker notes" look like this one.

What is it?

Progestin-only pills (POPs) are birth control pills. It uses a small amount of only one hormone to keep you from getting pregnant. That hormone is called progestin. Unlike the combined birth control pill, POPs have no estrogen in it.

POPs come in 28-day packs. To keep from getting pregnant, you take 1 pill every day at the same time — with no days off. That is because each pill has a hormone in it to keep you from getting pregnant. There are no sugar pills (placebos) in a POPs pack.

POPs

progestin-only pills (POPs) are also called Mini-pills.

Those who cannot use the combined birth control pill because of the estrogen may be able to use POPs. These include patients who:

▸ get headaches or nausea from the estrogen

▸ are breastfeeding

▸ smoke and are over 35 years old

POPs work well to keep you from getting pregnant. But it does not protect against HIV and other STIs. Use condoms every time you have sex to help protect against these STIs.

How does it work?

POPs work mostly by keeping the cervical mucus thick and sticky. This keeps sperm from getting into the uterus to meet with an egg.

You must take POPs at the same time every day to keep the mucus thick. If it is not taken at the same time every day, the mucus can get thinner. If that happens, sperm could then get through the cervix to meet an egg. **If you are even 3 hours late in taking POPs, you could get pregnant if an egg is ready.**

POPs may also:

▸ Keep the egg from leaving the ovaries. If there is no egg to meet with sperm, you can't get pregnant.

How well do POPs work?

When you talk to your patients, you will need to explain how well POPs work (how effective it is). Be sure to explain the difference between "perfect use" and "typical use." You can read more about this in the "Stage 3" section of Chapter 2.

Talk to your patients about Emergency Contraception.

Emergency Contraception (EC), in the form of EC pills or an IUD, can prevent pregnancy after sex. Patients can use EC up to 5 days after unprotected sex. Read more about it in the section on EC.

With perfect use, POPs are 99.7% effective.

That means that if 100 patients take POPs exactly the right way, only 1 (and probably none) of them may get pregnant in a year.

With typical use, POPs are 93% effective.

For those who don't always take their pill exactly the right way, 7 out of 100 may get pregnant in a year.

How do you use POPs?

Teach your patients these steps so they can use POPs correctly. Your provider's advice may differ from the advice given here. Be sure to give your patients the advice used at your health care site.

Taking POPs

Be sure your patient knows:

- They must *swallow* the pill.

- They must take one pill *every* day, even if they are not having sex that day.

1. **Talk to a health care provider about whether POPs are right for you.**

   The health care provider will ask you some questions. Talk to the provider about:

   - Any health problems you may have
   - Any medicine you may be taking
   - Any questions you may have

   Your health care provider will help you decide if POPs are right for you.

Always be sure to take your own POPs. Don't borrow from others. And don't give someone else your pills. All birth control pills are not the same.

Learn how your health care setting provides POPs for patients. Be sure to explain to your patient:

- How and where they will pick up the pills
- How much they can expect to pay

2. **Choose a second birth control method to use along with POPs when you first start using them.**

    You must take your POPs at the same time every day. It can take time to get into the habit of doing this. So it is a good idea to use this second method along with POPs during the first month to help make sure you don't get pregnant.

    Tip: Keep this second method around in case you need it later.

3. **Talk to your provider about how to start taking POPs.**

    There are a few different ways to start the first pack of POPs. Each way has something good about it. Your health care setting may use one way for all of your patients. Or the medical provider may decide which way will work best for each patient. Here are some ways to start POPs. Talk to your patient only about the way or ways you do it at your health care setting.

    - **You can start on the first day of your period.**

    - **If you are sure you are not pregnant, you can start any other day of the month.** If the day you start is not the first day of your period, you must use a second method, like the condom, along with POPs. Use this second method for 1 month after you start taking POPs.

    - **You can start right after childbirth, a miscarriage, or an abortion.**

> **Tell your patients about a back-up method.**
>
> For the first month they are using POPs, they should use a second method, like condoms. They should use it until they finish their first pack. It is not always easy to remember to take a pill *at the same time* every day. It takes time to get used to it.

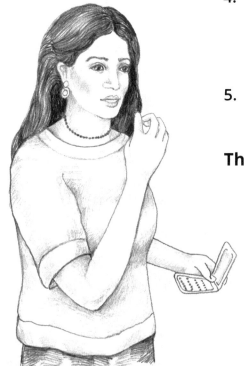

4. **Take 1 pill at the same time every day until the pack of pills is finished.**

    With POPs, if you don't take POPs *at the same time* every day, you may not be protected from pregnancy.

5. **Start a new pack of POPs the next day.**

    Do *not* skip any days between packs.

Things to remember when you use POPs

- Be sure to take your POPs *at the same time* every day. It may help to think of something you do at the same time every day. For example, you could take it when you brush your teeth, eat a meal, or go to bed.

- There are no "days off" when you use POPs. You must take a pill *every* day.

- Use a second birth control method until you get in the habit of taking the pill on time every day.

▶ If you see a doctor for any reason, tell the doctor you are taking POPs.

▶ If you miss one or more POPs, follow the provider's advice.

What will your periods be like when you are on POPs?

Most patients are curious about what to expect with their periods when they are on POPs. Here's what you can say.

▶ Your periods will probably be lighter and less regular.

▶ It is common to have light bleeding (spotting) between periods.

▶ Your periods may be less crampy.

▶ Some users skip one or more periods.

▶ Some users stop having periods while they are on POPs.

▶ Your periods will return to normal quickly once you stop using POPs.

Note: If you miss one or two periods after many months of regular periods, take a pregnancy test. There is a chance you could be pregnant.

What if you forget to take your POPs?

Teach your patients these steps so they will know what to do if they forget to take one or more POPs. Your provider's advice may differ from the advice given here. Be sure to give your patients the advice used at your health care site.

You need to take your POPs at the same time each day. But sometimes you may forget. Remember that if you are even 3 hours late in taking POPs, you have a greater chance of getting pregnant.

If you miss taking 1 pill on time, follow these steps:

▶ Take your missed POPs as soon as you remember it.

▶ Take your next POPs at your regular time — even if that means taking 2 pills in 1 day.

▶ If you are even 3 hours late taking your POPs, use a second birth control method, like condoms, withdrawal, spermicides or abstaining from reproductive sex, for the next 2 days to help protect you from pregnancy.

▶ Call the provider right away to ask about Emergency Contraception (EC).

If you miss 2 or more pills in a row follow these steps:

▶ Take your pill as soon as you can.

▶ Use EC as soon as you can. If you don't have any EC pills, you can get them from your provider or at a drug store.

▶ Use a second method of birth control like condoms, for 2 days.

▶ You may also need a pregnancy test if you had unprotected sex during those days that you missed your pills.

Important

If you miss any pills and have had sex within the past 5 days:

- Call the provider right away to ask about Emergency Contraception (EC). Or visit this website: **cecinfo.org** to learn more.

- It is important to ask about EC if you were even 3 hours late in taking your POPs.

- Follow the advice you are given about getting back on schedule with your POPs.

Get a pregnancy test if you don't get your period in the next 4 to 6 weeks.

Are there any side effects?

POPs are incredibly safe however some users have minor side effects when using POPs. Encourage your patients to talk to a health care provider if the side effects bother them. Here are some possible side effects to tell your patients about.

▶ **Changes in menstrual bleeding**

You may miss periods. You may also spot or bleed between periods. This is the most common side effect of POPs.

▶ **Other side effects**

Other side effects are rare, but may include headaches, nausea, mood changes and breast tenderness.

POPs and Weight Concerns

Q. Do POPs cause weight gain?

A. No.

Q. If someone is overweight, will POPs still work?

A. Most of the time, yes.

Q. Are there medical problems if someone is overweight and using POPs?

A. There could be. A patient should talk to their provider about the risk of blood clots, heart attack, or stroke while using POPs.

Research shows that POPs do not cause weight gain. Most people gain weight over time whether they take POPs or not, especially teens and young adults who are still growing.

What about complications and warning signs?

Serious complications are very rare with POPs. But here are some warning signs you should know about:

- ▸ **Abdominal pain.** Call your health care provider right away. It could be an ovarian cyst or a pregnancy outside of the uterus (an ectopic pregnancy).

- ▸ **Repeated, very severe headaches.** A severe headache or a headache that just doesn't go away can be a reaction to the progestin.

If you have any of these signs, call the provider right away or go to the emergency room.

POPs have not been shown to increase the risk of cancer, blood clots, stroke, or heart attack. Even so, some drug company inserts for the POPs may list these estrogen-related risks. Check with your provider about how to discuss this with patients.

Are there any precautions?

A health care provider may advise you to use a different method if any of the following is true:

- ▸ You have ever had breast cancer.
- ▸ You have unexplained bleeding from the vagina.
- ▸ You have liver disease.
- ▸ You have an intestinal problem that might keep POPs from working for you.
- ▸ You are taking medications that may keep POPs from working well.

Breastfeeding

Those who breastfeed can start using POPs right after childbirth.

The health care provider will talk with you about your health to make sure that there is no reason for you not to use POPs.

What are the advantages and disadvantages of POPs?

There are many things people like about taking POPs. And there are some things they don't like. Find out what your patient likes and encourage them to focus on those things.

What some people like about POPs:

▸ POPs are good at preventing pregnancy.

▸ POPs make periods very light and less crampy.

▸ It does not interrupt having sex.

▸ Those who can't take the combined pill because of the estrogen can use POPs.

▸ Those who are breastfeeding can use POPs.

▸ It does not cause serious health problems in most users.

Find out what your patient might not like about taking POPs.

Ask your patients if they have any concerns about using POPs. Then talk to them about their concerns. Help them think through how to solve any problems they might have while using POPs. Try to get them to come up with their own solutions first. Read the chart that follows for some ideas on how to deal with concerns. Keep in mind that POPs aren't the best method for everyone. It is the patient's choice.

POPs: Some Problems and Ways to Solve Them

Problem	Ways to Solve the Problem
It is hard for me to get to my appointment.	Perhaps your partner, family member, or friend could bring you.
I don't want to have an exam.	You may not need an exam. But if you do, it may help to know that an exam is a key part of keeping you healthy. Regular exams can help find things before they become a problem. Ask your patient what troubles them about getting an exam. Perhaps they don't know what to expect. It may help if you explain it to them.
I have to remember to take it at the same time every day.	▶ Think of something else you do at about the same time each day, like brushing your teeth or eating a meal. You could plan to take your POPs at that same time. ▶ You could set a watch or cell phone alarm to remind you when to take your POPs. ▶ Your partner can help remind you to take your POPs. If you do forget to take your POPs, be sure to use a second method of birth control. Follow instructions for getting back on schedule with your POPs.
What if I have sex around the time I forget to take my POPs?	Call the provider for advice. You can still try to prevent pregnancy after sex. Find out about EC pills.

POPs: Some Problems and Ways to Solve Them

Problem	Ways to Solve the Problem
I may get side effects.	If your side effects continue to bother you, talk to a health care provider.
I could get a serious complication.	Serious problems are **very** rare for those who are healthy when they start taking POPs. ▶ **Before** you start POPs, talk to your health care provider about any health problems you have. ▶ Call your health care provider right away if you have any of the warning signs.
POPs do not protect against HIV and other STIs.	When you are using POPs, also use condoms every time you have sex to help protect against STIs.

What if you want to stop using POPs?

You can stop using POPs whenever you would like. If you stop using them, you could become pregnant right away. Use another birth control method if you don't want to be pregnant.

There are no health problems to watch for when you stop this method.

Make sure your patient understands.

Before your patients leave, make sure they understand how to use POPs successfully. Here are some things you can ask to make sure they understand.

- ▸ Tell me what you know about POPs.
- ▸ How does POPs work?
- ▸ When will you start your first pack?
- ▸ What time will you take your POPs each day?
- ▸ What will help you remember to take it at that time?
- ▸ What will you do if you are late taking POPs?
- ▸ What will you do if you miss two or more POPs in a row?
- ▸ What might be the most difficult problem for you when using POPs?
- ▸ How would you solve that problem?

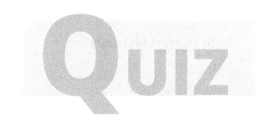

POPs

Directions. Read each of the following statements.
Is it true or false? Circle the best answer.

1. There are no sugar pills (placebos)   True   False
   in the pack of POPs.

2. POPs work mostly by making the cervical   True   False
   mucus thick and sticky.

3. It is okay if a user doesn't take the   True   False
   progestin-only pill at the same time
   each day.

4. A user should take 7 days off between   True   False
   their POP packs.

5. If a user is even 3 hours late taking a   True   False
   progestin-only pill, they have a greater
   chance of getting pregnant.

Directions. Read each of the following and write your best answer
in the spaces below.

6. List two possible side effects of using POPs.

   ▪ _____

     _____

   ▪ _____

     _____

Go on to the next page.

7. List two things some people like about using POPs.

   ▪ _____

   _____

   ▪ _____

   _____

8. List one concern that a patient may have about using POPs and what you might say to help them deal with that concern.

   Patient's concern:

   ▪ _____

   _____

   What you can say:

   ▪ _____

   _____

   Check your answers on the next page.

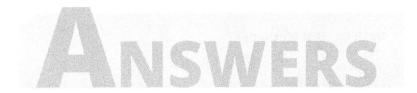

POPs

Check your answers.

1. **True**   There are no sugar pills (placebos) in the
POPs pack.

2. **True**   POPs do work mostly by making the cervical mucus
thick and sticky.

3. **False**   Patients must take their POP at the same time each
day. If they don't take it at the same time each day,
they could get pregnant.

4. **False**   A user should not take 7 days off between their
POP packs. If they skip **any** days between packs,
they could get pregnant.

5. **True**   If a user is even 3 hours late taking POP, they do
have a greater chance of getting pregnant.

6. Possible side effects of using POPs include:
   - Missed periods
   - Spotting or bleeding between periods
   - Mood changes, headaches, nausea, breast tenderness

7. Things that some people like about POPs include:
   - It is very good at preventing pregnancy.
   - It does not interrupt having sex.
   - It makes periods lighter and less crampy.
   - Those who can't take the combined pill
because of the estrogen can use POPs.
   - You can breastfeed while using POPs.
   - It does not cause serious health problems
in most users.

8. Here are two concerns a patient might have about using POPs and what you might say to help them. For other possible concerns and responses, please see "The POPs: Some Problems and Ways to Solve Them" chart near the end of POPs section.

- *Patient's concern.* "I have to remember to take it at the same time every day."

  What you could say. "Think of something you do at about the same time each day, like brushing your teeth or eating a meal. You could plan to take your pill at that same time. Or you could set a watch or cell phone alarm to remind you when to take your pill."

- *Patient's concern.* "I'm afraid of getting pregnant if I forget to take a pill on time and have sex."

  What you could say. "Always try to take your pill on time. But if you forget and have sex, call us for advice. You can still prevent pregnancy after sex. Find out about Emergency Contraception."

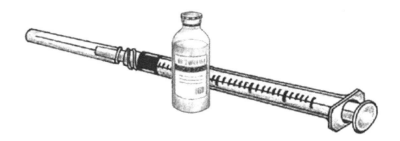

Birth Control Shot

This section is mostly written as though you were talking to your patients. It gives you an idea of how to explain the birth control shot in a way your patients can understand. This section also has notes written directly to you, the health worker. Those "health worker notes" look like this one.

What is it?

The birth control shot is a shot that you get every 12 weeks to keep from getting pregnant. The shot has one hormone in it to make it work. That hormone is progestin. The shot has no estrogen in it. That means that those who cannot take estrogen for some reason can use this shot.

The shot works well to prevent pregnancy. But it does not protect you against HIV or other STIs. Use condoms every time you have sex to help protect against these STIs.

How does it work?

The shot works mostly by keeping the egg from leaving the ovaries. If there is no egg to meet with sperm, you can't get pregnant. The shot may also:

> Keep the mucus of the cervix thick. This helps keep sperm from getting into the uterus to meet an egg.

Other terms for the Shot

The shot is also called:

- Depo-Provera
- Depo
- DMPA

How well does the Shot work?

When you talk to your patients, you will need to explain how well the shot works (how effective it is). Be sure to explain the difference between "perfect use" and "typical use." You can read more about this in the "Stage 3" section of Chapter 2.

With perfect use, the shot is 99.8% effective.

This means that if 100 patients use the shot exactly the right way, only 1 (and probably none) of them may get pregnant in a year.

With typical use, the shot is 96% effective.

For those who don't always use the shot exactly the right way, 4 out of 100 may get pregnant in a year.

Talk to your patients about Emergency Contraception.

Emergency Contraception (EC), in the form of EC pills or an IUD, can prevent pregnancy after sex. Patients can use EC up to 5 days after unprotected sex. Read more about it in the section on EC.

How do you use the Shot?

Teach your patients these steps so they can use the shot the right way. Your advice may need to differ from the advice given here. Be sure to give your patients the advice used in your health care setting.

1. **Talk to a health care provider about whether the shot is right for you.**

   The health care provider will ask you some questions. Talk to the provider about:

   ▸ Any health problems you may have

   ▸ Any medicine you may be taking

   ▸ Any questions you may have

Your health care provider will help you decide if the shot is right for you. If the shot is right for you, you can schedule a time for your first shot. Often you can get your first shot that very same day.

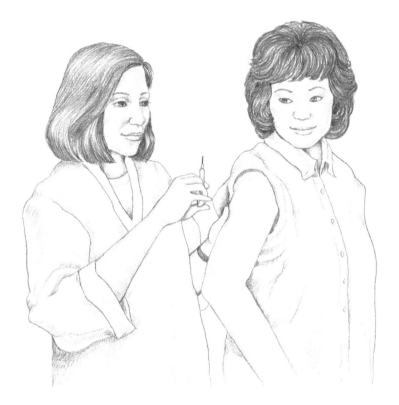

2. **Get your first shot.**

    You will need to come to the health care site for your shot. You will get the shot in your arm or hip. If you get your first shot during the first 5 days of your period, the shot starts preventing pregnancy right away. If you get your first shot at another time, you will need to use a second method of birth control method, like condoms, for 7 days after you get your first shot.

3. **Make an appointment for your next shot. Or set a reminder on your phone to make an appointment 2 or 3 weeks before your next shot is due.**

    To prevent pregnancy, you must get your shots on time. After your first shot, come back to the health care site every 12 weeks for another shot.

4. **If you see a doctor for any reason, tell the doctor that you are using the shot.**

If they forget...

- Be sure to tell your patients what to do if they forget to get their shot on time.

- Give them easy-to-read written materials about this to take home.

- Ask your patients what second method they would use for back-up if they needed one.

What if you are late getting a shot?

The Shot keeps working.

It's good to know that even if your patient is late for their shot, the shot keeps working for as long as 16 weeks. This gives them a "grace period" to get back for their next shot.

If you forget to get your shot on time, you could get pregnant. Follow these steps:

- ▸ Call us right away to make an appointment for your shot.

- ▸ If you had sex since your shot was due, ask about Emergency Contraception (EC). Or visit this website: **cecinfo.org** to learn more.

- ▸ Use a second method of birth control, like condoms, from the day you were due for your next shot until 7 days after you get your next shot.

Are there any side effects?

All users have one or more side effects with the shot. Your patients can talk to a provider if their side effects really bother them. Here is what you could say to your patients about possible side effects.

Changes in periods

At first, all those who use the shot have changes in their periods:

- ▸ You may not know when you will have your period.

- ▸ You may have spotting between periods. For most users, this lessens over time.

- ▸ You may have longer or shorter periods.

- ▸ They may have no periods at all after the first few weeks or months.

After using the shot for 12 months, some users stop having periods. Your periods will return to normal within 6-12 months after the last shot wears off.

Other common side effects

Some who use the shot may get one or more of these side effects:

- Weight gain (usually 5 pounds or less)
- Depression
- Headaches
- Nervousness
- Changes in sex drive
- Sore breasts

Some of these side effects may not go away until the shot wears off. It can take 3 to 4 months for the side effects to go away after you stop getting the shot.

If you have any problems, talk to a health care provider. There may be something that can be done to help. But you may have to wait until the shot wears off.

Bone density loss

While someone is using the shot, they may temporarily lose a small amount of bone density. This is because the shot temporarily turns the ovaries off, so they don't make estrogen. (This is like what happens during breastfeeding.) This is temporary and is not associated with any long-term effects. The shot is considered safe for most people of any age for as long as they chose to use it.

The Shot and Weight Gain

Make sure you talk about weight gain with your patients who are thinking about using the shot.

Research shows that the Depo shot can cause weight gain in a few users (approximately 15%) and some can gain quite a bit of weight.

If someone gains more than 5% of their body weight after the first one or two shots, they will likely keep on gaining weight as long as they are on the Shot.

Tell your patient to let the provider know if they gain 5 or more pounds in the first few months they are on the shot. They may want to use another method.

However, also tell them that it does not cause any weight gain in most (**85% do not gain weight while using the shot**). And, most people gain weight over time whether they use the shot or not, especially teens and young adults who are still growing.

355

A delay in getting pregnant

> Be sure to tell your patients that there may be a delay of up to a 18 months in getting pregnant after they quit using the shot.

You should be aware that you will not be able to get pregnant right away after you get your last shot.

- ▶ Some patients who use Depo may be able to get pregnant as soon as their last shot wears off (about 3 months).

- ▶ Others can take as long as 18 months.

What about complications and warning signs?

Serious problems are **very rare** with the shot. But here are some possible problems you should know about:

- ▶ **Heavy bleeding**

  This means heavy, bright red bleeding that fills a super maxi-pad in less than an hour. You may also feel faint or lightheaded. This is rare. But if it happens to you, call the provider right away or go to the Emergency Room.

  Be aware that bleeding that is dark red or brownish and usually not as heavy as a period is common when you first start using the shot. It is not a complication or warning sign.

- ▶ **Abdominal pain**

  Call your health care provider right away. It could be an ovarian cyst or a pregnancy outside of the uterus (an ectopic pregnancy).

- ▶ **Severe headache**

  A severe headache or a headache that just doesn't go away can be a reaction to the progestin. If you have this warning sign, call the provider right away.

- ▶ **Infection**

  Some users get an infection at the place on their arm or hip where they got the shot. Signs of infection include redness, swelling, heat, and tenderness. It may look like a large pimple. If you get this warning sign, call the provider right away.

> The shot has not been shown to increase the risk of cancer, blood clots, stroke, or heart attack. Even so, some drug company inserts for the shot may list these estrogen-related risks. Check with your provider about how to discuss this with patients.

Are there any precautions to using the Shot?

A health care provider may advise you to use a different method if any of the following is true:

- ▶ You have had breast cancer.
- ▶ You have liver disease.
- ▶ You have irregular bleeding from the vagina for no known reason.

The health care provider will talk with you about your health to make sure that there is no reason for you not to use the shot.

Breastfeeding

Those who breastfeed can use the shot, but they may have to wait awhile after childbirth. A provider can tell the patient how long they would have to wait.

What are the advantages and disadvantages of using the Shot?

There are many things people like about using the shot. And there are some things they don't like. Find out what your patient likes and encourage them to focus on those things.

What some people like about the shot:

- ▶ It is easy to use and lasts for 12 weeks.
- ▶ It is very good at preventing pregnancy.
- ▶ It may help prevent some health problems, like ovarian cancer and cancer of the lining of the uterus.
- ▶ Periods are lighter and less crampy.
- ▶ Some users like not having a period.

- ▶ It can be used by those who can't take estrogen.
- ▶ Using it doesn't interrupt sex.
- ▶ It may decrease symptoms from some health problems like uterine fibroids, endometriosis, painful periods and sickle cell anemia.
- ▶ It's private.

Find out what your patient might not like about using the shot.

Ask your patients if they have any concerns about using the shot. Then talk to them about their concerns. Help them think through how to solve any problems they might have while using the shot. Try to get them to come up with their own solutions first. Read the chart that follows for some ideas on how to deal with concerns.

Keep in mind that the shot isn't the best method for everyone. It is the patient's choice.

The Shot: Some Problems and Ways to Solve Them

Problem	Ways to Solve the Problem
I don't like getting shots.	You may be able to get used to getting shots. If not, you may want to choose another method.
I don't want to have an exam.	You may not need an exam. But if you do, it may help to know that an exam is a key part of keeping you healthy. Regular exams can help find things before they become a problem. Ask your patient what troubles them about getting an exam. Perhaps they don't know what to expect. It may help if you explain it to them.
It's hard for me to get to my appointment.	▶ Perhaps your partner or a friend can bring you to the health care site. ▶ Make your appointment early so you can schedule a time that works best for you.
I have to remember to go to the health care site every 12 weeks for a shot.	▶ Each time you get a shot, make an appointment for your next shot. Write it down. ▶ Find a way that will help you remember. It might help to put it on a calendar. ▶ Your partner can remind you.
I may get some side effects.	Some side effects will go away with time. But some won't. If your side effects bother you, talk to your health care provider.

The Shot: Some Problems and Ways to Solve Them

Problem	Ways to Solve the Problem
It would really bother me if the spotting kept going on and on.	In most people, there will be less spotting over time. But there is no way to know how long the spotting might go on for you. If that would bother you, the shot may not be the best method for you.
I want to have a period every month.	If having a period every month is important to you, the shot may not be the best method for you.
It can take a long time to get pregnant if I want to.	If you think you will want to get pregnant soon after stopping your method of birth control, the shot may not be the best method for you.
I could get a serious complication.	Serious problems are very rare with the shot. If you are ever worried about something you think is not normal, call the provider for advice.
What if I forget to get my shot on time and have sex?	Call the provider for advice. You may still try to prevent pregnancy after sex by taking emergency contraception.
The shot does not protect me from HIV and other STIs.	Use condoms every time you have sex to help protect against STIs.

What if you want to stop using the Shot?

You can stop using the shot whenever you would like to. But once you get a shot, you have to wait 3 months for it to wear off. Once you skip a shot, you could get pregnant if you don't use another birth control method.

There are no health problems to watch for when you stop this method.

Make sure your patient understands.

Before your patients leave, make sure they understand how to use the shot successfully. Here are some things you can ask to make sure they understand.

- ▶ Tell me what you know about the shot.
- ▶ How does the shot work?
- ▶ When will you get your first shot? Your second shot?
- ▶ What will help you remember to come in for your shot?
- ▶ What will you do if you forget to get your shot?
- ▶ What might be the most difficult problem for you when using the shot?
- ▶ How would you solve that problem?
- ▶ What warning signs will you look for while you are using the shot?

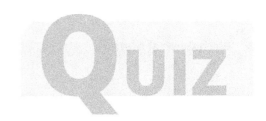

BIRTH CONTROL SHOT

Directions. Circle the best answer.

1. What is the best time for a patient to get their first Birth Control Shot?
   a. After their period ends
   b. When they ovulates
   c. During the first 5 days of their period
   d. Just before their next period

2. How long does each Shot work to prevent pregnancy?
   a. 12 weeks
   b. 20 weeks
   c. 24 weeks
   d. None of the above

3. Many patients who use the Shot for one year:
   a. Gain 20 to 30 pounds
   b. Stop having a period
   c. Become pregnant
   d. Become infertile

4. Which of the following can be a complication of using the Shot?
   a. Heavy bleeding
   b. Stroke
   c. Blood clots
   d. Toxic Shock Syndrome

Go on to the next page.

5. Which of the following is something that some patients like about using the Shot?

   a. It is easy to use.

   b. It is very good at preventing pregnancy.

   c. Periods are lighter and less crampy.

   d. All of the above

Directions. Read each of the following and write your best answer in the spaces below.

6. What is the main thing the Shot does to prevent pregnancy?

   _____

   _____

   _____

   _____

7. List one concern that a patient may have about using the Shot and what you might say to help them deal with that concern.

   - *Patient's concern:*

   _____

   _____

   - *What you can say:*

   _____

   _____

Check your answers on the next page.

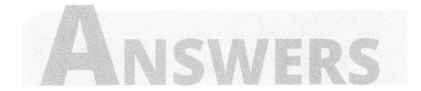

ANSWERS

BIRTH CONTROL SHOT

Check your answers.

1. **C**   The best time for a patient to get their first birth control shot is during the first 5 days of their menstrual period.

2. **A**   Each shot works to prevent pregnancy for 12 weeks.

3. **B**   Many but not all who use the shot for one year stop having a period.

4. **A**   One possible (but rare) complication of using the shot is heavy bleeding. This means heavy, bright red bleeding that fills a super maxi-pad in less than an hour.

5. **D**   All of the above. These are all things that some users like about the Shot:
    - It is easy to use.
    - It is very good at preventing pregnancy.
    - Periods are lighter and less crampy.

    Other things some users like about the Shot include:
    - It lasts for 12 weeks.
    - Using it doesn't interrupt sex.
    - It may help prevent some health problems, like ovarian cancer and cancer of the lining of the uterus.
    - Periods may stop after one year and some people like not having a period.
    - Those who can't take estrogen may be able to use it.

Go on to the next page.

6. The Shot mainly prevents pregnancy by keeping the egg from leaving the ovaries. The Shot may also:
   - Make the mucus of the cervix thick.

7. Here are two concerns a patient might have about using the Shot and what you might say to help. For other possible concerns and responses, please see "The Shot: Some Problems and Ways to Solve Them" chart near the end of the Birth Control Shot section.

   - *Patient's concern.* "I don't like getting shots."

     What you could say. "You may be able to get used to getting shots. If not, you may want to choose another method."

   - *Patient's concern.* "It could be hard to remember to go to the health care site every 12 weeks for a shot."

     What you could say. "What are some things you think you could do to help you remember?" You could offer these suggestions:
     - Each time you get a shot, make an appointment for your next shot. And write it down.
     - Add an alarm on your phone or download an app with reminder notifications.
     - Your partner can help you remember.

Tier Two or Three: Information-Based Methods

This section is about birth control methods that use only the patient's knowledge about their body and about how pregnancy can happen. That is why they are called "information-based methods." They include:

- Abstinence (not having reproductive sex)
- Fertility Awareness-Based (FAB) Methods
- Withdrawal
- Lactation Amenorrhea Method (LAM)

These methods are safe, basically free, and work well to prevent pregnancy. But they are often not mentioned to patients. We encourage you to make sure your patients know about these options.

Patients may want to use these methods at different times of their lives. For example:

- A young teen may choose abstinence until they are ready for sex.
- A couple may choose Fertility Awareness (not having sex during the fertile days) to prevent pregnancy until they feel ready to have a child.
- Someone who knows how to use withdrawal can use it at any time to prevent pregnancy. They may choose to use withdrawal when there is no other method to use or use as a back-up method. They may also use withdrawal with other birth control methods to be extra sure to avoid an unintended pregnancy.
- Someone who is breastfeeding can use the Lactation Amenorrhea Method (LAM) for up to 6 months after the baby is born. This gives them time to think about other birth control methods they would like to use later.

Topics in this section

▸ Abstinence

▸ Fertility Awareness-Based (FAB) Methods

▸ Withdrawal

▸ Lactation Amenorrhea Method (LAM)

Objectives

After reading this section, you will be able to:

▸ Explain how the different information-based methods work to prevent pregnancy.

▸ Describe the advantages and disadvantages of these methods.

▸ Discuss any side effects and complications of each method.

▸ Tell how well each method works to prevent pregnancy.

Some words you may need to know

Words	Description
Abstinence	Not having reproductive sex (abstaining)
Vaginal sex	Having sex with the penis in the vagina (also called reproductive sex)
Anal sex	Having sex with the penis in the anus
Withdrawal	A birth control method in which the penis is pulled out of the vagina or anus before ejaculation ("coming")
Ovulation	When the egg leaves an ovary
Fertile mucus	A mucus that helps keep sperm alive. This mucus is made by the cervix around the time that an egg leaves an ovary.
Lactation	Breastfeeding/Chestfeeding

Abstinence

Abstinence means to *not* have sex. The problem with this is that there are many definitions for the word "sex." For some people, "sex" only means when a penis enters a vagina (**"vaginal sex" or "vaginal intercourse"**). For others, "sex" may mean any contact between one person and another person's penis, vagina, mouth, or anus.

When talking about preventing pregnancy, **abstinence is when partners choose not to put the penis in or near the vagina or anus. In other words, they are choosing not to have reproductive sex or sex that may cause a pregnancy.**

Make sure your patients understand that vaginal sex is **not** the only way a person can get pregnant. A person who ovulates can get pregnant by doing *anything* that lets sperm get near the opening of their vagina. This includes *anal sex*, which is when a penis enters an anus. It also includes ejaculating ("coming") **near** the vagina, anus, or thigh.

There are many forms of sexual pleasure partners using abstinence can enjoy. Make sure your patients understand this as well. You can ask your patients if they can think of other ways to enjoy each other if they choose abstinence.

What is Abstinence?

Abstinence means to *not* have sex. But "sex" means something different to different people. When talking about *preventing pregnancy*:

> **Abstinence is when partners choose not to put the penis in or near the vagina or anus or not to have reproductive sex.**

This kind of abstinence can prevent pregnancy. And it can lower the chances of getting HIV or other STIs. But if you and your partner have other kinds of close sexual contact, like oral sex or touching each other's penis or vagina, you can still spread an STI. When talking about *preventing STIs:*

> **Abstinence is when partners choose not to have sex of any kind using the vagina, anus, penis, or mouth.**

To help protect yourself from STIs, use a condom whenever you have sex of any kind using the vagina, anus, penis, or mouth.

How does your patient define "Abstinence"?

Be sure to ask your patients what abstinence means to them.

Make sure they understand which types of sex can cause a pregnancy and which cannot.

If patients want to use abstinence, ask them these questions:

- What do you mean when you say that you choose not to have sex?

- If you want to prevent pregnancy, what **can** you do with your partner sexually?

- If you decide to stop using abstinence and have sex, what is your backup plan? What will you do to prevent pregnancy?

Why do people choose Abstinence?

People choose abstinence for many personal, religious, and practical reasons. Maybe:

▸ You don't have another birth control method at the time.

▸ You don't feel ready for sex at the time.

▸ You want to wait to have sex until a certain age or relationship status or you get married.

▸ You are worried about pregnancy or getting an STI.

▸ You feel it is important to follow your personal or religious beliefs.

Everyone has the right to choose when they do or don't want to have sex. You need to make choices that are right for you. Some people choose not to have sex (to abstain) for a certain time or for specific reasons. Others choose to abstain from sex their whole lives.

You can still express yourself sexually when you choose not to have sex with the penis, anus, or vagina. Some of these ways are:

▸ Holding hands

▸ Flirting

▸ Touching other parts of your partner's body

▸ Kissing

▸ Massage

▸ Sharing fantasies

How does Abstinence work?

Here is one way to explain to your patient how abstinence works.

For a person to get pregnant, a sperm must meet with an egg.

About the time the egg leaves the ovary (**ovulation**), the body makes what is called **fertile mucus.** This mucus helps keep sperm alive. It also helps the sperm get to the egg. This mucus is made by the cervix and flows out of the vagina. That means this mucus can also be found just outside the vagina and near the anus. So, when there is fertile mucus:

▸ If ejaculate ("come") is anywhere *near* a vagina or anus, sperm can swim into the fertile mucus and travel up the vagina. This may cause a pregnancy.

▸ If ejaculation does not happen anywhere near a vagina or anus, it *cannot* cause a pregnancy.

So, if the penis is not placed in or near the vagina or anus and there is no ejaculation, it cannot cause a pregnancy.

How well does Abstinence work?

When you talk to your patients, you will need to explain how well abstinence works (how effective it is). Be sure to explain the difference between "perfect use" and "typical use." You can read more about this in the "Stage 3 of a Patient Education Session" covered in Chapter 2.

Abstinence is the only method that can always work to prevent pregnancy. Of course, this is only true when "abstinence" means doing nothing that lets sperm get near a vagina.

With perfect use, abstinence is 100% effective.

This means that if 100 people do not have any reproductive sex at all, none of the them will get pregnant in a year.

With typical use, no one is sure.

Talk to your patients about

Emergency Contraception (EC), in the form of EC pills or an IUD, can prevent pregnancy after sex. Patients can take EC up to 5 days after unprotected sex. Read more about EC at the end of this chapter.

How do you use Abstinence?

If you choose to prevent pregnancy by *not* having sex, you can't do anything that lets sperm anywhere in or near the opening of the vagina or anus.

Choosing not to have sex isn't always easy. It is important that you know what you really want to do:

▸ Define what abstinence means to you.

▸ Decide if you want any kind of sexual activity.

▸ Decide what kind of sexual activity you do and don't want to do.

You will want to:

▸ Know and understand why you have made the choice not to have reproductive sex.

▸ Talk to your partner about what you want and don't want. Ask your partner what they want.

▸ Make a decision about what kinds of things are right for both of you. If you don't both agree, one of you might pressure the other into having sex.

Here are a few suggestions on talking about sex with your partner:

▸ First, write down your thoughts and feelings. This can help you think about them very carefully. You may want to share these feelings with your partner.

▸ Talk about what you want *before* being sexual with your partner.

▸ Bring up the subject by talking about a romantic movie you saw and talk about your feelings.

▸ Talk about sex in a general way. Then talk about what you think and feel.

Here are some things that can help you use abstinence:

▸ Be careful about using alcohol and other drugs. They can affect your judgment. This might make it hard for you to not have sex.

▸ Think about (and talk about) other forms of sexual pleasure the two of you can enjoy.

▸ Stay out of situations that might be hard to handle.

Breastfeeding

Those who are breastfeeding can use abstinence as their birth control method.

▸ If you are finding it hard *not* to have sex, think about the long-term effects of having sex. What would it be like to have a baby before you are ready? How would having sex change your relationship? How might you feel about yourself?

▸ Learn about effective birth control methods as back-up methods to abstinence. If or when you decide to have sex, you can still avoid pregnancy and STIs.

Are there any side effects, complications, or precautions?

Abstinence is safe for anyone. It causes no side effects or health problems. Some people say that if someone who is sexually aroused doesn't have sex, it can harm them. This is *not* true.

What are the advantages and disadvantages of using Abstinence?

There are many things people like about choosing abstinence. And there are some things they don't like. Find out what your patients like. Encourage them to focus on those things.

What some people like about abstinence:

▸ It is free.

▸ It causes no harmful side effects or health problems.

▸ It always works to prevent pregnancy when used correctly.

▸ A couple can still enjoy each other sexually in ways that can't cause a pregnancy.

▸ It can lower the chances of getting STIs.

Find out what your patients might not like about choosing abstinence.

Ask your patients if they have any concerns about using abstinence. Then talk to them about their concerns. Help them think through how to solve any problems they might have while using abstinence. Try to get them to come up with their own solutions first. Read the chart that follows for some ideas on how to deal with concerns.

Keep in mind that abstinence isn't the best method for everyone. It is the patient's choice.

Abstinence: Some Problems and Ways to Solve Them

Problem	Ways to Solve the Problem
Abstinence can be sexually frustrating.	Know that you can express yourself sexually without having vaginal or anal (reproductive) sex. You can find other ways of sexually pleasuring each other.
My partner really puts a lot of pressure on me to have vaginal sex.	It is your choice whether or not to have vaginal sex. Explain to your partner why it is important for you to abstain from vaginal sex.
What if we get caught up in the moment?	You can still stop at any time. But, in case you don't stop, always have a back-up method of birth control, like condoms, on hand. If you change your mind and want to have sex, use that back-up method.
My partner thinks I don't love them because I've decided not to have vaginal or anal sex.	Talk to your partner about how you really feel. You can show your love for your partner in other ways. And, for more intimate connection, you can still use your hands or mouth to pleasure each others bodies and your own.
We go out drinking every weekend. I'm worried that when we drink and get turned on, we might have sex.	It is a good idea to limit the amount of drugs or alcohol you use. Alcohol and drugs make it hard to abstain. They also make it hard to use other kinds of birth control methods correctly.
I've already had sex with my partner. Can I still use this as a method?	You can choose *not* to have sex anytime. Just because you've had sex before doesn't mean you have to keep having it if you don't think it is the best choice for you.
What if we end up having reproductive sex after all?	Call the provider for advice. You can still try to prevent pregnancy after sex. Find out about EC.
Abstinence to prevent pregnancy isn't the same as abstinence to prevent HIV and other STIs. How do I protect myself?	You can use abstinence to protect yourself from STIS, too. Do not have sex with the penis, vagina, anus or mouth. If you do have sex using the vagina, penis, anus, or mouth, use a condom or another barrier like dental dams every time.

What if you want to stop using this method?

You can stop using abstinence whenever you want to. But if you stop using it (have reproductive sex) you could become pregnant right away. Use another birth control method if you don't want to be pregnant.

There are no health problems to watch for when you stop this method.

Make sure your patient understands.

Before your patients leave, make sure they understand how to use abstinence successfully. Here are some things you can ask to make sure they understand.

- Tell me what you know about abstinence.
- Does abstinence mean you have to avoid all intimacy or pleasure with a partner?
- How does abstinence work?
- What do you like about abstinence?
- What don't you like about abstinence?
- What might be the most difficult problem for you when using abstinence?
- How would you solve that problem?

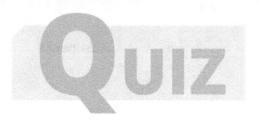

ABSTINENCE

*Directions: Read each of the following statements.
Is it true or false? Circle the best answer.*

1. There is only one definition for the
   word "sex."   **True   False**

2. One definition of using abstinence for   **True   False**
   pregnancy prevention is: "When partners
   choose not to put the penis in or near the
   vagina or anus."

3. Partners using abstinence can enjoy   **True   False**
   many forms of sexual pleasure.

4. There are some types of sex that can't   **True   False**
   get you pregnant but can spread sexually
   transmitted infections (STIs).

5. If ejaculate is near the vagina, but not in the   **True   False**
   vagina, a pregnancy cannot happen.

Directions: Circle <u>all</u> the answers that apply.

6. Which of the following can patients do to help them
   successfully use abstinence?

   a. Drink alcohol.

   b. Talk with their partner about other forms of sexual
      pleasure the two of them can enjoy.

   c. Stay out of situations that might be hard to handle.

   d. If they are starting to get caught up in the moment,
      think about the long-term effects of having unprotected
      reproductive sex.

   e. Do drugs.

Go on to the next page.

Directions: *Write your best answer to each of the following.*

7. List two things some people like about abstinence.

    ▪ _____

    ▪ _____

8. List one concern that patients may have about using abstinence. What could you say to help them deal with that concern?

    _____

    _____

    _____

Check your answers on the next page.

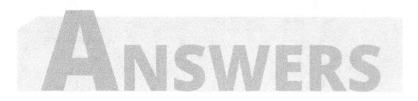

ABSTINENCE

Check your answers.

1. **False**   There are *many* definitions for the word "sex."
For some people, sex means vaginal intercourse
only. For others, sex may mean any contact
between one person and another person's penis,
vagina, or anus. Some might think that deep kissing
(French kissing) is sex.

2. **True**   One definition of abstinence for pregnancy
prevention is: "When partners choose not to put the
penis in or near the vagina or anus." A pregnancy
can happen if any sperm get *near* the opening of a
vagina.

3. **True**   Partners using abstinence can enjoy many
forms of sexual pleasure.

4. **True**   There are some types of sex that can't get you
pregnant but can spread STIs. Sex with the mouth
(oral sex) or even touching each other's penis,
vagina, or anus, can spread some STIs.

5. **False**   If ejaculate is anywhere *near* a vagina or anus,
pregnancy can happen. This is because fertile
mucus, the type of mucus that keeps sperm alive,
can be outside the vagina. If sperm touch the fertile
mucus, they can travel up the vagina, into the
uterus and fallopian tubes and fertilize an egg. The
fertilized egg may travel to the uterus and implant
causing a pregnancy.

Go on to the next page.

6. **B, C, D**   These are things patients can do to help them successfully use abstinence:

   - Talk with their partner about other forms of sexual pleasure the two of them can enjoy.
   - Stay out of situations that might be hard to handle.
   - If they are starting to get caught up in the moment, think about the long-term effects of having reproductive sex.

   Drinking alcohol or using drugs might make it hard for a patient to not have reproductive sex because they affect a person's judgment.

7. Here are things that some people like about abstinence:

   - It is free.
   - It causes no harmful side effects or health problems.
   - It always works to prevent pregnancy when used correctly.
   - Partners can still enjoy each other sexually in ways that can't cause a pregnancy.
   - It can lower the chances of getting any sexually transmitted infections.

8. Here are two concerns patients might have about using abstinence and what you might say to help them. For other possible concerns and responses, please see the "Abstinence: Some Problems and Ways to Solve Them" chart in the Abstinence section.

   - *Patient's concern:* "Abstinence can be sexually frustrating."

     What you could say: "You can express yourself sexually without having vaginal or anal sex. You can find other ways of sexually pleasuring each other."

   - *Patient's concern:* "My partner puts a lot of pressure on me to have sex."

     What you could say: "It is your choice whether or not to have sex. Explain to your partner why it is important for you to abstain from reproductive sex."

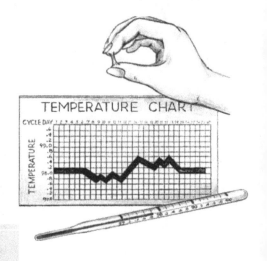

Fertility Awareness-Based (FAB) Methods

This information about FAB methods is mostly written as though you were talking to your patients. It gives you an idea of how to explain these methods in a way your patients can understand. This section also has notes written directly to you, the health worker. Those "health worker notes" look like this one.

What are FAB Methods?

Fertility Awareness-Based (FAB) Methods including Natural Family Planning (NFP) and Fertility Awareness Methods (FAM), are birth control methods based on:

▶ Knowing how human reproduction works and how pregnancy starts;

▶ Understanding that you or your partner can become pregnant only about one week during a menstrual cycle;

▶ Knowing how to tell when you or your partner can and cannot get pregnant;

▶ Learning what to do during the times that pregnancy can happen:

- You may decide not to have reproductive sex during the time that you or your partner could get pregnant. This is also known as *Natural Family Planning (NFP)*.

- You may choose to use a barrier or other information-based birth control method during the time that pregnancy is possible. These include condoms, the diaphragm, cap, sponge, spermicides or withdrawal. These are known as *Fertility Awareness Methods (FAM)*.

> **FAM and NFP What's the difference?**
>
> When using *Fertility Awareness Methods (FAM)*, the patient may use a barrier or information-based birth control method during the fertile times in their cycle to avoid pregnancy.
>
> When using *Natural Family Planning (NFP)*, the patient will ONLY abstain from reproductive sex during their fertile times. No birth control methods will be used.

If you choose a FAB method, you will need to learn more about how to use it correctly. The information given here will give you a basic idea of what to expect.

FAB methods help prevent pregnancy, but they do not protect you from HIV or other STIs. Use a condom every time you have sex to help protect yourself from these STIs.

How do FAB methods work?

With FAB methods, a couple learns to know when pregnancy is possible. You can then choose *not* to have sex during the days that pregnancy can happen. Or you can choose to use a birth control method, like condoms or withdrawal, during those days. Either way, the sperm need to be kept from meeting with an egg. This prevents pregnancy.

You could use these methods even without your partner's support. You will need to be able to have no reproductive sex or use a barrier or information-based birth control method on the days you could get pregnant. Of course, this is a lot easier if your partner is supportive and understands how the method works too.

Note: Once you learn when you can and cannot get pregnant, you can also use this information to help you get pregnant.

Here are some of the basics behind why FAB methods work:

Fertile days. A person can get pregnant only about 5 to 7 days during each menstrual cycle. Those days are called their **fertile days.** Fertile days include the day the egg leaves the ovary **(ovulation).** It also includes a few days before ovulation when live sperm may be present.

Infertile days. The other days of the menstrual cycle are called the **infertile days.** These are the days a person cannot become pregnant.

Fertile mucus. Around the time the egg leaves the ovary, the cervix (the opening to the uterus) makes a special kind of mucus called "fertile mucus." This mucus is wet, slippery, and stretchy. It helps sperm live up to 5 days in the body. It also helps sperm travel through the uterus to the tubes where the egg is. The rest of the menstrual cycle, the mucus is sticky or dry. It helps block sperm from getting into the uterus and sperm can't live in it.

Sperm. Sperm can live in fertile mucus for up to 5 days. Sperm can live in infertile mucus for only a few minutes to a few hours.

Eggs. An egg can live and be able to meet with the sperm up to one day (12-24 hours).

Fertility signs. A person's body will give them signs that show when they can and cannot get pregnant. These are called **fertility signs.** When a person understands the fertility signs and how they change, they can use them to make sure the sperm do not meet with an egg. This keeps them from getting pregnant. NFP and FAM are based on learning about and keeping track of the fertility signs.

Fertility signs

Here are the three major fertility signs. You can read more about these signs in Chapter 3.

Cervical mucus:

- ▸ Cervical mucus is made in the cervix.

- ▸ During infertile days, there may not be any cervical mucus or the mucus does not feel wet. It may feel sticky or dry.

- ▸ As the egg is getting ready to leave an ovary, this mucus starts to feel wet. It may also be stretchy and slippery. This type of mucus helps keep sperm alive for up to 5 days. This means if you have reproductive sex up to 5 days before the egg leaves the ovary, the sperm can live in your body until the day you ovulate. This is why the fertile days start a few days before the egg leaves the ovary.

- ▸ After the egg leaves the ovary, the mucus loses its wet feeling. It gets sticky or even dry. Sperm can't live in this mucus.

- ▸ You can check your mucus by wiping the vaginal opening with toilet tissue or reaching into your vagina with a finger or two. You do this for a few days every menstrual cycle.

- ▸ You will use a special chart or app to record these changes in your cervical mucus.

The cervix:

▸ As the time nears for an egg to leave an ovary, the cervix feels higher in the vaginal canal.

▸ The area around the opening of the cervix softens and the opening gets wider.

▸ You can check these changes in your cervix by feeling them with your finger. You do this for a few days every cycle.

▸ You will use a special chart to record these changes.

Basal body temperature (BBT):

▸ Basal body temperature is the temperature of the body at rest. It is the temperature of your body when you first wake up in the morning.

▸ Around the time an egg leaves an ovary, the BBT goes up. You can use your BBT to know when an egg has left an ovary and when the fertile days for that cycle are over.

▸ The BBT is usually lowest from the day your period starts until just before an egg comes out of your ovary. It then rises and stays high for about two weeks or until you start your period.

▸ You take your temperature for several mornings each menstrual cycle when you first wake up.

▸ You write your temperature on a special chart.

▸ You will be taught how to read this chart to know when an egg leaves an ovary and when your fertile days have ended. You can then avoid pregnancy when having reproductive sex without birth control until your next period starts.

Some patients may ask you to tell them more about certain types of natural family planning or fertility awareness methods. Read the box that follows called "Types of Fertility Awareness-Based Methods" to learn what you might say. Find out if your health care site has a list of FAB instructors. If it doesn't, patients may be able to find an instructor by calling another family planning or Planned Parenthood clinic, a local department of public health, or a church. If they can't find a class, they can learn more about the methods by reading a book on FAB Methods.

Types of Fertility Awareness-Based Methods

Cervical Mucus FAB Methods:

▶ Billings Ovulation Method

▶ TwoDay Method

These methods involve checking your cervical mucus a few days during each cycle. By tracking the mucus changes, you will know when you can and cannot get pregnant. If you don't want to become pregnant, you don't have reproductive sex during the days you could get pregnant or use a barrier or information-based birth control method.

With perfect use, cervical mucus FAB methods are 94-97% effective.

That means that if 100 patients use a cervical mucus method exactly the right way, only 3-4 of them may get pregnant in a year.

With typical use, cervical mucus FAB methods are 77-86% effective.

For those who don't always use a cervical mucus method exactly the right way, 14-23 out of 100 may get pregnant in a year.

Symptothermal FAB Methods

With this method, you use two signs to know when your fertile days may be: cervical mucus and basal body temperature. This method tells you when your fertile days begin and end.

With perfect use, the symptothermal FAB method is 99.6% effective.

That means that if 100 patients use the symptothermal method exactly the right way, only 1 (and probably none) of them may get pregnant in a year.

With typical use, the symptothermal FAB method is 98% effective.

For those who don't always use the symptothermal method exactly the right way, 2 out of 100 may get pregnant in a year.

Menstrual Cycle Tracking Methods:

▸ Standard Days Method (includes: Cycle Beads)

▸ Calendar Rhythm Method

These methods involve counting the days of your menstrual cycle to determine which days you could be fertile and which days you are not fertile.

If you have regular 26 to 32-day cycles, you can use the **Standard Days Method**. Day 1 of your cycle is the first day of your period. To avoid pregnancy you do not have reproductive sex on days 8 through 19. Or, you can use Cycle Beads (plastic beads to show what days you can get pregnant and which days you cannot get pregnant. Each day of your cycle is marked by either a brown or white bead). Cycle Beads is also available as an app.

For the **Calendar Rhythm Method** you keep a record of the length of your previous 6-12 menstrual cycles to determine the longest and shortest cycles. Subtract 18 from the shortest cycle to find out the 1st cycle day you could get pregnant. Subtract 11 from the longest cycle to find out the last cycle day you could get pregnant. The days in between are all the days you could get pregnant. These are all the days you would not have reproductive sex to avoid pregnancy.

When you use these methods, there may be more days each month when you *can't* have reproductive sex than with other FAB methods.

With perfect use, the menstrual cycle tracking Standard Days method is 95% effective (there is no perfect use rate for the Calendar Rhythm Method).

That means that if 100 patients use the Standard Days method exactly the right way, only 5 of them may get pregnant in a year.

With typical use, the menstrual cycle tracking FAB methods are 86-88% effective.

For those who don't always use a menstrual cycle tracking method exactly the right way, 12-14 out of 100 may get pregnant in a year.

How well do FAB methods work?

When you talk to your patients, discuss how well FAB methods work (how effective they are). Be sure to explain the difference between "perfect use" and "typical use." You can read more about this in the "Stage 3" section of Chapter 2.

Talk to your patients about Emergency Contraception.

Emergency Contraception (EC), in the form of EC pills or an IUD, can prevent pregnancy after sex. Patients can use EC up to 5 days after unprotected sex. Read more about it in the section on EC.

For patients who chart the signs carefully and follow all the rules, these methods can work very well.

With perfect use, these methods are 95% to 99% effective.

This means that if 100 patients use FAB methods perfectly, 5 to 9 of them may get pregnant in a year. It depends on which method they are using.

With typical use, these methods are as low as 77% effective.

For those who don't use the methods perfectly, 23 out of 100 may get pregnant in a year.

How can you learn to use NFP or FAM?

The best way to learn about these methods is to take a class from a trained, qualified NFP/FAM instructor. In class, you will learn about the following:

▶ The names of the fertility signs, why and when they happen, and how to keep track of them.

▶ How to use the fertility signs to prevent pregnancy or to get pregnant.

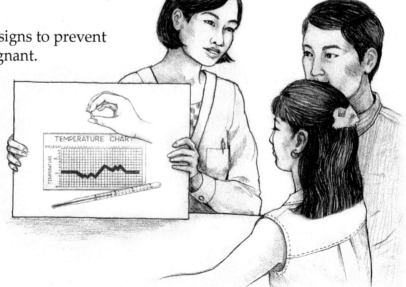

Are there any side effects, complications, or precautions?

There are no side effects. It does not cause any health problems, so there are also no warning signs.

Breastfeeding

Those who breastfeed can use NFP or FAM as their method.

There may be side effects if another birth control method is used during your fertile days.

Not everyone can always use these methods the right way. If you have irregular periods, or your cycles are longer than 35 days, you will not be able to use these methods.

What are the advantages and disadvantages of using NFP and FAM?

There are many things people like about FAB Methods. And there are some things they don't like. Find out what your patients like. Encourage them to focus on those things. To teach patients about these methods, you need more training than this manual can give. For now, you can help your patients see NFP and FAM as choices for birth control. If they are interested in using these methods, you can refer them to FAB Methods classes in your area.

What some people like about NFP and FAM:

▸ They enjoy learning about the body and how reproduction works.

▸ They feel closer to their partner by talking about family planning.

▸ They may like these methods for religious or other personal reasons.

▸ These methods do not cause any health problems.

Find out what your patient might not like about NFP or FAM.

Ask your patients if they have any concerns about using FAB methods. Then talk to them about their concerns. Help them think through how to solve any problems they might have while using these methods. Try to get them to come up with their own solutions first. Read the chart that follows for some ideas about how to deal with concerns.

Keep in mind that these aren't the best methods for everyone.
It is the patient's choice

NFP or FAM: Some Problems and Ways to Solve Them

Problem	Ways to Solve the Problem
It takes time to learn how to use these methods.	It may take one or more months to be really comfortable with these methods. You will need to talk with your partner to decide what you will do sexually while you are learning the method.
I don't know if I will like having to chart my temperature and mucus.	With practice, you will start to feel more aware of changes in your body. There are fertility tracking apps available to help you such as DOT, Clue, Cycle Beads and Natural Cycles.
With FAB methods, we can't have sex during the fertile days.	If you want to have sex during the fertile days, you can use FAM instead of NFP. You will just need to use a barrier or temporary method of birth control during the days you could get pregnant.
It is hard to remember when my fertile days are.	That is what is good about charting, using cycle beads or an app. Checking the chart, calendar, app or cycle beads can become part of your routine.
What if we make a mistake and have reproductive sex on a fertile day?	If that happens, you may still be able to prevent pregnancy even after sex. Call the provider for advice. Find out about emergency contraception.
FAB Methods do not protect me from HIV or other STIs.	True, but you can also use a condom every time you have sex to help protect yourself from STIs.

What if you want to stop using your FAB Method?

You can stop using NFP or FAM whenever you want to. But if you stop using it, you could become pregnant right away. Use another birth control method if you don't want to be pregnant.

There are no health problems to watch for when you stop these methods.

Make sure your patient understands.

Before your patients leave, make sure they understand how to use NFP or FAM successfully. Here are some things you can ask to make sure they understand.

- ▸ Tell me what you know about FAB methods.
- ▸ How do FAB methods work?
- ▸ What's the difference between Fertility Awareness Method and Natural Family Planning?
- ▸ What do you like about FAB methods?
- ▸ What don't you like about FAB methods?
- ▸ What might be the most difficult problem for you when using FAB methods?
- ▸ How would you solve that problem?
- ▸ Where will you go to learn more about FAB methods?

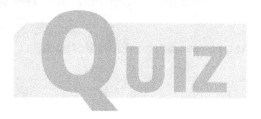

FERTILITY AWARENESS-BASED
(FAB METHODS)

Directions: Circle the best answer.

1. Which of the following are FAB Methods based on?
   a. Knowing how the human reproduction works and how pregnancy happens.
   b. Understanding that pregnancy can happen only about one week out of a menstrual cycle.
   c. Learning what to do to avoid pregnancy during the fertile times.
   d. All of the above

2. Which of the following are fertility signs (signs of a body that show when someone can and cannot get pregnant)?
   a. Changes in the basal body temperature
   b. How heavy the last period was
   c. Changes in the cervical mucus
   d. Both A and C

3. The Standard Days method:
   a. Works well for those who have cycles between 26 and 32 days long.
   b. Is easy for most people to learn.
   c. Works only for those who check their cervical mucus every day.
   d. Both A and B.

Go on to the next page.

4. During the fertile days, the mucus made by the cervix:

    a. Feels wet, stretchy, or slippery

    b. Feels dry or sticky

    c. Blocks sperm from getting into the uterus

    d. None of the above

5. What happens to the basal body temperature (BBT) around the time an egg leaves an ovary?

    a. It goes up.

    b. It goes down.

    c. It stays the same.

    d. None of the above

Directions: Write your best answer to each of the following.

6. With typical use, how well do FAB methods work?

    _____

    _____

7. List two things some people like about FAB methods.

    ■ _____

    _____

    ■ _____

    _____

Check your answers on the next page.

ANSWERS

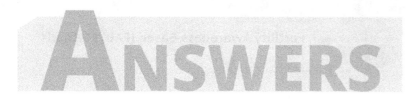

FAB METHODS

Check your answers.

1. **D** All of the above. Both FAB Methods are based on:
   - Knowing how human reproduction works and how pregnancy happens
   - Understanding that pregnancy can happen only about one week out of each menstrual cycle
   - Learning what to do to avoid pregnancy during the fertile times.
2. **D** Both A and C. Both of the following are fertility signs:
   - Changes in the body temperature
   - Changes in the cervical mucus
3. **D** Both A and B. The Standard Days Method works well for those who have a 26- to 32-day cycle and is easy for most people to learn to use.
4. **A** During the fertile days, the mucus made by the cervix feels wet, stretchy, or slippery.
5. **A** Around the time an egg leaves an ovary, the basal body temperature (BBT) goes up.
6. With typical use, FAB Methods are as low as 77% effective. This means that, among typical users of FAB Methods, about 23 users out of 100 may get pregnant in a year.
7. Here are things that some people like about FAB methods:
   - They enjoy learning about human reproductive anatomy and how it works.
   - They feel closer to their partner by talking about family planning.
   - They may like these methods for religious or other personal reasons.
   - These methods do not cause any health problems.

Withdrawal

What is it?

Other words for withdrawal

Your patient may refer to withdrawal as:

- Pulling out
- Coitus interruptus (interrupting vaginal sex)

Withdrawal is an effective birth control method. When you use withdrawal, your partner does not ejaculate (come) in or near your vagina.

During vaginal sex, at some point before your partner comes, they need to pull their penis out of your vagina. They need to move their penis away from your vagina, inner thigh or anus, before they ejaculate.

Withdrawal helps prevent pregnancy, but it does not protect against HIV and other STIs. Use condoms every time you have sex to help prevent these STIs.

Why withdrawal has a bad reputation

Withdrawal can be a good method of birth control. When used right, it is safe, works well, and is free. And it is always available to a couple.

But withdrawal has a bad reputation for two reasons:

- Some people think that partners with penises can't or won't use it well.
- Some think that withdrawal does not work.

The fact is that many partners **are** willing and able to use withdrawal if they understand how to use it the right way and if they practice alone before having reproductive sex.

How does it work?

Withdrawal works by keeping sperm away from the vagina. Before ejaculating ("coming"), the partner must pull their penis out of the vagina and makes sure not to ejaculate anywhere near the vaginal opening.

If sperm don't enter the vagina, they can't travel to an egg and you cannot get pregnant.

To use withdrawal the right way, the partner who makes sperm must be aware of their body's sexual responses. They must know when they are about to ejaculate from their penis (when they are about to "come").

This means that each time you have sex, the partner with the penis must pay attention to when they are close to coming and be able to pull out their penis and ejaculate somewhere away from the vaginal opening.

What about pre-come?

Pre-come is the fluid that leaves the penis before an ejaculation ("come"). It is made when a body that makes sperm is sexually excited, but *before* sperm enter the penis. Pre-come leaves the penis *before* the ejaculation.

Ejaculate ("come") must have millions of sperm in it to cause a pregnancy. Most of those sperm are killed before they get to the tubes to meet an egg. For example, if there are 100 million sperm in the semen, only about a million would make it up the tubes to meet with an egg. It takes all these sperm to help one sperm get to and fertilize an egg.

In pre-come, there may be a few hundred sperm left behind from a previous ejaculation. There is rarely enough sperm in pre-come to cause a pregnancy. However, most of this leftover sperm may be washed out of the urethra by urinating after each ejaculation.

Some facts about withdrawal

- It can be used with all of the other birth control methods making them even more effective.

- It can be used when sex is unplanned, and no other birth control method is available.

- It is used by some people for religious or cultural reasons.

- It is used by some who have trouble with other birth control methods.

How well does Withdrawal work?

When you talk to your patients, you will need to explain how well withdrawal works (how effective it is). Be sure to explain the difference between "perfect use" and "typical use." You can read more about this in the "Stage 3" section of Chapter 2.

Talk to your patients about Emergency Contraception.

Emergency Contraception (EC), in the form of EC pills or an IUD, can prevent pregnancy after sex. Patients can use EC up to 5 days after unprotected sex. Read more about it in the section on EC.

For withdrawal to work really well, the penis must be pulled out of the vagina before any semen comes out. When pulling out, you must also be sure that no sperm gets near the vagina or anus. It is also important to clear out any old semen from the penis by urinating before sex and after each ejaculation. This is called "perfect use."

With perfect use, withdrawal is 96% effective.

This means that if 100 patients use withdrawal perfectly, 4 of them may get pregnant in a year.

But the penis is not always pulled out before ejaculating in the vagina. Or sperm gets near the vagina or anus, such as on the inner thigh or just outside of the vagina. This is called "typical use." As you might guess, with typical use, the pregnancy rate is higher.

With typical use, withdrawal is 80% effective.

When they don't use withdrawal the right way every time, 20 out of 100 of them may get pregnant in a year.

Note: Some studies show that pre-ejaculate ("pre-cum") fluid does NOT contain sperm but a few other studies have found small amounts of sperm in pre-ejaculate fluid (even if the urethra was "cleaned out" by urinating since a previous ejaculation). This means that theoretically the sperm in the pre-cum could cause a pregnancy. However, with perfect use the theoretical risk of pregnancy is very low.

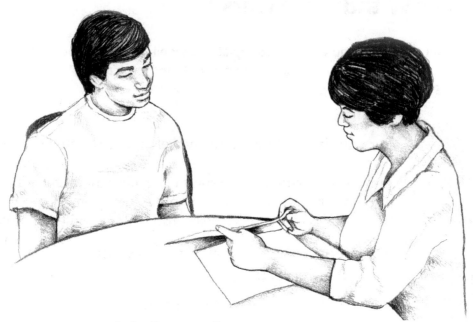

How do you use Withdrawal?

Teach your patients with a penis who make sperm these steps so they can use withdrawal successfully.

Know your body. Be aware of how you feel as you have sex. When you are aware, you are able to withdraw from the vagina before you start to ejaculate.

1. Before sex, urinate (pee) and wipe off the tip of your penis.

2. When you feel you are about to ejaculate or anytime before ejaculation, pull your penis out of the vagina or anus and continue stimulation with a hand or sex toy if you still want to ejaculate.

3. Ejaculate away from the vagina, anus and inner thighs. Be careful not to come in a place where sperm could drip onto or near the vagina.

4. Wipe the penis tip before it touches your partner again.

5. **Before you have sex again,** urinate and wipe off the tip of your penis. This helps wash away any sperm that might still be inside your penis from the last time you ejaculated.

Are there any side effects, complications, or precautions?

Withdrawal is safe for anyone. It causes no side effects or health problems.

Breastfeeding

Those who breastfeed can use withdrawal as their method.

Withdrawal and Weight Concerns

Q: Does withdrawal cause weight gain?

A: No.

Q: Does withdrawal still work if the user is overweight?

A: Yes.

Q: If a user is overweight, would using withdrawal cause any medical problems?

A: No.

Research shows that withdrawal does not cause weight gain. Most people gain weight over time whether they are using withdrawal or not. This is especially true for teens and young adults who are still growing.

What are the advantages and disadvantages of using Withdrawal?

There are many things people like about using withdrawal. And there are some things they don't like. Find out what your patients like about this method. Encourage them to focus on those things.

What some couples like about withdrawal:

▸ Withdrawal is always available when a couple needs birth control. No supplies are needed, and it is free.

▸ It works well when used right.

▸ It causes no health problems.

▸ It is a great option when no other method is available.

▸ It can be used with and enhances the effectiveness of other birth control methods.

Find out what your patients might not like about using withdrawal.

Ask your patients if they have any concerns about using withdrawal. Then talk to them about their concerns. Help them think through how to solve any problems they might have while using this method. Try to get them to come up with their own solutions first. Read the chart that follows for some ideas about how to deal with concerns.

Keep in mind that withdrawal is not the best method for everyone. It is the patient's choice.

Withdrawal: Some Problems and Ways to Solve Them

Problem	Ways to Solve the Problem
I'm afraid I won't be able to pull out in time.	With practice, you can learn how to pull out in time. You can practice by having sex while wearing a condom and pulling out before you come. You can practice while masturbating to learn how it feels when you are about to ejaculate and practice stopping stimulation to delay or stop coming.
I think I'll worry too much about when I should pull out.	With practice, you will start to feel more aware of when you are going to come. The more confident you become, the less you will worry.
My partner is really worried about whether I'll pull out in time.	This method takes trust and practice. Perhaps your partner can use another method while you are learning to use this method. If your partner is still too nervous, withdrawal may not be a good method for you. You can also use withdrawal with all other methods.
What if I don't pull out in time?	If that happens, you may still be able to prevent pregnancy even after sex. Call the provider for advice. Find out about emergency contraception.
Withdrawal doesn't protect us from HIV and other STIs.	Use condoms every time you have sex to help protect yourself from these STIs.

What if you want to stop using Withdrawal?

You can stop using this method whenever you want to. But if you stop using it, you are able to cause pregnancy right away. Use another birth control method if you don't want a pregnancy.

There are no health problems to watch for when you stop this method.

Make sure your patient understands.

Before your patients leave, make sure they understand how to use withdrawal successfully. Here are some things you can ask to make sure they understand.

▶ Tell me what you know about withdrawal.

▶ How does withdrawal work?

▶ How can you practice using withdrawal?

▶ What other birth control methods can you use with the withdrawal method?

▶ What do you like about withdrawal?

▶ What don't you like about withdrawal?

▶ What might be the most difficult problem for you when using withdrawal?

▶ How would you solve that problem?

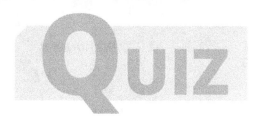

WITHDRAWAL

Directions: Read each of the following statements.
Is it true or false? Circle the best answer.

1. Withdrawal never protects against pregnancy.   **True**   **False**

2. Withdrawal does not protect against STIs.   **True**   **False**

3. There is usually not enough sperm in pre-come to cause a pregnancy.   **True**   **False**

4. To prevent a pregnancy, the penis must be pulled out of the vagina right *after* ejaculation ("coming").   **True**   **False**

5. Many partners who make sperm would be willing to use withdrawal if they understood how to use it the right way.   **True**   **False**

Directions: Circle all the answers that apply.

6. Which of the following are things you would tell someone who wants to use withdrawal?

   a. Be aware of how you feel as you have sex.

   b. Pull the penis out of the vagina or anus before you "come."

   c. Wipe off your penis before letting it touch your partner.

   d. Urinate (pee) before you have sex again.

   e. Don't "come" in a place where sperm might be able to travel to the vagina.

Go on to the next page.

Directions: Read each of the following and write your best answer in the spaces below.

7. If 100 patients use withdrawal perfectly, how many of them might get pregnant in a year?

_____

8. List two things some people like about using withdrawal.

- _____

- _____

Check your answers on the next page.

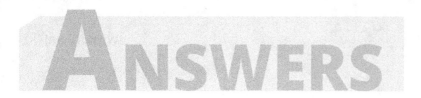

WITHDRAWAL

Check your answers.

1. **False**   Withdrawal does protect against pregnancy. In fact, when done correctly, it works well to prevent pregnancy.

2. **True**   Withdrawal does not provide protection from STIs.

3. **True**   There is usually not enough sperm in pre-come to cause a pregnancy.

4. **False**   To prevent pregnancy, the penis must be pulled out of the vagina *before* ejaculation ("coming"). This is to make sure no sperm get into the vagina.

5. **True**   Many partners who make sperm would be willing to use withdrawal if they understood how to use it the right way.

6. **A, B, C, D, E**   You would tell someone who wants to use withdrawal all of these things:
   - Be aware of how you feel as you have sex.
   - Pull the penis out of the vagina or anus before you "come."
   - Wipe off your penis before letting it touch your partner.
   - Urinate (pee) before you have sex again.
   - Don't "come" in a place where sperm might be able to get near the vagina.

7. If 100 patients use withdrawal perfectly, *4* of them may get pregnant in a year.

8. Here are things that some people like about withdrawl:
   - Withdrawal is always available when you need birth control. No supplies are needed, and it is free.
   - It works well when done right.
   - It causes no health problems.
   - It helps partners be more aware during sex.

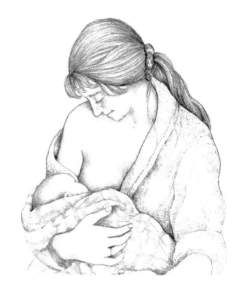

Lactation Amenorrhea Method (LAM)

This information on LAM is mostly written as though you were talking to your patients. It gives you an idea of how to explain LAM in a way your patients can understand. This section also has notes written directly to you, the health worker. Those "health worker notes" look like this one.

What does LAM mean?

L stands for lactation. This means breastfeeding.

A stands for amenorrhea (a-menor-REE-uh). This is when a person stops having a period.

M stands for method.

What is it?

LAM stands for Lactation Amenorrhea Method. It is a method of birth control where you breastfeed a certain way to keep from getting pregnant. It only works for up to 6 months after the baby is born.

LAM works well to prevent pregnancy. But it does not protect against HIV and other STIs. Use condoms every time you have sex to help protect against these STIs.

How does LAM work?

When you breastfeed, your body makes a special hormone that helps keep you from getting pregnant. When you follow the LAM directions, breastfeeding keeps your eggs from leaving your ovaries each month. If no egg leaves the ovaries, you can't get pregnant.

Who can use LAM?

▶ If your patient is pregnant now and interested in breastfeeding, you can tell them about LAM. They could use it as a birth control method.

▶ If your patient has already given birth and is breastfeeding now, they may still be able to use LAM as a birth control method.

▶ They will *not* be able to use LAM if either of these is true:

- They have been breastfeeding for more than 56 days in a way different from the LAM directions.
- They have already gotten their period after giving birth. (This is not the bleeding that happens to everyone for 2 to 8 weeks after giving birth.)

How well does LAM work?

When you talk to your patients, you will need to tell them how well LAM works (how effective it is). Be sure to explain the difference between "perfect use" and "typical use." You can read more about this in the "Stage 3" section of Chapter 2.

For those who follow these directions carefully, LAM can work very well for the first 6 months after the baby is born.

With perfect use, LAM is 98% effective.

This means that if 100 patients use LAM perfectly, 2 of them may get pregnant during the 6 months of LAM use.

With typical use, LAM is 95% effective.

For those who don't use LAM exactly the right way, 5 of 100 may get pregnant during the 6 months of LAM use.

LAM may not work at all for those who use a breast pump.

Talk to your patients about Emergency Contraception.

Emergency Contraception (EC), in the form of EC pills or an IUD, can prevent pregnancy after sex. Patients can use EC up to 5 days after unprotected sex. Read more about it in the section on EC.

Talk about Emergency Contraception (EC).

EC can prevent pregnancy after sex. Patients can take EC, in the form of pills or have an IUD inserted, up to 5 days after unprotected sex. Read more about EC at the end of this chapter.

If your patients use LAM the right way, they should not need EC. Tell them to call the provider for advice if any of the following happens:

- They start to feed their baby something other than breast milk.
- They feed less often than LAM guidelines.
- They start their period.

Note: If a breastfeeding patient needs EC pills, let them know that there are EC pills that are not likely to affect their milk supply. They should talk to their health care provider about their choices.

LAM and Weight Concerns

Q: Does LAM cause weight gain?

A: No.

Q: Does LAM work if a patient is overweight?

A: Yes.

Q: If a patient is overweight, would LAM cause any medical problems?

A: No.

Research shows that LAM does not cause weight gain. Most people gain weight over time whether they are using LAM or not. This is especially true for teens and young adults who are still growing.

How do you use LAM?

Teach your patients these rules so they can use LAM successfully.

To use LAM as a birth control method, you must:

- Start breastfeeding the day your baby is born.
- Breastfeed every time your baby wants to be fed or wants the breast for comfort (this is usually 8-12 times per day)
- Feed the baby only breast milk, nothing else.
- Breastfeed at least every 4 hours during the day and at least every 6 hours at night.

You can use this as a method until your baby is 6 months old.

Once you get your period, that means the ovaries are releasing eggs again. You must use another birth control method if you don't want to get pregnant.

If you are not sure you are breastfeeding the right way, meet with a Breastfeeding Consultant (Lactation Consultant) to learn more.

Find out if your health care site has a list of breastfeeding consultants that you can share with your patients.

Are there any side effects?

There are no side effects to using LAM as a birth control method.

When can you not use LAM?

You *can't* use LAM as a method if:

- Your baby is more than 6 months old.
- You have already gotten your period, even if your baby is less than 6 months old.
- You do not feed your baby at least every 4 hours during the day and every 6 hours at night.
- You feed your baby more than 2 mouthfuls a day of juice, water, or other foods.
- You use a breast pump often.

What about complications and warning signs?

Breastfeeding is natural. It does not cause any serious health problems.

Are there any precautions?

A provider may advise you not to breastfeed if any of the following is true:

- ▸ You are HIV positive.
- ▸ You are taking certain drugs or medicines. (Some drugs and medicines may get in the breast milk and may be bad for the baby.)
- ▸ You have a serious illness.

What are the advantages and disadvantages of using LAM?

There are many things people like about using LAM. And there are some things they don't like. Find out what your patient likes. Encourage them to focus on those things.

What some people like about LAM:

- ▸ It is free.
- ▸ You can have sex whenever you want.
- ▸ You don't have to use any other method of birth control.
- ▸ LAM is healthy for you and your baby.

Using LAM gives you time to learn about other birth control methods. You will want to choose a method you can use when you are finished with LAM.

Find out what your patients might not like about LAM.

Ask your patients if they have any concerns about using LAM. Then talk with them about those concerns. Help them think through how to solve any problems they might have while using LAM. Have them come up with their own solutions first. Read the following chart for some ideas about how to deal with some specific concerns.

Keep in mind that LAM isn't the best method for everyone. It is the patient's choice.

LAM: Some Problems and Ways to Solve Them

Problem	Ways to Solve the Problem
Breastfeeding takes time. I don't know if I can breastfeed at least every 4 hours during the day and every 6 hours at night.	Using LAM correctly is a real commitment. But many find it is easier than they thought it would be. You can always switch to another birth control method if it becomes too hard for you to breastfeed as often as needed with LAM.
I don't know if I want to just breastfeed my baby.	When you want to start giving your baby other liquids or food, you will need to switch to another birth control method to avoid pregnancy.
I don't like that it can only be used for 6 months after the baby is born.	If you want a method you can use for more than 6 months, LAM may not be the best method for you.
LAM does not protect us from HIV and other STIs.	Use condoms every time you have sex to help protect against these STIs.

What if you want to stop using LAM?

If you stop using this method, you could become pregnant right away. Use another birth control method if you don't want to get pregnant.

There are no health problems to watch for when you stop this method.

Make sure your patient understands.

Before your patients leave, make sure they understand how to use LAM successfully. Here are some things you can ask to make sure they understand.

- ▸ Tell me what you know about LAM.
- ▸ How does LAM work?
- ▸ What do you like about LAM?
- ▸ What don't you like about LAM?
- ▸ What might be the most difficult problem for you when using LAM?
- ▸ How would you solve that problem?

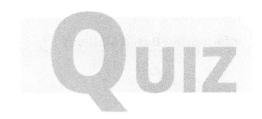

LACTATION AMENORRHEA
METHOD (LAM)

Directions: Circle the best answer.

1. If a patient wants to use LAM, when do they need to start breastfeeding their baby?

    a. One or two weeks after labor and delivery

    b. Right after the baby is born

    c. It doesn't matter when they start

    d. None of the above

2. How often does a person using LAM need to breastfeed their baby?

    a. At least every 4 hours during the day
        and at least every 6 hours during the night

    b. At least once a day

    c. At least 4 times a day

    d. It doesn't matter how often they breastfeed.

3. You cannot use LAM if:

    a. Your baby is more than 6 months old.

    b. You have already gotten your period.

    c. You regularly give your baby juice, water, or other foods in addition to breastfeeding.

    d. All of the above

Go on to the next page.

4. Which one of the following is a side effect, complication, or warning sign that can be caused by LAM?

    a. Nausea

    b. Headaches

    c. Breast cancer

    d. None of the above

Directions: Write your best answer to each of the following in the spaces below.

5. List two things some people like about LAM.

    ▪ _____

    ▪ _____

6. List one concern that patients may have about using LAM. Then write what you could say to help them deal with that concern.

    ▪ *Patient's concern:* _____

    _____

    ▪ *What you could say:* _____

    _____

Check your answers on the next page.

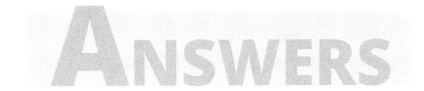

LACTATION AMENORRHEA METHOD (LAM)

Check your answers.

1. **B**   To use LAM, a patient needs to start breastfeeding their baby right after the baby is born.

2. **A**   A person using LAM needs to breastfeed their baby at least every 4 hours during the day and every 6 hours during the night.

3. **D**   All of the above. You cannot use LAM if:
   - Your baby is more than 6 months old.
   - You have already gotten your period.
   - You regularly give your baby juice, water, or other foods in addition to breastfeeding.

4. **D**   None of the above. Breastfeeding is natural. It does not cause any serious health problems, so there are no warning signs to watch for.

5. Here are things that some people like about LAM:
   - You can have sex whenever you want. You don't have to use any other method of birth control.
   - LAM is healthy for you and your baby.
   - LAM doesn't cost anything.
   - Using LAM gives you time to learn about other birth control methods. You will want to choose a method you can use when you are finished with LAM.

Go on to the next page.

6. Here are two concerns patients might have about using LAM and what you might say to help them. For other possible concerns and responses, please see the "LAM: Some Problems and Ways to Solve Them" chart in the LAM section.

   - *Patient's concern:* "Breastfeeding takes time. I don't know if I can breastfeed at least every 4 hours during the day and every 6 hours at night."

     What you could say: "Using LAM correctly is a real commitment. But many people find it is easier than they thought it would be. You can always switch to another birth control method if it becomes too hard for you to breastfeed as often as needed with LAM."

   - *Patient's concern:* "I don't know if I want to just breastfeed my baby."

     What you could say: "When you want to start giving your baby other liquids or food, you will need to switch to another birth control method."

Tier Three: Barrier Methods

Barrier methods help prevent pregnancy. Some barrier methods also help lower the chances of getting some STIs.

Barrier methods keep sperm from traveling through the cervix and into the uterus. By doing this, they keep sperm from meeting with an egg.

Spermicides are a type of chemical barrier method that works best when used along with another barrier method. Spermicides kill sperm before they can meet with an egg. They are put in the vagina before sex.

Topics in this section

▸ External Condom

▸ Internal Condom

▸ Diaphragm

▸ Birth Control Cap

▸ Birth Control Sponge

▸ Spermicides

    ▪ Birth Control Foam

    ▪ Birth Control Jelly or Cream

    ▪ Vaginal Suppositories

    ▪ Vaginal Film

Objectives

After reading this section, you will be able to:

▸ Explain how each barrier method works.

▸ Tell how well each method works to prevent pregnancy.

▸ Describe how to use each method correctly.

▸ List a side effect, complication, and warning sign for each method.

▸ Discuss some advantages of each method.

▸ Describe some problems people may have with each method and how they could deal with these problems.

Words you may need to know

Here are some words you may need to know when you talk with your patients about barrier methods.

Words	Definition
Spermicide (SPUR-muh-side)	A spermicide is a chemical that kills sperm. "Spermicides" is also the word used to describe the sperm-killing creams, gels, jellies, foam, and film used for birth control. These different forms of spermicide are known by many names. For example, a cream containing a spermicide might be called a spermicidal cream, a birth control cream, or a contraceptive cream.
Nonoxynol-9 (nah-NAHK-si-nuhl 9)	One chemical that kills sperm (a spermicide). It is the chemical used in most forms of spermicide.
Lubricant	Also called "lube." A special liquid or gel used for extra moisture during sex. It can make sex more comfortable or make the condom easier to use. Examples of lubricants are K-Y Gel, AquaLube, or AstroGlide.
Latex	A type of rubber. Most external condoms are made from this. Some people are allergic to latex.
Polyisoprene	A synthetic latex that is thin and soft.
Polyurethane (pah-lee-YUR-uh-thayn)	A thin, soft plastic. Some external condoms are made from this plastic. People who are allergic to latex can use condoms made of polyurethane. The sponge is also made of polyurethane.

Nitrile
A type of synthetic rubber used to make the internal condom. Internal condoms made out of nitrile are able to be used with non water soluble personal lubricants. Also, in medical facilities, gloves made from nitrile are used for patients or health care providers who are allergic to latex.

Cervix
The opening to the uterus. It is at the back of the vagina. The diaphragm, cap and sponge are designed to cover the cervix.

Silicone rubber
A type of rubber. The cap and the diaphragm are made from this. This type of rubber does not cause allergies. Silicone-based lubes should not be used with the cap or the diaphragm.

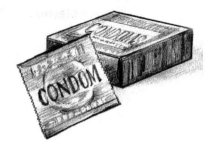

External Condom

What is it?

Condoms are known by many names.

Patient may refer to external condoms as:

- male condoms
- rubbers
- hats
- jimmies
- raincoats

You can write down other names you hear.

The external condom is a thin covering that fits over an erect penis. Condoms can be made out of four kinds of material:

- ▸ Latex, a thin kind of rubber
- ▸ Polyurethane, a thin, soft plastic
- ▸ Polyisoprene, a synthetic latex that is thin and soft
- ▸ Animal membranes, such as lambskin

Latex, polyurethane and polyisoprene condoms can help prevent pregnancy and STIs, including HIV. Sperm and STI germs cannot pass through these types of condoms. You can use these condoms to help protect yourself from STIs when you have sex using a penis, vagina, mouth, or anus.

Condoms made from lambskin help prevent pregnancy. But they do not protect against STIs. This is because STI germs are much smaller than sperm. STI germs can get through lambskin condoms.

In this manual, when we say that condoms protect against HIV and other STIs, we are talking about *latex, polyurethane,* or *polyisoprene* external condoms or internal condoms made from nitrile. Lambskin condoms do *not* protect against these infections.

Condoms come in different textures, colors, and sizes. Here are some other differences in condoms:

- ▶ Some are lubricated. Lubricants make the condom more slippery. They can also make them more comfortable to use during sex.

- ▶ Some have spermicide on them. Spermicides are chemicals that kill sperm.

- ▶ Some condoms have both a lubricant and a spermicide on them.

- ▶ Some have a special tip at the end for the semen.

How does it work?

During sex, sperm stay inside the condom. This keeps sperm from getting into the vagina. If no sperm get into the vagina, the sperm can't meet with an egg and you can't get pregnant.

The condom also helps protect against HIV and STIs. It does this by keeping some STI germs from passing from one person to the other. Without an external condom:

- ▶ Any STI germs in the semen can get into the sex partner's vagina, anus, or mouth.

- ▶ Any STI germs in the partner's vagina, anus, or mouth can get on the penis.

Questions from a counselor

Q: My patient only uses condoms to keep from getting pregnant. Do they need to worry about pregnancy when they have anal sex?

A: Yes. We know that sperm travel. The anus is very close to the vagina. Any sperm around the anus can get to the vagina. It is not the easiest way to get pregnant, but it does happen. So, they should also use an external or internal condom to prevent pregnancy when they have anal sex.

Note about herpes and genital warts

Condoms can't always help prevent the spread of herpes or genital warts. This is because herpes sores or genital warts can be anywhere in the genital area. That means the sore or wart may not be covered or protected by the condom.

You should still encourage patients who have herpes or genital warts to use condoms when they have sex. This will help protect them from warts or sores in areas covered or protected by the condom.

You can also tell your patient that the internal condom does a better job than the external condom of providing protection from herpes and warts because it covers a larger area.

How well does it work?

You will need to explain to your patients how well the external condom works (how effective it is). Be sure to explain the difference between "perfect use" and "typical use." You can read more about this in the "Stage 3" section of Chapter 2.

Talk to your patients about Emergency Contraception.

Emergency Contraception (EC), in the form of EC pills or an IUD, can prevent pregnancy *after* sex. Patients can use EC up to 5 days after unprotected sex. Read more about it in the section on EC.

With perfect use, the external condom is 98% effective.

This means that if 100 people use the external condom exactly the right way *every* time they have sex, 2 of them may get pregnant in a year.

With typical use, the external condom is 87% effective.

For those who *don't* use it the right way every time they have sex, 13 out of 100 may get pregnant in a year.

How do you use the External Condom?

Be sure to use a new condom every time you have sex. Whether you have sex with the mouth, anus, penis, or vagina, use a new condom every time.

Put the condom on the erect penis before the penis is near the vagina, mouth, or anus.

1. **Before you open the condom package:**
    -   Get consent for the safe sexual act you will be doing.
    -   Check the expiration date. If too old, use a new one.
    -   Check for holes or rips in the package. You should feel a small pillow of air in the package. If there is none, the condom may have dried out.

2. **Be careful not to tear the condom when you take it out of its package.**
    -   Don't use teeth or scissors to open the package.
    -   If you have long fingernails, be careful not to rip the condom.
    -   Slide the condom out and see which way it unrolls.

3. **Put the condom on the erect penis before the penis is near the vagina, mouth, or anus.**

    ▸ Squeeze the tip of the condom while you put it on. This leaves room for the semen. If the condom does not have a special tip, squeeze the air out of an inch of space at the tip of the condom.

    ▸ Roll the condom down as far as it will go.

    ▸ If you want to add a lubricant to the outside of the condom, be sure to use a water-based or silicone based lubricant. Some people find this makes the condom easier to use and may add pleasure.

    ▸ Do not add lubricant to the inside of the condom. It could cause the condom to slip off the penis.

    ### Remember

    If sperm is near the vagina (like the upper inner thighs or anus), it could travel into the vagina and it could cause a pregnancy.

4. **After you have sex, hold the condom on at the base of the penis as you pull out of the vagina anus, or mouth.**

    After sex, hold the condom on at the base of the penis. Pull the penis with the condom out of the vagina, anus, or mouth. Do this while the penis is still hard. That way if there is any semen, it won't spill out. Move away from your partner to slide the condom off. Make sure not to spill semen anywhere near the vagina. Throw the used condom in the trash.

5. **If you want to have sex more than once, use a new condom every time you have sex.**

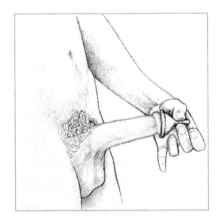

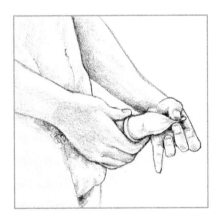

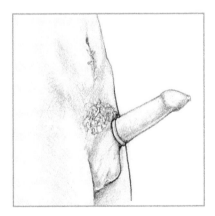

Step 1:

Place the unrolled condom on the end of the penis, with the rolled rim on the outside.

Step 2:

Keep holding the tip as you unroll the condom to the base of the penis. This keeps empty space at the tip for possible semen.

Step 3:

Either partner may put the condom on the penis or sex toy and remove it.

Using lubes

Some lubes are water-based. Other lubes are silicone-based. Both are safe to use with external and internal condoms. Silicone-based lubes are NOT safe to use with the Cap or with some sex toys. Do not use silicone-based lubes with anything made out of silicone.

The External Condom and Weight Concerns

Q: Do external condoms cause weight gain?

A: No.

Q: If someone is overweight, will the external condom still work well?

A: Yes!

Q: Are there medical problems if someone using the external condom is overweight?

A: No, none at all.

Tips to keep External Condoms from breaking

Here are some things you can tell your patients to help them make sure their external condoms won't break.

▶ **Always check the expiration date on the condom package.** Make sure the condom isn't too old.

▶ **Squeeze the tip of the condom while putting it on.** If there is air in the tip when you put the condom on, it may break.

▶ **Store your condoms in a cool, dry place.** You may be able to keep condoms in the glove box of your car or your wallet for a short period of time when kept away from heat and sunlight. The pressure and heat can cause some condoms to break.

▶ **Use water-based lubes on the outside of the condom.** That way there won't be too much friction. Too much friction can cause a condom to break.

▶ **If you use a lubricant, make sure it is water-based or silicone based.** Examples of water-based lubricants are AstroGlide or a birth control jelly. Don't use an oil-based lubricant like Vaseline, cooking oil, baby oil, or hand lotion. These can make a latex condom break.

Are there any side effects?

Some people are allergic to the latex in a condom. Others may be allergic to the lubricant or spermicide. If you are allergic, your skin may itch, burn, or turn red. Or you may get a rash near the vagina, penis, or anus.

You can try other brands to find a condom or lubricant that doesn't bother you. If the spermicide in the condom is the problem, you can try a condom without spermicide. If you are allergic to latex, you can try the polyurethane or polyisoprene external condom or the nitrile internal condom.

Any complications/warning signs?

The external condom causes no serious health problems.

Are there any precautions?

Some people are allergic to latex, the lubricant, or the spermicide used. If you know you have this allergy, tell the medical provider. You may need to use a different brand or type of condom.

Breastfeeding

Those who are breastfeeding can use condoms when they have sex.

What are the advantages and disadvantages of using Condoms?

There are many things people like about using condoms. And there are some things they don't like. Find out what your patient likes. Encourage them to focus on those things.

What some people like about External Condoms:

▶ Condoms help prevent some STIs, including HIV.

▶ They cause no serious health problems.

▶ You can find condoms in many places, like drugstores and vending machines.

▶ They are easy to carry around.

▶ Condoms may help a penis stay erect longer.

▶ You only use condoms when you need them.

▶ You can use them to cover sex toys. That helps keep from spreading germs.

Condoms and Sex Toys

You can let your patients know that condoms can be used on sex toys. It helps prevent spreading germs between partners who share the toys. It also protects someone who wants to use a toy in more than one place in their body.

Find out what your patient may not like about Condoms.

Ask your patients if they have any concerns about using condoms. Then talk to them about their concerns. Help them think through how to solve any problems that they might have while using condoms. Try to get them to come up with their own solutions first. Read the chart that follows for some ideas about how to deal with concerns.

Keep in mind that condoms may not be the best birth control method for every patient. It is the patient's choice.

The External Condom: Some Problems and Ways to Solve Them

Problem	Ways to Solve the Problem
I have to stop what I'm doing to put it on.	Make putting on condoms part of the sex play.
I might not have any condoms with me when I need them. Or I might run out.	<ul><li>Carry extra condoms in your bag, purse, or backpack.</li><li>Have extra condoms stored in a cool, dry place.</li><li>Go to the store for more.</li><li>Decide to wait for another time to have sex.</li></ul>
My partner or I may be allergic to the latex, lubricant, or spermicide.	If you are, you can try using different types of condoms, lubes, or spermicides to find one that doesn't bother you.
I'm afraid sex won't feel as good with condoms.	<ul><li>You can try using a lubricant.</li><li>Try a different brand or style. Find one that fits the penis well. Some condoms may feel more natural than others.</li></ul>
My partner doesn't want to bother using them.	<ul><li>Talk to your partner about why it is important to use condoms.</li><li>Have condoms with you when you need them. If you have them ready, your partner may be willing to use them.</li></ul>
The condom could break or slip off.	If you follow the tips for using condoms correctly, condoms seldom break or slip off. But if one does, you can still try to prevent pregnancy after sex. Find out about emergency contraception.

Help your patients talk with their partners about using condoms.

Anyone may find it hard to talk about using condoms. Some of the reasons for this include:

- ▸ In some cultures, people don't talk with each other about sex.
- ▸ In some relationships, using condoms may be seen as a sign of distrust.
- ▸ People with partners who try to control them may be afraid to bring it up.
- ▸ Some people may not know how to bring it up or talk about it.

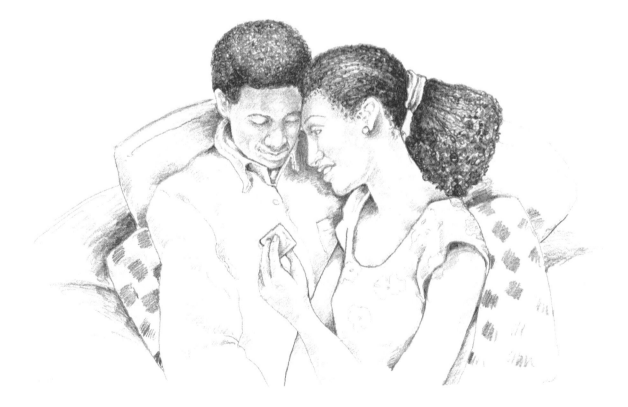

You can help your patients think through problems they may have talking with their partners. Help them come up with ways to solve the problems. Perhaps you could practice with them by doing a role-play.

You could brainstorm possible solutions with your patients. First, ask your patients for ideas. If they need help, here are a couple of examples you could suggest. Use the spaces below these examples to write in a few ideas of your own.

▸ I really want to have sex with you. But only if we use condoms. Condoms will help protect both of us.

▸ You know, I'd feel a lot better knowing we are protected. Let's use condoms.

▸ _____

_____

▸ _____

_____

▸ _____

_____

What if you want to stop using the External Condom?

You can stop using the external condom whenever you want to. If you stop using it, use another birth control method if you don't want a pregnancy. Be aware that if you have sex without a condom, you will not be protected from HIV or other STIS.

There are no health problems to watch for when you stop using condoms for birth control.

Make sure your patient understands.

Before your patients leave, you will want to make sure they understand how to use a condom successfully. Some of these questions may help.

▸ Tell me what you know about external condoms.

▸ How do external condoms work?

▸ What infections can condoms help prevent?

▸ What can you do to keep external condoms from breaking or slipping?

▸ What might be the most difficult thing for you when using external condoms?

▸ How could you get around that problem?

▸ How will you store your external condoms?

▸ How will you talk with your partner about using condoms?

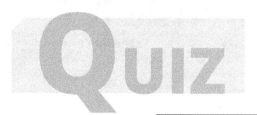

EXTERNAL CONDOM

Directions: Read each of the following statements. Is it true or false? Circle the best answer.

1. Condoms made from latex, polyurethane or polyisoprene will help protect against pregnancy and some STIs, including HIV.   True   False

2. External condoms made from lambskin will help protect against pregnancy, but not against HIV and other STIs.   True   False

3. Condoms work by keeping sperm out of the vagina.   True   False

4. Condoms can only be used once.   True   False

5. Condoms can be used for oral, anal, or vaginal sex.   True   False

6. Someone needs to hold the condom onto the penis when the penis is pulled out of the mouth, anus, or vagina.   True   False

Directions: Read the following question. Circle all of the answers that apply.

7. What should you do to help keep an external condom from breaking during sex?

   a. Always check the expiration date on the condom package.

   b. Squeeze the tip of the condom while putting the condom on.

   c. Store condoms in a cool, dry place.

   d. Put a few drops of water-based lube on the outside of the condom after you put the condom on.

   e. Use only water or silicone based lubricants.

Go on to the next page.

Directions: Read each of the following statements or questions, and write your best answer in the space below.

8. Your patient is allergic to the latex in a condom. What kind of condom could you suggest the patient might use to protect against pregnancy and STIs?

_____

9. A patient tells you that sex doesn't feel as good when they use an external condom. What could you tell them that might help?

_____

_____

_____

_____

Check your answers on the next page.

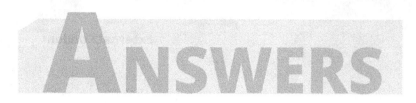

EXTERNAL CONDOM

Check your answers.

1. **True**   Condoms made from latex, polyurethane or polyisoprene *will* help protect against pregnancy and some STIs, including HIV.

   Sperm and STI germs cannot pass through these types of condoms. You can use these condoms to help protect yourself from STIs when you have sex using a penis, vagina, mouth, or anus.

2. **True**   External condoms made from lambskin *will* help protect against pregnancy, but will *not* help protect against HIV and other STIs.

   STI germs are much smaller than sperm. STI germs can pass through lambskin and other animal skin condoms.

3. **True**   Condoms work by keeping sperm out of the vagina. During sex, sperm stay inside the condom. If no sperm get into the vagina, sperm can't meet with an egg.

4. **True**   Condoms can only be used once. Never use a condom more than once.

5. **True**   Condoms can be used for oral, anal, or vaginal sex.

6. **True**   Someone needs to hold the external condom onto the penis when the penis is pulled out of the mouth, anus, or vagina.

   If the condom is not held onto the penis, semen could spill out and the partner could get pregnant or get an STI.

Go on to the next page.

7. **A, B,** You should do all of these things to help keep an
   C, D, external condom from breaking during sex:
   E
   - Always check the expiration date on the condom package.
   - Squeeze the tip of the condom while putting the condom on.
   - Store condoms in a cool, dry place.
   - Put a few drops of water-based lube on the outside of the condom after you put the condom on.
   - Use only water-based lubricants.

8. If your patient is allergic to latex, you could suggest the patient try the *polyurethane or polyisoprene condom*.

9. If a patient says sex doesn't feel as good when they use an external condom, two things you could tell them that might help are:
   - You could try using a lubricant.
   - You could try a different brand or style of condom.
   - Find one that fits the penis well. And there are some condoms that may feel more natural than others.

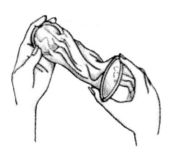

Internal Condom

What is it?

The internal condom is a loose-fitting condom. You put it in your vagina before you have sex. It is made of a thin but strong plastic called nitrile. It comes in one size that fits most vaginas.

The internal condom is open at one end and closed at the other. It has a firm, flexible ring at each end. One ring (the inner loose ring) holds the closed end of the condom in the vagina. The ring at the open end (the outer ring) hangs outside of the vagina. The penis enters the vagina through the open end of the condom. During sex, the internal condom also covers the lips of the vulva and the base of the penis.

The internal condom is lubricated with silicone based lube to make it easier to use.

Internal condoms can help prevent pregnancy and STIs, including HIV. Sperm and STI germs cannot pass through the internal condom. You can use internal condoms to help protect against STIs.

Note about herpes and genital warts

Internal condoms can't always help prevent the spread of herpes or genital warts. This is because herpes sores or genital warts can be anywhere in the genital area. That means the sore or wart may not be covered or protected by the internal condom.

You should still encourage patients who have herpes or genital warts to use condoms (internal or external) when they have sex. This will help protect them from warts or sores in areas covered or protected by the condom.

"How well does it work?"

During sex, sperm stay inside the condom and can't get into the vagina. If no sperm get into the vagina, the sperm can't meet with the egg and cause a pregnancy.

The internal condom also helps protect against HIV and other STIs. It helps keep STI germs from passing from one person to the other.

How well does the Internal Condom work?

You will need to explain to your patients about how well the internal condom works (how effective it is). Be sure to explain the difference between "perfect use" and "typical use." You can read more about this in the "Stage 3" section of Chapter 2.

With perfect use, the internal condom is 95% effective.

That means that if 100 people use the internal condom exactly the right way every time they have sex, 5 of them may get pregnant in a year.

With typical use, the internal condom is 79% effective.

For who don't use the internal condom the right way every time, 21 out of 100 may get pregnant in a year.

How do you use the Internal Condom?

Here are the steps to teach patients to use the internal condom correctly.

Talk to your patients about Emergency Contraception.

Emergency Contraception (EC), in the form of EC pills or an IUD, can prevent pregnancy after sex. Patients can use EC up to 5 days after unprotected sex. Read more about EC at the end of this chapter.

Be sure to use a new condom every time you have sex.

You can put the internal condom in right before you have sex or up to 8 hours before you have sex. Be sure to put it in before the penis is near the vagina or anus.

1. **Before you open the internal condom package:**

    ▸ Get consent for the safe sexual act you will be doing.

    ▸ Check the expiration date. If too old, use a new one.

    ▸ Check for holes or rips in the package. If you find any, the condom could be damaged so do not use it.

2. **Be careful not to tear the condom when you take it out of its package.**

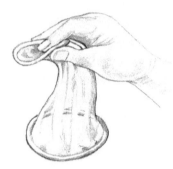

3. **You can put a few drops of the lubricant on the outside of the condom.**

    With the internal condom, you can use water-based, oil-based, or silicone based lubes.

4. **Hold the closed end of the internal condom.**

    Squeeze the ring at the closed end (the inner ring) together.

5. **Slide the condom into your vagina.**

Follow these steps:

-   Sit or lie down with your legs apart. Or you could stand with your foot on a chair.

-   Use your free hand to open the lips of the vagina.

-   While squeezing the inner ring, slide the closed end of the condom into the vagina.

-   Place one finger inside the condom to push the inner ring in as far as it will go. The other ring should hang down outside of the vagina.

6. **Check to make sure the internal condom is in right.**

    -   The inner ring of the condom should be just past the pubic bone. Put your fingers into your vagina to check. The condom should hang down straight.

    -   The outer ring and about 1 inch of the open end will stay outside your body.

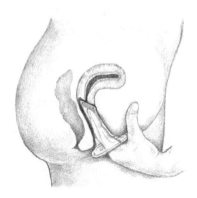

7. **When the penis is hard, you or your partner can use your hand to guide it into the condom.**

    The penis doesn't have to be fully erect to use the internal condom successfully.

8. **After sex, take the internal condom out right away.**

To take the condom out, follow these steps:

- Squeeze and twist the outer ring of the condom to keep any semen inside.

- Then gently pull the condom out of the vagina.

- Throw the condom away. Don't use the same condom more than once.

Remember

If sperm is anywhere near the vagina (like the upper inner thighs, or anus), it could travel into the vagina. You could get pregnant.

What if you want to have sex more than once?

Use a new internal condom every time you have sex.

Things to remember when you use the Internal Condom

Help your patients understand how they can make the internal condom work for them.

▶ **Make sure the condom stays in the right place during sex.**

During sex, the internal condom may move from side to side. Or it may move up and down on the penis. To prevent this, put lubricant inside the condom or on the penis before sex.

▶ **Stop having sex if:**

- You feel the outer ring of the condom start to go into the vagina.

- You feel the penis start to go in the vagina outside of the condom.

If either of these things happens, take the condom out and put in a new one.

The Outer Ring

The outer ring may touch/rub sensitive areas (like the clitoris). That can be pleasurable for some partners.

▶ *Never* **use the internal condom and the external condom at the same time.**

- They will rub together.

- This can make them break or move out of place.

Help your patients understand all the steps to using the internal condom. That way, they can talk about it with their partner.

▶ Tell them that they can put the internal condom inside their partner as a part of sex play. Help them find ways to talk about this with their partner.

▶ Make sure they know that they should tell their partner if they feel the penis start to go into the vagina outside of the condom.

Are there any side effects?

There are no side effects to using the internal condom.

Any complications or warning signs?

The internal condom causes no serious health problems.

Breastfeeding

Those who are breastfeeding can use internal condoms when they have sex.

Are there any precautions?

A health care provider may suggest that you choose a different method of birth control if the internal condom doesn't fit well in your vagina. However, this is extremely rare.

What are the advantages and disadvantages of using the Internal Condoms?

There are many things people like about using the internal condom. And there are some things they don't like. Find out what your patient likes. Encourage them to focus on those things.

What some people like about the internal condom:

▶ It is a method a person with a vagina can use to help prevent HIV and other STIs.

▶ It does not cause any serious health problems.

▶ During sex, it almost never breaks or tears.

▶ It is easy to carry around.

▶ You only use them when you need them.

▶ You can put it in for up to 8 hours before having sex.

▶ It can be used for vaginal or anal sex.

▶ It warms to body temperature so sex may feel more natural.

▶ You can use the internal condom with water-based, oil-based, or silicone-based lubricants.

▶ More of the outside parts of the genitals are covered. This may give more protection.

Find out what your patient may not like about internal condoms.

Ask your patients if they have any concerns about using internal condoms. Then talk to them about their concerns. Help them think through how to solve any problems they might have while using internal condoms. Have them think of their own solutions first. Read the chart that follows for some ideas about how to deal with concerns.

Keep in mind that internal condoms may not be the best birth control method for some patients. It is the patient's choice.

The Internal Condom and Weight Concerns

Q: Do internal condoms cause weight gain?

A: No.

Q: If someone is overweight, will the internal condom still work well?

A: Yes!

Q: Are there medical problems if someone using the internal condom is overweight?

A: No, none at all.

The Internal Condom: Some Problems and Ways to Solve Them

Problem	Ways to Solve the Problem
It seems like it would be hard to use.	Practice putting it in when you are alone. It may help to get used to it before you have sex.
I don't like putting my fingers inside my vagina.	<ul><li>You may get more used to this with time.</li><li>Your partner may be able to put the condom in for you. It can be part of sex play.</li></ul>
I might not have any internal condoms with me when I need them.	<ul><li>You could carry extra internal condoms in your purse.</li><li>Go to the store for more.</li><li>Decide to wait for another time to have sex.</li></ul>
I don't like how the outer ring looks outside my vagina.	You and your partner may not notice it while you are having sex. This is likely something you can get used to. Some users find it pleasurable or stimulating because it can rub on the clitoris during sex.
The internal condom can be noisy.	You can put extra lubricant inside the condom to reduce any noise the condom may make during sex.
What if my partner's penis enters the vagina outside the internal condom?	If this happens, stop having sex and put in a new internal condom. If they ejaculated into your vagina, you can still try to prevent pregnancy after sex. Find out about EC.
What if the internal condom breaks or tears?	If you follow the tips for using the internal condom, they will rarely break or tear. But if one does, you can still try to prevent pregnancy after sex. Find out about EC.

What if you want to stop using the Internal Condom?

You can stop using the internal condom whenever you want to. If you stop using it, use another birth control method if you don't want a pregnancy. Be aware that if you have sex without a condom, you will not be protected from HIV or other STIs.

There are no health problems to watch for when you stop using the internal condom for birth control.

Make sure your patient understands.

Before your patients leave, you will want to make sure they understand how to use an internal condom successfully. Some of these questions might help.

▸ Tell me what you know about internal condoms.

▸ How do you insert an internal condom?

▸ What infections can the internal condoms help prevent?

▸ What might be the most difficult thing for you about using internal condoms?

▸ How would you get around that problem?

▸ How will you store your internal condoms?

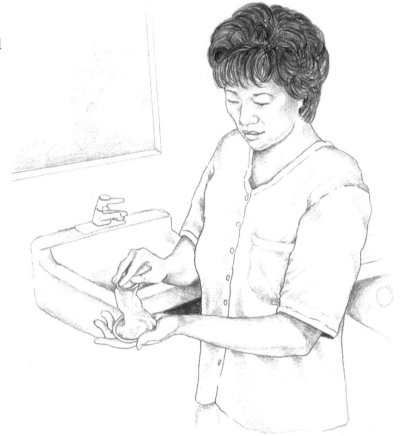

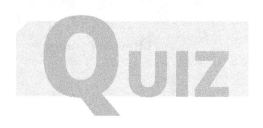

INTERNAL CONDOM

Directions: Circle the best answer.

1. How do internal condoms help prevent pregnancy?
    a. Internal condoms make the cervical mucus thicker.
    b. During sex, sperm stay inside the internal condom and can't get into the vagina.
    c. Internal condoms stop sperm production.

2. Before you use an internal condom, you should:
    a. Check the expiration date.
    b. Check for holes or rips in the package.
    c. Fill the internal condom with water.
    d. Both A and B

3. When you use an internal condom, you should:
    a. Be careful not to tear the condom when you open the package.
    b. Guide the penis into the condom.
    c. Take the internal condom out of the vagina right after sex and before standing up.
    d. All of the above

4. To put an internal condom into the vagina, you could:
    a. Sit or lie down with your legs apart.
    b. Stand with one foot on a chair.
    c. Sit in a chair with your feet on the ground.
    d. A or B

Go on to the next page.

5. What are the side effects of using a internal condom?

a. The internal condom has no side effects.

b. Some users get headaches when they use it.

c. Some users get heavier periods after using it.

d. All of the above

Directions: Write your best answer in the spaces below.

6. What are two things some people like about the internal condom?

- _____

- _____

7. List one concern that a patient may have about using the internal condom and what you might say to help them deal with that concern.

Patient's concern:
- _____

_____

What you can say:
- _____

_____

Check your answers on the next page.

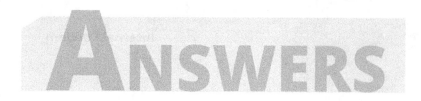

INTERNAL CONDOM

Check your answers.

1. **B** Internal condoms help prevent pregnancy because during sex, sperm stay inside the condom and can't get into the vagina. If no sperm get into the vagina, the sperm can't meet with an egg and cause a possible pregnancy.

2. **D** Both A and B. Before you use an internal condom, you should check the expiration date and check for holes and rips in the package. You should not fill the internal condom with water to check for holes.

3. **D** All of the above. When you use an internal condom, you should do all of the following:
   - Be careful not to tear the condom when you open the package.
   - Guide the penis into the condom.
   - Take the internal condom out of the vagina right after sex and before standing up.

4. **D** Both A and B. To put an internal condom into the vagina, you can either sit or lie down with your legs apart or stand with one foot on a chair.

   You would then:
   - Slide the closed end of the condom into the vagina while squeezing the inner ring.
   - Place one finger inside the condom to push the inner ring in as far as it will go.

5. **A** The internal condom has no side effects.

Go on to the next page.

6. Here are some things that some people like about the internal condom.

   - It is a method a person with a vagina can use to help prevent HIV and other STIs.
   - It does not cause any serious health problems.
   - During sex, it almost never breaks or tears.
   - It is easy to carry around.
   - You only use them when you need to.
   - You can put it in up to 8 hours before having sex.

   Remember, what one patient likes about a method, another patient might not like. Every patient is different.

7. Here are two concerns a patient might have about using the internal condom and what you might say to help them. For other possible concerns and responses, please see the "Internal Condoms: Some Problems and Ways to Solve Them" chart near the end of the Internal Condom section.

   - *Patient's concern:* "It seems like it would be hard to use."

     What you could say: "Practice putting it in when you are alone. It may help to get used to it before you have sex."

   - *Patient's concern:* "I don't like putting my fingers inside my vagina."

     What you could say: "You may get more used to this with time. Also, your partner may be able to put the condom in for you. It can be part of sex play."

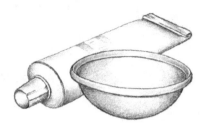

Diaphragm

Caya Diaphragm

In the United States, the Caya silicone diaphragm is starting to replace the traditional dome-shaped versions.

Caya comes in one size and a prescription is needed to receive one (it may become available over the counter). It is reuseable for up to 2 years.

Caya should be fitted by a provider to ensure patient's can place, use and remove it. Caya has a fingertip removal dome making it easier to remove than traditional diaphragms.

Learn more: www.caya.us.com

What is it?

The diaphragm is a round piece of soft, thin silicone rubber with a firm, flexible ring. It is used along with a birth control cream or jelly.

You put the diaphragm in your vagina so that it covers the opening to your uterus (the cervix). You should not notice the diaphragm once it is in place. Most partners with a penis won't feel the diaphragm during sex.

You will see a health care provider to make sure the diaphragm is a good fit for you. They will show you how to insert and remove the diaphragm. They will also make sure you know how to use it properly with each act of reproductive sex.

The diaphragm does not help protect you from HIV or other STIs. Use a condom every time you have sex to help protect yourself from these STIs.

How does it work?

The diaphragm helps prevent pregnancy in two ways:

▶ It covers the cervix to help block the sperm from entering the uterus. That way, sperm cannot meet with an egg.

▶ It holds the birth control cream or jelly in place. The cream or jelly kills any sperm that may get past the diaphragm.

How well does it work?

You will need to explain to your patients about how well the diaphragm works (how effective it is). Be sure to explain the difference between "perfect use" and "typical use." You can read more about this in the "Stage 3" section of Chapter 2.

With perfect use, the diaphragm is 84% effective.

That means that if 100 patients use the diaphragm exactly the right way every time they have sex, 16 of them may get pregnant in a year.

With typical use, the diaphragm is 77% effective.

For those who don't use the diaphragm the right way every time they have sex, 23 out of 100 may get pregnant in a year.

How do you use the Diaphragm?

Teach your patients these steps so they can use the diaphragm correctly.

Talk to your patients about Emergency Contraception.

Emergency Contraception (EC), in the form of EC pills or an IUD, can prevent pregnancy after sex. Patients can use EC up to 5 days after unprotected sex. Read more about it in the section on EC.

First, a health care provider will fit you for the diaphragm. The provider will help you practice putting it in and taking it out. You can get the birth control cream or jelly to use with it at a clinic, drugstore, or supermarket.

You can put the diaphragm in right before you have sex or up to 6 hours before. Be sure to put it in before the penis is put in or near the vagina or anus.

Practice first

It is a good idea to practice putting the diaphragm in a few times when you are not planning to have sex.

How to put the diaphragm in:

1. **Wash your hands.**

2. **Wash the diaphragm with mild soap and cool water. Rinse and dry it.**

3. **Check it for holes:**
    - Fill it with water to see if it leaks.
    - Hold it in front of a bright light to look for holes or tears.

    If there are any leaks, holes, or tears, use a different birth control method until you get a new diaphragm.

4. **Put the birth control jelly or cream in the diaphragm.**
    - Check the expiration date on the tube of cream or jelly. If the date has passed, use a newer tube.
    - Squeeze about 1 teaspoon (about the size of a quarter) of the cream or jelly into the diaphragm.
    - Spread it around to cover the inside of the diaphragm with a thin layer. Add more if you need to.

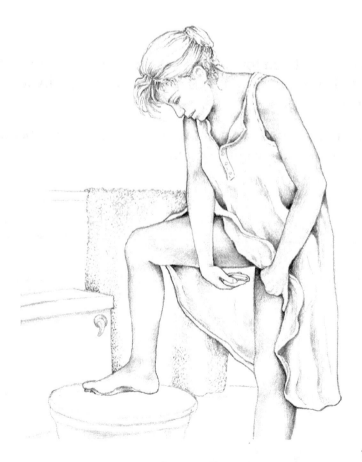

5. **Put the diaphragm in the vagina.**

   You can put one foot on a chair, or you can squat or lie down while you put it in. Follow these steps:

   - Squeeze the sides of the diaphragm rim until the sides are together. The Caya diaphragm has grip dimples on both sides so you know how to hold it during insertion.
   - Slide the diaphragm into the vagina. Push it in and back as far as it will go.
   - Tuck the front of the diaphragm rim behind your pubic bone.

6. **Check that the diaphragm is in the right place.**

   Put your finger in the vagina to feel the diaphragm.

   - The dome of the diaphragm should cover the cervix.

   Note: Be aware that during your most fertile days, your cervix is higher in the vagina. The cervix may be harder to reach at those times.

   - The front of the rim should be tucked behind the pubic bone. This is the bony area near your cervix.

7. **You can have sex right away if you want to.**

8. **Leave the diaphragm in for at least 6 hours after you have reproductive sex with ejaculation or "pre-come."**

   This is to make sure there are no live sperm in the vagina when you take the diaphragm out.

   But make sure that you do NOT leave the diaphragm in for more than 24 hours.

How to take the diaphragm out:

1. **Wash your hands.**

2. **You can put one foot on a chair or you can squat or lie down.**

3. **Use your finger to check that the diaphragm has stayed in the right place.**

   If the diaphragm has moved out of place, you may get pregnant. You can talk to your health care provider about Emergency Contraceptive (EC).

4. **Take the diaphragm out.** Follow these steps:

   - Hook your finger under the rim of the diaphragm. The Caya diaphragm has a fingertip removal dome for easier removal.
   - Gently pull the diaphragm down and out of the vagina.

5. **Wash the diaphragm with plain soap and water.**

   Be sure to rinse and dry it.

6. **Hold it to the light to check for holes or tears.**

7. **Store the diaphragm in its case in a cool, dry place and out of direct sunlight.**

What if the diaphragm is in more than 6 hours before you have sex?

If this happens, you can do either of the following:

▶ Take the diaphragm out. Rinse and dry it. Add cream or jelly just as you did the first time, then put the diaphragm back in.

▶ Leave the diaphragm in. Use the birth control cream or jelly applicator to put cream or jelly into your vagina just before you have sex.

What if you want to have sex more than once?

You must leave the diaphragm in place at least 6 hours after you have sex. If you want to have sex again during those 6 hours, you need to add more birth control jelly or cream.

Follow these steps:

▶ *Don't* remove the diaphragm.

▶ Use the birth control cream applicator to add more cream or jelly to the vagina just before you have sex.

▶ Remember to keep the diaphragm in place *at least 6 hours* after the last time you have sex.

Things to remember when you use the diaphragm:

▶ Use the diaphragm every time you have sex. Be sure to use birth control cream or jelly with it.

▶ If the diaphragm feels uncomfortable, it may be out of place. Take it out, add more birth control cream or jelly, and try again.

▶ If you need extra lubrication during sex, use your birth control cream or jelly. It is okay to use a water-based lubricant instead. Do NOT use silicone-based lubricants.

▶ Don't use petroleum jelly, hand lotion, creams to treat vaginal infections, or other oil-based products in the vagina. They can damage the diaphragm.

▶ You can safely leave the diaphragm in a total of *24 hours,* unless you are having your period. You can go to the bathroom, fall asleep, or do any activities you want with the diaphragm in place.

   ▪ If you are having your period, do not leave the diaphragm in the vagina more than *8 hours.* This is to protect you from Toxic Shock Syndrome (TSS). TSS is a rare but serious illness.

Have the diaphragm checked.

The diaphragm may not be the right size for you. If it does not fit well, it may not work for you. You may need to see your provider to check the fitting each year. You may also need it checked if:

▸ You have bladder infections often.

▸ You feel the diaphragm move out of place during sex.

▸ You have pain in the vagina or pelvic area when you use the diaphragm.

▸ The diaphragm hurts your partner's penis.

▸ You give birth.

▸ You have pelvic surgery.

The Diaphragm and Weight Concerns

Q: Does the diaphragm cause weight gain?

A: No.

Q: If a patient is overweight, will the diaphragm still work well?

A: Yes!

Q: Are there medical problems if a patient is overweight and uses the diaphragm?

A: No, none at all.

Are there any side effects?

Some people may have the following side effects:

▸ **Allergy to the silicone rubber or to the birth control cream or jelly:** This can cause skin rashes, itching, burning, or redness in or around the vagina or penis. Also, irritation of the vagina caused by spermicides can give you a higher chance of getting STIs or HIV if you are exposed. You can try changing brands of cream or jelly. Allergies to silicone are not common.

You may have the following side effects if your diaphragm doesn't fit well. If you have any of these side effects, go to your health care provider to get refitted:

▸ **Bladder infection:** This can happen if the diaphragm presses against the urethra (the thin tube that your urine flows through).

▸ **Pelvic cramps or discomfort**

▸ **Irritation of the vagina**

What about complications and warning signs?

Be sure to tell your patients about the warning signs for Toxic Shock Syndrome.

The only serious problem that the diaphragm may cause is Toxic Shock Syndrome (TSS). This is very rare. But it is serious. The bacteria that causes TSS can grow during your period if the blood stays in the vagina too long. Tampons keep the blood from flowing out. That is why you need to change your tampons often. The diaphragm also keeps the blood from flowing out. That is why you should never leave a diaphragm in longer than 8 hours during your period.

Toxic Shock Syndrome Warning Signs

Warning Signs

- ▶ Sudden high fever
- ▶ Vomiting or diarrhea
- ▶ Feeling dizzy, faint, or weak
- ▶ Sore throat
- ▶ Aching muscles and joints
- ▶ A rash that looks like a sunburn

If you have any of these warning signs, take the diaphragm out. **Call your health care provider right away.**

Breastfeeding

A patient who breastfeeds can use the diaphragm. But before they can use it they must:

- Wait 4 to 6 weeks after childbirth.
- Be refitted for the diaphragm.

They should use a different method of birth control until then.

Are there any precautions?

A health care provider may advise you to use a different birth control method if any of the following is true:

- ▶ You or your partner has an allergy to the silicone rubber in the diaphragm or to the birth control cream or jelly.
- ▶ You can't be properly fitted with the diaphragm.
- ▶ You have bladder infections often or have ever had TSS.

What are the advantages and disadvantages of using a Diaphragm?

There are many things people like about using the diaphragm. And there are some things they don't like. Find out what your patient likes. Encourage them to focus on those things.

What some people like about the diaphragm:

- ▶ Diaphragm causes few health problems.
- ▶ It can be put in up to 6 hours before sex. It can be left in for up to 24 hours for convenience.
- ▶ You only use it when you need it.
- ▶ It is mostly under the patient's control.

Find out what your patient might not like about the diaphragm.

Ask your patients if they have any concerns about using the diaphragm. Then talk to them about their concerns. Help them think through how to solve any problems they might have while using the diaphragm. Have them think of their own solutions first. Read the chart that follows for some ideas about how to deal with their concerns.

Keep in mind that the diaphragm isn't the best method for everyone. It is the patient's choice.

What if you want to stop using the Diaphragm?

You can stop using the diaphragm whenever you want to. If you stop using it, you could become pregnant right away. Use another birth control method if you don't want to be pregnant.

There are no health problems to watch for when you stop using the diaphragm.

Make sure your patient understands.

Before your patients leave, make sure they understand how to use a diaphragm successfully. Some of these questions may help.

- ▸ Tell me what you know about the diaphragm.
- ▸ How will you use the diaphragm?
- ▸ How long after reproductive sex do you need to leave the diaphragm in your vagina?
- ▸ How does the diaphragm work?
- ▸ What might be the most difficult thing for you when using a diaphragm?
- ▸ How could you get around that problem?
- ▸ How will you take care of your diaphragm?

ubbleЇЇ

Diaphragm

The Diaphragm: Some Problems and Ways to Solve Them

Problem	Ways to Solve the Problem
I have trouble putting it in.	Practice putting it in. Do this when you are not planning to have sex. After a few tries, it will be easier. If you still have trouble, come back for a refitting. The diaphragm may be too large.
I don't like putting my fingers inside my vagina to put it in or remove it.	▪ Many patients feel this way at first. With practice, you may get used to it. ▪ Your partner can put it in and remove it for you.
It seems messy.	After you get used to how to put it in and how much birth control gel you need, it may seem less messy.
I am (or my partner is) allergic to the birth control cream or jelly (or silicone rubber).	▪ You can try different brands of cream or jelly. ▪ If the allergy is to the rubber, you may need to choose a different method. Allergies to silicone are not common.
What if I don't have my diaphragm or my birth control cream or jelly with me when I need it?	▪ You could have non-reproductive sex or be intimate in ways that can not cause a pregnancy. ▪ You could use condoms, withdrawal or another birth control method at those times. ▪ You could decide to wait for another time to have sex.
What if, after sex, I find out my diaphragm slipped out of place or had a hole in it?	You can help prevent this problem if you: ▪ Check your diaphragm for holes or tears before you use it. ▪ Make sure your diaphragm is in right before you have sex. If you do find the diaphragm has slipped or had a hole in it, you can still try to prevent a possible pregnancy after sex. Find out about EC.
The diaphragm does not protect against HIV and other STIs.	To help protect yourself against HIV and other STIs, use an external condom along with the diaphragm every time you have sex.

© Essential Access Health

449

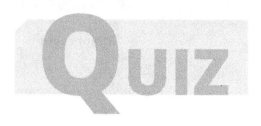

DIAPHRAGM

Directions: Read each of the following statements. Is it true or false? Circle the best answer.

1. The diaphragm is a round piece of soft, thin, silicone rubber with a firm, flexible ring.　　　True　　False

2. You do not need to use a spermicide with the diaphragm.　　　True　　False

3. The diaphragm holds spermicide close to the cervix to kill sperm before they can enter the uterus.　　　True　　False

4. A diaphragm must be fitted by a provider.　　　True　　False

5. It may take practice to use a diaphragm well.　　　True　　False

Directions: Read the following question. Circle all of the answers that apply.

6. Which of these are steps for putting in a diaphragm?

   a. Wash your hands.

   b. Wash the diaphragm with soap and warm water.

   c. Check it for holes.

   d. Put the birth control jelly or cream in the diaphragm.

   e. Put the diaphragm in the vagina.

   f. Have the size of your diaphragm checked.

   g. Check that the diaphragm is in the right place.

Go on to the next page.

Directions: Read each of the following statements or questions, and write your best answer in the space below.

7. List two possible side effects of using the diaphragm.

   ▪ _____

   _____

   ▪ _____

   _____

8. What is the one serious problem that a diaphragm could cause?

   _____

   _____

Check your answers on the next page.

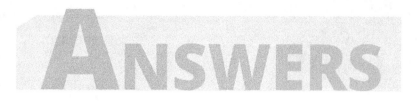

DIAPHRAGM

Check your answers.

1. **True**   The diaphragm is a round piece of soft, thin, silicone rubber with a firm, flexible ring.

2. **False**   You do need to use a spermicide with the diaphragm. The diaphragm is used along with a birth control cream or jelly. The diaphragm holds the cream or jelly in place.

3. **True**   The diaphragm does hold the spermicide close to the cervix to kill sperm before they can enter the uterus. That way, sperm cannot meet with an egg.

4. **True**   A diaphragm must be fitted by a provider.

5. **True**   It may take practice to use a diaphragm well. It is a good idea to practice putting the diaphragm in a few times when you are not planning to have reproductive sex.

6. **A, B, C, D, E, G**   All of these are steps in putting in a diaphragm:
   - Wash your hands.
   - Wash the diaphragm with soap and warm water.
   - Check it for holes.
   - Put the birth control jelly or cream in the diaphragm.
   - Put the diaphragm in the vagina.
   - Check that the diaphragm is in the right place.

   Only F it not a step in putting in a diaphragm.
   - Your provider should check the size of your diaphragm at least once a year.

Go on to the next page.

7. The possible side effects of using the diaphragm include:
   - Allergy to the rubber or to the birth control cream or jelly
   - Vaginal infection
   - Bladder infection
   - Pelvic cramps or discomfort
   - Irritation of the vagina

8. The only serious problem that the diaphragm may cause is Toxic Shock Syndrome (TSS). This is very rare. But it is serious.

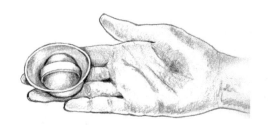

Birth Control Cap

What is it?

The birth control cap (also known as FemCap) is a small, hat-shaped piece of silicon rubber. This is a non-latex material. People who are allergic to latex can use this method. It has a large brim that helps it fit well in the vagina. It is used with a birth control cream or jelly.

You put the cap in your vagina so that it fits over the opening to your uterus (the cervix). You should not notice the cap once it is in place. Most partners with a penis won't feel it during sex.

There are three sizes. A health care provider will fit you with the right one. The same cap may be used for up to one year. Then you have to get a new one.

The cap does not help protect you from HIV or other STIs. Use a condom every time you have sex to help protect yourself from these STIs.

How does it work?

The cap helps prevent pregnancy in two ways:

- ▶ It covers the cervix to help block the sperm from entering the uterus. That way, sperm cannot meet with an egg.
- ▶ The birth control cream or jelly that is used with the cap kills any sperm that get past the cap.

How well does the Cap work?

The effectiveness of the cervical cap (FemCap) is affected by whether or not a patient has given birth.

For patients who have never given birth, the cervical cap is 86% effective.

> ▶ That means if 100 patients who have never given birth use the cap every time they have sex, 14 of them may get pregnant in a year.

For patients who have given birth, the cervical cap is 71% effective.

> ▶ That means if 100 patients who have given birth use the cap every time they have sex, 29 of them may get pregnant in a year.

Talk to your patients about Emergency Contraception.

Emergency Contraception (EC), in the form of EC pills or an IUD, can prevent pregnancy after sex. Patients can use EC up to 5 days after unprotected sex. Read more about it in the section on EC.

How do you use the Cap?

Teach patients these steps so they can use the cap correctly.

First, a health care provider will fit you for the right size cap. The provider will also help you practice putting it in and taking it out. You must use the birth control cream or jelly with the cap. You can get cream or jelly to use with the cap at your clinic, drugstore, or supermarket.

You can put the cap in right before you have sex or up to 48 hours before. Be sure to put it in before a penis is put in or near the vagina or anus. Be sure to leave the cap in place for 6 hours after the last time you have sex.

Practice first.

It is a good idea to practice putting the cap in a few times when you are not planning to have sex.

How to put the cap in:

1. **Wash your hands.**

2. **Wash the cap with plain soap and water.**

   Rinse and dry it.

3. **Check the cap for holes, tears, or cracks:**

   Hold the cap in front of a bright light to look for holes. If you see any holes, tears, or cracks, use a different birth control method until you get a new cap.

4. **Put the birth control cream or jelly in the cap.**

   - Check the expiration date on the tube of cream or jelly. If the date has passed, use a newer tube.

   - Put a small amount, about the size of a dime, on the inside of the cap. If you use too much, the cap won't stay on your cervix.

   - Spread a thin layer on the outside of the brim. Don't put any where your thumb and finger are. This will help prevent the cap from slipping out of your hand.

   - Turn the cap over. Put the cream or jelly in the groove between the dome and the brim. Put in about a half a teaspoon of the cream.

5. **Place the cap on the cervix.**

   You can put one foot on a chair, squat, or lie down. Then, follow these steps:

   - You can use your finger to feel inside your vagina to find where the cervix is. It will feel like the end of your nose. That is where the cap will go.

   Note: Be aware that during your most fertile days, your cervix is higher in the vagina. The cervix may be harder to reach at those times.

   - Squeeze the cap between your thumb and forefinger.

   - Slide the cap into your vagina. The bowl should be facing upward and the long brim should go in first. Push it down toward the back wall of your vagina, then downward and back as far as it can go. The walls of your vagina will hold it in place.

   - Use your finger to press the cap against the cervix for 10 seconds. This will help make sure it is in place.

6. **You can have sex right away if you want to.**

7. **Leave the cap in for at least 6 hours after you have sex.**

   This is to make sure there are no live sperm in the vagina when you take the cap out.

How to take the cap out:

1. **Wash your hands.**

2. **You can put one foot on a chair, squat, or lie down.**

3. **Take the cap out.**

   - Push your finger on the dome of the cap. This will break the suction and allow room for your finger to fit in the removal strap.

   - Hook the removal strap with the tip of your finger.

   - Gently pull the cap out of your vagina.

4. **Wash the cap with plain soap and water.**

5. **Rinse and dry it well.**

   Let the cap air dry or gently pat it dry with a clean, soft towel.

6. **You can dust it with cornstarch to help keep it dry.**

   Don't use powders with talc or perfume in them. And don't use petroleum jelly or silicone-based lubricants. These can damage the silicone rubber.

7. **Store it in its case in a cool, dry place.**

What if you want to have sex more than once?

You can have sex as many times as you want while the cap is in. Do not remove the cap to have more sex. Use the special applicator to add more cream or jelly each time you have sex.

Be sure to leave the cap in for *at least 6 hours* after the last time you have sex.

Things to remember when you use the cap:

Do's

- ▸ Use the cap *every* time you have sex. Remember to use birth control cream or jelly with the cap.
- ▸ Be sure the cap is in the right place before you have sex. If it is not in right, take it out. Rinse and dry it and follow the steps to put it in.
- ▸ When you put the cream or jelly on the inside of the cap, don't put any where your thumb and finger are. This will help prevent the cap from slipping out of your hand.
- ▸ If you need extra lubrication during sex, you can use your birth control cream or jelly. Or you can use another water-based lube.
- ▸ The cap can safely stay in place for up to 48 hours (2 days). Do not douche (rinse the vagina) while the cap is in. Showers and baths are okay. You can go to the bathroom, fall asleep, or do any activities you want with the cap in place.
- ▸ If you have cramping while the cap is in, it may be too tight. Come to the health care site to have the size of your cap checked.

Don'ts

- ▸ Do not use silicone-based lubricants.
- ▸ Don't use the cap if it looks like it is getting worn out.
- ▸ Don't use the cap during your period. Use a different method of birth control. This is to protect you from Toxic Shock Syndrome (TSS). TSS is a rare but serious illness.

You can read more about Toxic Shock Syndrome under "What about complications and warning signs."

Are there any side effects?

Some who use the cap may have one or more of the following side effects:

▸ **Allergy to the birth control cream or jelly.** This can cause skin rashes, itching, burning, or redness. You can try changing brands of cream or jelly.

▸ **Irritation from the birth control cream or jelly:** This can give you a higher chance of getting STIs or HIV if you are exposed.

▸ **Vaginal infection.** This can happen if the cap is left in too long or if it is not cleaned and dried well after use.

▸ **Irritation of the cervix.** This can happen if the cap doesn't fit well or is left in too long.

What about complications and warning signs?

The only serious problem that the cap may cause is Toxic Shock Syndrome (TSS). This is very rare. But it is serious. The bacteria that causes TSS can grow during your period if the blood stays in the vagina too long. Tampons keep the blood from flowing out. That is why you need to change your tampons often. The cap also keeps blood from flowing out.

That is why you should use a different birth control method during your period.

The Cap and Weight Concerns

Q: Will using the cap cause weight gain?

A: No.

Q: If someone is overweight, will the cap still work well?

A: Yes.

Q: Are there medical problems if a cap user is overweight?

A: No.

Toxic Shock Syndrome Warning Signs

▸ Sudden high fever

▸ Vomiting, diarrhea

▸ Feeling dizzy, faint, or weak

▸ Sore throat

▸ Aching muscles and joints

▸ A rash that looks like a sunburn

If you have any of these warning signs, take the cap out. **Call your health care provider right away.**

Breastfeeding

Those who breastfeed should check with their provider before using the cap. This is for two reasons:

- The cap does not work as well for those who have had a baby.

- If this is their first delivery, they will need to be refitted for the cap 8 weeks after childbirth. Until then, they should use a different form of birth control.

Are there any precautions?

A health care provider may advise you to use a different birth control method if any of the following is true:

▶ You or your partner has an allergy to the birth control cream or jelly.

▶ You have an infection in your vagina or have an abnormal Pap smear.

▶ You have bladder infections often or have ever had TSS.

You may be advised to use a different method of birth control until about 8 weeks after childbirth or having an abortion.

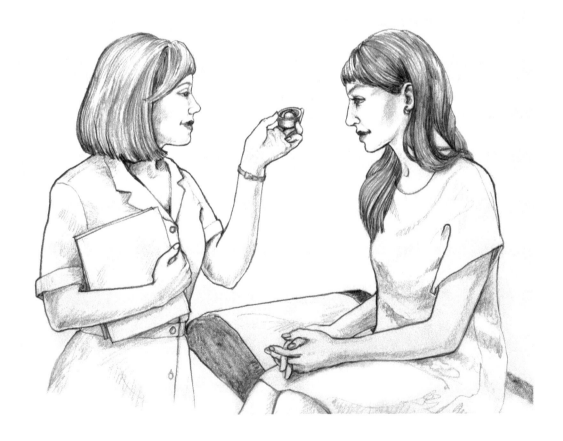

What are the advantages and disadvantages of using the Cap?

There are many things people like about using the cap. And there are things some they don't like. Find out what your patient likes. Encourage them to focus on those things.

What some people like about the cap:

- ▸ It causes few health problems.
- ▸ It is not made of latex, so those with allergies to latex can use it.
- ▸ You can have sex as many times as you want for up to 48 hours.
- ▸ You only use it when you need it.
- ▸ It doesn't have hormones in it.
- ▸ It is under the patient's control.

Find out what your patient might not like.

Ask your patients if they have any concerns about using the cap. Then talk to them about their concerns. Help them think through how to solve any problems they might have while using the cap. Have them think of their own solutions first. Read the chart that follows for some ideas about how to deal with their concerns.

Keep in mind that the cap isn't the best method for everyone. It is the patient's choice.

The Cap: Some Problems and Ways to Solve Them

Problem	Ways to Solve the Problem
I have trouble putting it in.	Practice putting it in when you are not going to have sex. After a few tries, it will be easier.
I don't like putting my fingers inside my vagina to put it in or remove it.	Many patients feel this way at first. With practice, you may get used to it. You can ask your partner to insert and remove it for you.
I am (or my partner is) allergic to the birth control cream or jelly.	You can try different brands of cream or jelly.
What if I don't have my cap or birth control cream or jelly with me when I need it?	▪ You could have non-reproductive sex or be intimate in ways that can not cause a pregnancy. ▪ You could use condoms, withdrawal or another birth control method at those times. ▪ You could decide to wait for another time to have sex.
What if, after sex, I find out my cap slipped out of place or had a hole in it?	You can help prevent this problem if you: ▪ Check your cap for holes or tears before you use it. ▪ Make sure the cap is in right before you have sex. If you do find that the cap has slipped or had a hole in it, you can still try to prevent pregnancy after sex. Find out about EC.
My partner can feel the cap during sex.	Most partners with a penis don't feel it during sex. But if your partner does and if it is painful to them, you may want to use a different method.
The cap does not protect against HIV and other STIs.	To help protect yourself against HIV and other STIs, also use a condom every time you have sex.

What if you want to stop using the Cap?

You can stop using the cap whenever you want to. If you stop using it, you could become pregnant right away. Use another birth control method if you don't want to be pregnant.

There are no health problems to watch for when you stop using the cap.

Make sure your patient understands.

Before your patients leave, make sure they understand how to use the cap successfully. Some of these questions may help.

- ▸ Tell me what you know about the birth control cap.
- ▸ How does the cap work?
- ▸ How will you use the cap?
- ▸ How long after reproductive sex do you need to leave the cap in your vagina?
- ▸ What might be the most difficult thing for you about using the cap?
- ▸ How would you get around that problem?
- ▸ How will you take care of your cap?

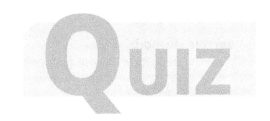

BIRTH CONTROL CAP

Directions: Circle the best answer.

1. The Birth Control Cap:

    a. Is a small, hat-shaped piece of silicon rubber.

    b. It has a large brim that helps it fit well in the vagina.

    c. It is used with a birth control cream or jelly.

    d. All of the above.

2. The Cap helps prevent pregnancy because:

    a. It changes the lining of the uterus so that sperm can't live.

    b. It covers the cervix to help block the sperm from entering the uterus.

    c. The birth control cream or jelly that is used with the cap kills any sperm that get past the cap.

    d. B and C

3. If you want to have sex more than once while using the Cap:

    a. Take the Cap out and add more spermicide.

    b. You can't. The Cap can only be used once.

    c. Use the special applicator to add more cream or jelly each time you have sex.

    d. None of the above

4. After taking the Cap out of the vagina, you should:

    a. Wash the Cap with plain soap and water.

    b. Rinse and dry it.

    c. Store it in its case in a cool, dry place.

    d. All of the above

Go on to the next page.

5. You hould not leave the Cap in the vagina for more than:

    a. 16 hours

    b. 24 hours

    c. 48 hours

    d. 60 hours

Directions: Read each of the following questions. Write your best answers in the space below.

6. What are two warning signs to watch for when you use the Cap?

    ▪ _____

    ▪ _____

7. List one concern that a patient may have about using the Cap and what you might say to help them deal with that concern.

    ▪ *Patient's concern:* _____

    _____

    ▪ *What you can say:* _____

    _____

    _____

Check your answers on the next page.

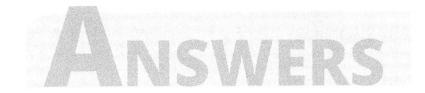

BIRTH CONTROL CAP

Check your answers.

1. **D**   All of the above. The Birth Control Cap is a small, hat-shaped piece of silicon rubber. It has a large brim that helps it fit well in the vagina. It is used with a birth control cream or jelly.

2. **D**   B and C. The Cap helps prevent pregnancy because it covers the cervix to help block the sperm from entering the uterus. Also, the birth control cream or jelly that is used with the Cap kills any sperm that get past it.

3. **C**   You can have sex as many times as you want while the Cap is in. Do not take the Cap out to have more sex. Use the special applicator to add more cream or jelly each time you have sex.

4. **D**   All of the above. After you the Cap out of the vagina, you should:
   - Wash the cap with plain soap and water
   - Rinse and dry it well.
   - Store it in its case in a cool, dry place.

5. **C**   Don't leave the Cap in the vagina for more than 48 hours.

Go on to the next page.

6. Warning signs to watch for when you use the Cap are:
   - Sudden high fever
   - Vomiting, diarrhea
   - Feeling dizzy, faint, or weak
   - Sore throat
   - Aching muscles and joints
   - A rash that looks like a sunburn

   If you have any of these warning signs, take the Cap out. **Call your health care provider right away.**

7. Here are two concerns a patient might have about using the Cap and what you might say to help them. For other possible concerns and responses, please see "The Cap: Some Problems and Ways to Solve Them" chart near the end of the Birth Control Cap section.
   - *Patient's concern:* "I have trouble putting it in."

     What you could say: "Practice putting it in when you are not going to have sex. After a few tries, it will be easier."

   - *Patient's concern:* "My partner feels the cap during sex."

     What you could say: "Most partners don't feel it during sex. But if your partner does and if it is painful to them, you may want to use a different birth control method."

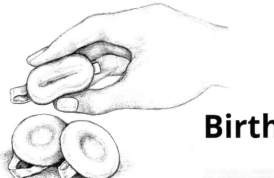

Birth Control Sponge

This section is mostly written as though you were talking to your patients. It gives you an idea of how to explain the sponge in a way your patients can understand. This section also has notes written directly to you, the health worker. Those "health worker notes" look like this one.

What is it?

The birth control sponge is a piece of soft foam made out of polyurethane (a type of plastic). It is round and has a dimple on one side and a strap on the other. The sponge has a spermicide in it called Nonoxynol-9. The spermicide is a chemical that kills sperm.

The sponge will cover the cervix (the opening of the uterus). You should not notice the sponge once it is in place. Most partners with a penis won't feel it during sex.

The sponge comes in one size. It can be purchased at pharmacies, supermarkets and clinics. You do not need to see a health care provider to start using the sponge.

The sponge does not help protect you from HIV or other STIs. Use a condom every time you have sex to help protect yourself from these STIs.

How does it work?

The sponge helps prevent pregnancy in three ways:

- ▶ It covers the cervix to help block the sperm from entering the uterus. That way, sperm cannot meet with an egg.
- ▶ It soaks up sperm and traps them to keep them from going into the cervix.
- ▶ The spermicide in the sponge kills the sperm.

How well does the sponge work?

You will need to explain to your patients about how well the sponge works (how effective it is). Be sure to explain the difference between "perfect use" and "typical use." You can read more about this in the "Stage 3" section of Chapter 2.

The sponge works best for patients who have never given birth.

> ▸ **With perfect use, the sponge is 91% effective for those who have never given birth.**
>
> That means that if 100 of those patients use the sponge exactly the right way every time they have sex, 9 of them may get pregnant in a year.

> ▸ **With typical use, the sponge is 88% effective for those who have never given birth.**
>
> For those patients who don't use the sponge the right way every time they have sex, 12 out of 100 may get pregnant in a year.

The sponge does not work as well for patients who have given birth.

> ▸ **With perfect use, the sponge is only 80% effective for those who have given birth.**
>
> That means that if 100 of those patients use the sponge exactly the right way every time they have sex, 20 of them may get pregnant in a year.

> ▸ **With typical use, the sponge is only 71% effective for those who have given birth.**
>
> For those patients who don't use the sponge the right way every time they have sex, as many as 29 out of 100 may get pregnant in a year.

Talk to your patients about Emergency Contraception.

Emergency Contraception (EC), in the form of EC pills or an IUD, can prevent pregnancy after sex. Patients can use EC up to 5 days after unprotected sex. Read more about EC at the end of this chapter.

How do you use the Sponge?

Teach patients these steps so they can use the sponge correctly.

You can put the sponge in right before you have sex or up to 24 hours before. Be sure to put it in before the penis is put in or near the vagina or anus.

Before you take out the sponge:

> ▸ **Check the expiration date on the box.**
> If the date has passed, don't use it. Use a newer package. Or use a different method of birth control.

> ▸ **Open the air-tight package.**
> When you open the box, the sponge will be inside an air-tight bag. Be careful not to damage the sponge when you open the bag.

How to put the sponge in:

1. **Wash your hands.**

2. **Wet the sponge with clean tap water.** Make sure it is wet all the way through.

3. **Gently squeeze the sponge until it gets sudsy.**
   - Hold the sponge with the dimple up. The strap will hang down.
   - As you squeeze, the sponge suds up. Don't worry about making too many suds. There is plenty of spermicide in the sponge.

4. **Put the sponge in the vagina.**
   You can put one foot on a chair, squat, or lie down. Follow these steps:
   - Hold the sponge so that the strap is under the sponge. Squeeze the sides of the sponge together.
   - Squeeze the sponge in half. Slide the sponge into the vagina. Push it back as far as it will go.
   - The dimple should face the cervix.

5. **Check that the sponge is in the right place.**
   Put your finger in the vagina to feel the sponge. If it doesn't push any farther back, then it is in correctly.

6. **You can have sex right away if you want to.**

7. **Leave the sponge in for at least 6 hours after you have sex.**
   This is to make sure there are no live sperm in the vagina when you take the sponge out.

How to take the sponge out:

1. **Wash your hands.**

2. **You can put one foot on a chair, squat, or lie down.**

3. **Take the sponge out.**

    Follow these steps:

    -   Hook your finger around the strap of the sponge. You can also grab the sponge between your thumb and finger.

    -   Gently pull the sponge out of your vagina. Be careful! It can tear.

4. **Toss the sponge away.**

    Do not flush the sponge down the toilet.

What if you can't get the sponge to come out?

Only the pressure from the muscles in the vagina will keep it from coming out. Relaxing the muscles of the vagina will help it to come out.

Stuck sponge
If the sponge seems stuck, it is probably due to suction around the cervix. Run your finger between the sponge and your cervix. Pull one side up to break the seal. It should now move normally. You can also squat and bear down as if you were going to have a bowel movement. This will will bring the sponge down lower in the vagina. You should be able to hook your finger around the strap more easily.

Upside down sponge
Sometimes the sponge might turn around in the vagina. This may make it hard to find the strap to help pull it out. If this happens, run your finger around the back of the vagina. You should feel the strap and can pull out the sponge. If you can't find the strap, you can squeeze the sponge between your thumb and finger to pull it out. It can help if you squat and bear down like you're having a bowel movement.

Torn sponge
It is important to treat the sponge gently. It can easily be torn. Pull it out gently. If it does tear, be sure to get every piece out.

What if you want to have sex more than once?

You can have as much sex as you want for 24 hours after putting in the sponge. You must leave the sponge in place at least 6 hours after you have sex.

Do not leave the sponge in for more than 30 hours!

Things to remember when you use the sponge:

Do's

- Use the sponge every time you have sex.

- Be sure the sponge is in the right place before you have sex. Put a finger in the vagina and make sure the sponge is pushed all the way back.

- Store the sponge in a cool, dry place.

- If you need extra lubrication during sex, you can use your birth control cream or jelly. Or you can use other water-based lubes.

- The sponge can safely stay in place for up to 30 hours. Do not douche (rinse the vagina) while the sponge is in. Showers and baths are okay. You can go to the bathroom, fall asleep, or do any activities you want with the sponge in place.

Don'ts

- Don't leave the sponge in for more than 30 hours. It can increase your chance of irritation in the vagina.

- Don't use the sponge during your period. This is to protect you from Toxic Shock Syndrome (TSS). TSS is a rare but serious illness.

You can read more about Toxic Shock Syndrome under "What about complications and warning signs."

The Sponge and Weight Concerns

Q: Does the sponge cause weight gain?

A: No.

Q: If a user is overweight, will the sponge still work well?

A: Yes.

Q: Are there medical problems if a sponge user is overweight?

A: No, not at all.

Are there any side effects?

Some patients may have one or more of the following side effects:

▸ **Allergy to the sponge:** The sponge contains sulfites. Some people are allergic to sulfites.

▸ **Allergy to the spermicide in the sponge:** This can cause skin rashes, itching, burning, or redness.

▸ **Irritation from the spermicide to the vagina:** People using a sponge may or may not feel the irritation at all. The more often you use the sponge, the more likely you will have an irritation. This could give you a higher chance of getting an STI or HIV, if you are exposed.

What about complications and warning signs?

Be sure to tell your patients about the warning signs for Toxic Shock Syndrome.

The only serious problem that the sponge may cause is Toxic Shock Syndrome (TSS). This is very rare. But it is serious. The bacteria that causes TSS can grow during your period if the blood stays in the vagina too long. For example, tampons keep the blood from flowing out. That is why you need to change your tampons often. The sponge also keeps blood from flowing out. That is why you should not use the sponge during your period.

Toxic Shock Syndrome Warning Signs

▸ Sudden high fever

▸ Vomiting, diarrhea

▸ Feeling dizzy, faint, or weak

▸ Sore throat

▸ Aching muscles and joints

▸ A rash that looks like a sunburn

If you have any of these warning signs, take the sponge out. **Call your provider right away.**

Are there any precautions?

A medical provider may advise you to use a different birth control method if any of the following is true:

▸ You or your partner has an allergy to the sulfites in the sponge, or to the birth control cream or jelly.

▸ You have bladder infections often or have had TSS.

▸ You have certain problems with your uterus or vagina.

▸ You may be advised to use a different method of birth control until about 6 weeks after childbirth or after having an abortion.

Breastfeeding

Those who breastfeed can use the sponge. But before they can use it, they must wait 6 weeks after childbirth.

They should use a different method of birth control until then.

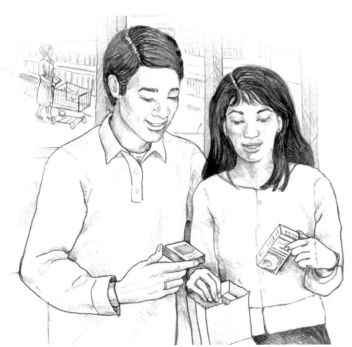

What are the advantages and disadvantages of using the sponge?

There are many things people like about using the sponge. And there are some things they don't like. Find out what your patient likes. Encourage them to focus on those things.

What some people like about the sponge:

- ▶ It causes few health problems.
- ▶ It is not made of latex, so patients with allergies to latex can use it.
- ▶ You can have sex as many times as you want for up to 24 hours.
- ▶ You only use it when you need it.
- ▶ It doesn't have hormones in it.
- ▶ It is under the patient's control.

Find out what your patient might not like about the sponge.

Ask your patients if they have any concerns about using the sponge. Then talk to them about their concerns. Help them think through how to solve any problems they might have while using the sponge. Have them think of their own solutions first. Read the chart that follows for some ideas about how to deal with their concerns.

Keep in mind that the sponge isn't the best method for everyone. It is the patient's choice.

The Sponge: Some Problems and Ways to Solve Them

Problem	Ways to Solve the Problem
I have trouble putting it in.	Practice putting it in when you are not going to have sex. After a few tries, it will be easier.
I don't like putting my fingers inside my vagina to put it in and remove it.	Many patients feel this way at first. With practice, you may get used to it. Your partner can put it in and remove it for you.
It seems messy.	You only need to get it a little sudsy for it to work.
I am (or my partner is) allergic to the spermicide.	This may not be the best method for you.
What if I don't have my sponge with me when I need it?	■ You could have non-reproductive sex or be intimate in ways that can not cause a pregnancy. ■ You could use condoms, withdrawal or another birth control method at those times. ■ You could decide to wait for another time to have sex.
What if, after sex, I find out my sponge slipped out of place?	You can help prevent this problem if you: ■ Make sure the sponge is in the right place before you have sex. If you do find that the sponge has slipped, you can still try to prevent pregnancy after sex. Find out about EC.
My partner is worried they will feel the sponge during sex.	Most partners with a penis don't feel it during sex. It is very soft and feels like the inside of the vagina.
The sponge does not protect against HIV and other STIs.	To help protect yourself against HIV and other STIs, use a condom along with the sponge every time you have sex.

What if you want to stop using the sponge?

You can stop using the sponge whenever you want to. If you stop using it, you could become pregnant right away. Use another birth control method if you don't want to be pregnant.

There are no health problems to watch for when you stop using the sponge.

Make sure your patient understands.

Before your patients leave, make sure they understand how to use the sponge successfully. Some of these questions may help.

Things you can ask your patient:

- ▸ Tell me what you know about the sponge.
- ▸ How does the sponge work?
- ▸ Tell me how to use the sponge.
- ▸ What might be the most difficult thing for you about using the sponge?
- ▸ How would you get around that problem?

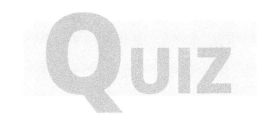

BIRTH CONTROL SPONGE

Directions: Circle the best answer.

1. The Birth Control Sponge is made of:
   a. Latex, a type of rubber
   b. Polyurethane, a type of plastic
   c. Sea sponge
   d. None of the above

2. The Sponge helps prevent pregnancy because:
   a. It covers the cervix to help block the sperm from entering the uterus.
   b. It soaks up sperm and traps them to keep them from going into the cervix.
   c. The spermicide in the Sponge kills any sperm that get past it.
   d. All of the above

3. Do not leave the Sponge in for more than:
   a. 12 hours.
   b. 6 hours.
   c. 30 hours.
   d. None of the above

4. Which of the following is true about the Sponge?
   a It can get torn or stuck in the vagina.
   b. It should not be used during your period.
   c. You have to use a new Sponge every time you have sex, even within the same 24 hour period.
   d. A and B

Go on to the next page.

5. This is a warning sign for the Sponge:

    a.   Shortness of breath

    b.   Sudden high fever

    c.   Blurred vision

    d.   Bleeding changes

Directions: Read the following and write your best answer in the space below.

6. List one concern that a patient may have about using the Sponge and what you might say to help them deal with that concern.

    ▪ *Patient's concern:*
    _____

    _____

    ▪ *What you can say:*
    _____

    _____

Check your answers on the next page.

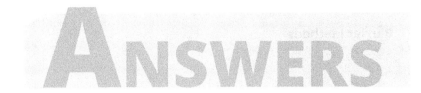

BIRTH CONTROL SPONGE

Check your answers.

1. **B**   The Birth Control Sponge is made of polyurethane, a type of plastic.

2. **D**   All of the above. The Sponge helps prevent pregnancy in three ways:
   - It covers the cervix to help block the sperm from entering the uterus. That way, sperm cannot meet with an egg.
   - It soaks up sperm and traps them to keep them from going into the cervix.
   - The spermicide in the sponge kills any sperm that get past it.

3. **C**   Do not leave the Sponge in for more than 30 hours.

4. **D**   A and B. It is true that the Sponge can get stuck in the vagina or torn. Also it should not be used during menstruation. You can leave the Sponge in and have sex as many times as you want in a 24 hour period without using a new Sponge.

5. **B**   Sudden high fever is a warning sign for the Sponge. These are other warning signs for the Sponge:
   - Vomiting, diarrhea
   - Feeling dizzy, faint, or weak
   - Sore throat
   - Aching muscles and joints
   - A rash that looks like a sunburn

   If a patient has any of these warning signs, they should take the Sponge out. **They should call their health care provider right away.**

Go on to the next page.

6. Here are two concerns a patient might have about using the Sponge and what you might say to help them. For other possible concerns and responses, please see "The Sponge: Some Problems and Ways to Solve Them" chart near the end of the Birth Control Sponge section.

- *Patient's concern:* "It seems messy."

  What you could say: "You only need to get it a little sudsy for it to work."

- *Patient's concern:* "What if, after sex, I find out my sponge slipped out of place?"

  What you could say: "You can help prevent this problem if you make sure the sponge is in right before you have sex. If you do find that the sponge has slipped, you can still try to prevent pregnancy after sex. Let me tell you about EC."

Spermicides

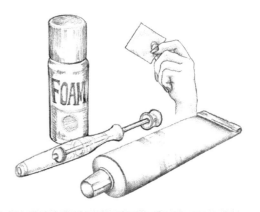

This section is mostly written as though you were talking to your patients. It gives you an idea of how to explain spermicides in a way your patients can understand. This section also has notes written directly to you as a health worker. Those "health workers notes" look like this one.

What are they?

Spermicides come in many forms:

- Foam
- Cream
- Jelly (or gel)
- Suppositories
- Vaginal film

They are put into the vagina before you have sex. All spermicides contain a chemical to kill sperm. The most common chemical used is nonoxynol-9.

Spermicides do not help protect against HIV and other STIs. Use a condom every time you have sex to help protect yourself from these STIs.

How do they work?

Spermicides kill sperm in the vagina. This keeps sperm from entering the uterus and meeting with an egg. Spermicides work best when they are used along with another barrier method such as condoms.

How well do they work?

Note: When spermicides are used alone, they are not as effective as other methods. If your patient chooses spermicides as a method, encourage them to also use a condom every time they have sex.

Also, let patients know that using a spermicide with nonoxynol-9 more than twice a day could increase their chances of getting an STI. You will need to explain to your patients about how well spermicides work (how effective they are). Be sure to explain the difference between "perfect use" and "typical use." You can read more about this in the "Stage 3" section of Chapter 2.

Talk to your patients about Emergency Contraception.

Emergency Contraception (EC), in the form of EC pills or an IUD, can prevent pregnancy after sex. Patients can use EC up to 5 days after unprotected sex. Read more about it in the section on EC.

With perfect use, spermicides are 82% effective.

That means that if 100 patients use spermicides exactly the right way every time they have sex, 18 of them may get pregnant in a year.

With typical use, spermicides are 72% effective.

For those who don't use spermicides the right way every time they have sex, 28 out of 100 may get pregnant in a year.

How do you use Spermicides?

Teach your patients these steps so they can use spermicides correctly.

The basics for using any type of spermicide

▸ **Check the expiration date on the package or can.**

If the date has passed, don't use it. Use a newer package or can. Or use a different method of birth control.

▸ **Wash your hands before you put the spermicide in.**

▸ **Put the spermicide in before the penis is put in or near the vagina or anus.**

Follow the instructions about when you need to put your spermicide in. To kill sperm, the spermicide must be put in before you have sex. Most spermicides can be put in up to 1 hour before sex.

▪ If more than 1 hour goes by before you have sex, add more spermicide.

▸ **Before each time you have sex, add more spermicide.**

▸ **Don't rinse out the vagina (douche) after sex.**
Rinsing can wash out the spermicide before it kills all of the sperm. Showers and baths are OK. If you want to rinse the vagina, you need to wait at least 6 hours after the last time you had sex.

▸ **If you use an applicator, wash and dry it after each use.** Use plain soap and water.

At the end of this section you will find the basic steps for each type of spermicide. Teach your patients the steps for the type or types of spermicide they would like to use. Make sure patients know that it is a good idea to read the instructions that come with the package. That is because each brand may be a little different.

Are there any side effects to using spermicides?

There are few side effects to using spermicides.

▸ **Irritation to the skin of the vagina:** You may or may not feel the irritation at all. The more often someone uses the spermicide, the more likely they are to have irritation.

▸ **Allergy to the spermicide:** It can cause skin rashes, itching, burning, or redness in or around the vagina or penis. Patients should not use a spermicide with nonoxynol-9 more than twice a day because their chances of getting an STI go up.

What about complications and warning signs?

Research shows that the irritation caused by spermicides can put a patient at higher risk of getting STIs or HIV if they are exposed.

Are there any precautions?

A health care provider may advise you to use a different birth control method if you or your partner is allergic to or is having irritation from the spermicide.

Spermicides and Weight Concerns

Q: Does using spermicides cause weight gain?

A: No.

Q: If a user is overweight, do spermicides still work well?

A: Yes.

Q: Are there medical problems if a spermicide user is overweight?

A: No.

What are the advantages and disadvantages of using Spermicides?

Breastfeeding

Those who breastfeed can use spermicides when they have sex.

There are many things people like about using spermicides. And there are some things they don't like. Find out what your patient likes. Encourage them to focus on those things.

What some people like about spermicides:

- They cause few health problems.
- You can find them at most drugstores.
- You can put them in up to 1 hour before you have sex.
- You only use them when you need them.
- They provide lubrication during sex.
- You can use them with many other methods.

Find out what your patient might not like about using spermicides.

Ask your patients if they have any concerns about using spermicides. Then talk to them about their concerns. Help them think through how to solve any problems they might have while using spermicides. Have them think of their own solutions first. Read the chart that follows for some ideas about how to deal with their concerns.

Keep in mind that spermicides are not the best method for everyone. It is the patient's choice.

Spermicides: Some Problems and Ways to Solve Them

Problem	Ways to Solve the Problem
I don't like having to touch my vagina.	▪ Many patients feel this way at first. You may get used to it over time. ▪ Your partner could put the spermicide in your vagina as part of sex play.
It seems messy to use.	Some spermicides can be messier than others. For example, if you think birth control foam is too messy, you might want to try film or suppositories.
I don't like having to put it in right before sex.	Try making the spermicide easy to get to during sex. You may want to keep it in a bedside drawer. Remember that you can put it in up to 1 hour before you have sex.
With some spermicides, you have to wait before you can have sex. I don't like having to wait.	You can use that "wait" time for sex play. Or you might try a type of spermicide that doesn't make you wait.
What if I forget to wait for the spermicide to melt before having sex or if I forget to put more spermicide in?	You can still try to prevent pregnancy after sex. Find out about Emergency Contraception (EC).
Spermicides don't protect me or my partner from HIV or other STIs.	To help protect yourself and your partner from these infections, use a condom every time you have sex.
It doesn't taste good during oral sex.	You may want to have oral sex before you put the spermicide in.
I am (my partner is) allergic to the spermicide.	You may need to use a different method.

What if you want to stop using spermicides?

You can stop using spermicides whenever you would like to.   If you stop using them, you could become pregnant right away. Use another birth control method if you don't want to be pregnant.

There are no health problems to watch for when you stop using spermicides.

Make sure your patient understands.

Before your patients leave, make sure they understand how to use spermicides successfully. Some of these questions may help.

Things you can ask your patient:

- ▸ Tell me what you know about spermicides.
- ▸ How do spermicides work?
- ▸ How long to spermicides last?
- ▸ What can you do to make spermicides work better?
- ▸ What might be the most difficult thing for you about using spermicides?
- ▸ How would you get around that problem?

Birth Control Foam

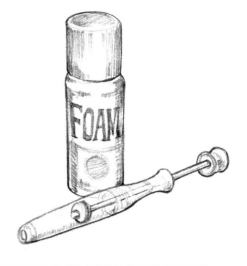

How do you use it?

Teach your patients these steps so they can use birth control foam correctly.

Always check the expiration date on the can. Don't use it after that date.

Put the foam in before the penis is in or near the vagina or anus. You can put the foam in right before you have sex or up to 1 hour before.

1. **Wash your hands.**

2. **Shake the can at least 20 times.**

3. **Fill the applicator with foam.**

    Follow these steps:

    - Stand the can up on a level surface.

    - Put the applicator on the can's nozzle.

    - Press the applicator down very gently until it is full.

    - Take the applicator off the can to stop the flow of foam.

4. **Put the foam in the vagina.**

    Follow these steps:

    - Gently slide the applicator into the vagina as far back as it will go.

    - Press gently on the applicator's plunger to push the foam into the vagina.

    - Take the applicator out.

5. **You can have sex right away.**

   ▪ Don't wait more than 1 hour to have sex.

   ▪ If more than 1 hour goes by and you haven't had sex, put in more foam before you do have sex. Use a full applicator of foam just as you did the first time.

What if you want to have sex more than once?

Every time you want to have sex, put another full applicator of foam in your vagina. Be sure to add the foam *before* each time you have sex.

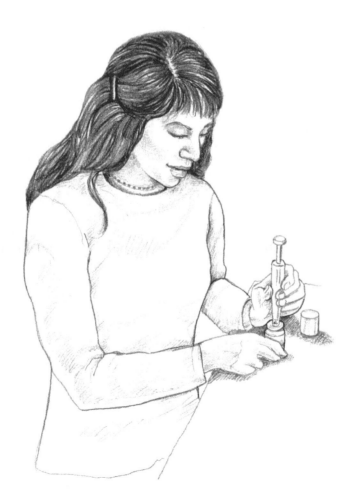

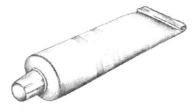

Birth Control Cream or Jelly (Gel)

How do you use it?

Teach your patients these steps so they can use birth control cream or jelly correctly.

Always check the expiration date on the tube of cream or jelly. Don't use it after that date.

Put the cream or jelly in before the penis is in or near the vagina or anus. You can put the cream or jelly in right before you have sex or up to 1 hour before.

1. **Wash your hands.**

2. **Fill the applicator with the birth control cream or jelly.**

    Follow these steps:

    - Take the cap off the tube of cream or jelly.
    - Screw the applicator onto the tube.
    - Squeeze the tube until the applicator is full.
    - Unscrew the applicator and put the cap back on the tube.

Note: Some brands of birth control jelly or cream come with an applicator that is already filled.

3. **Put the birth control cream or jelly in the vagina.**

    This is a lot like putting in a tampon. Follow these steps:

    - Gently slide the applicator into the vagina as far back as it will go.
    - Gently press the applicator's plunger to push the cream or jelly into the vagina.
    - Take the applicator out.

4. **You can have sex right away.**

    - Don't wait for more than 1 hour to have sex.
    - If more than 1 hour goes by and you haven't had sex, put more cream or jelly in *before* you have sex. Use a full applicator of cream or jelly just as you did the first time.

What if you want to have sex more than once?

Every time you want to have sex, put another full applicator of cream or jelly in your vagina. Be sure to add the cream or jelly *before* each time you have sex.

Birth Control Suppositories

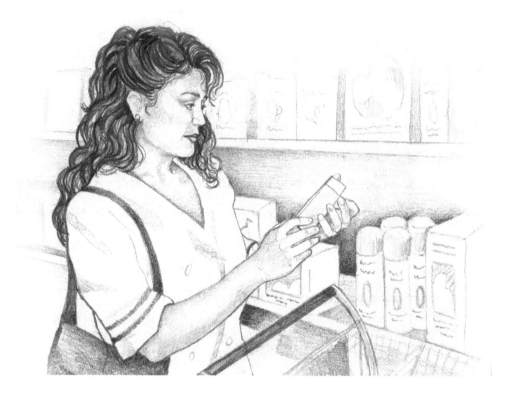

How do you use it?

Teach your patients these steps so they can use birth control suppositories correctly.

Always check the expiration date on the suppository package. Don't use it after that date.

Put the suppository in the vagina at least 10 minutes before the penis is in or near the vagina or anus. Some suppositories must be put in 20 minutes before. It is a good idea to read the instructions for the brand of suppositories you use. You can put the suppository in up to 1 hour before you have sex.

1. **Wash your hands.**

2. **Take the cover off the suppository.**

3. **Slide the suppository into the vagina.**

   Use your finger or an applicator to slide it into your vagina as far back as it will go.

4. **Wait until the suppository is completely melted before you have sex.**

   - The suppository has to melt before it will work. You may need to wait 20 minutes.
   - Do not have sex before the suppository is completely melted.

5. **You can have sex as soon as the suppository has melted.**

   - Don't wait more than 1 hour after you put it in to have sex.
   - If more than 1 hour goes by and you haven't had sex, put in a new suppository. Wait until it has melted before you have sex.

What if you want to have sex more than once?

▸ Every time you want to have sex, put in a new suppository. Be sure you put it in before you have sex.

▸ Wait until it has melted before you have sex.

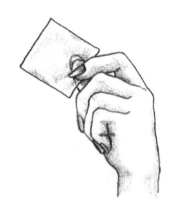

Birth Control Film

How do you use it?

Teach your patients these steps so they can use birth control film correctly.

Always check the expiration date on the film's package. Don't use it after that date.

Put the birth control film in the vagina about 15 minutes before the penis is in or near the vagina or anus. The film usually needs 15 minutes to melt and cover the cervix.

1. **Wash your hands.**

2. **Put the film in your vagina.**

   Follow these steps:

   - With dry hands, take 1 piece of film from its package.
   - Fold the film in half. Then fold it over your middle finger.
   - Use your middle finger to push the film into your vagina as far back as it will go.

   Note: Once the film is on your finger, put it in the vagina right away. This keeps the heat of your hand from melting the film

3. **Wait to have sex until the film has melted (about 15 minutes).**

4. **You can have sex as soon as the film has melted or up to 1 hour after you put it in.**

   - Don't wait more than 1 hour to have sex after you put the film in.
   - If more than 1 hour goes by and you haven't had sex, put in a new piece of film. Wait until it has melted before you have sex.

What if you want to have sex more than once?

   ▸ Every time you want to have sex, put a new piece of film in the vagina. Be sure to put it in before you have sex.

   ▸ Wait until it has melted before you have sex.

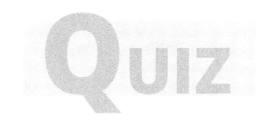

SPERMICIDES

*Directions: Read each of the following statements.
Is it true or false? Circle the best answer.*

1. Spermicides are chemicals that kill sperm. **True** **False**

2. Spermicides work best when they are
   used with another barrier method, like the
   external or internal condom or a diaphragm
   or cap. **True** **False**

3. Most spermicides can be put into the vagina
   up to one hour before sex. **True** **False**

4. After you put spermicide in once,
   you can have sex as often as you
   would like in 24 hours. **True** **False**

5. Rinsing out the vagina after sex washes
   away spermicide before it can kill all of
   the sperm. **True** **False**

*Directions: Read the following question.
Circle all of the answers that apply.*

6. Which of these spermicides must melt in a vagina before you
   can have sex?
   a. Foam
   b. Jelly
   c. Film
   d. Cream
   e. Suppositories

Go on to the next page.

Directions: Read each of the following, and write your best answer in the space below.

7. List one possible side effect of using spermicides.

   ▪ _____

   _____

8. What are two things some people like about using spermicides?

   ▪ _____

   _____

   ▪ _____

   _____

Check your answers on the next page.

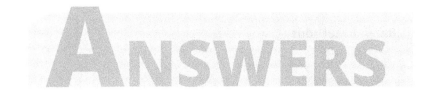

SPERMICIDES

Check your answers.

1. **True**   Spermicides are chemicals that kill sperm.

2. **True**   Spermicides work best when they are used with another barrier method, like the external or internal condom or a diaphragm or cap.

   When spermicides are used alone, they are not as effective as other methods. If your patient chooses spermicides as a method, encourage them to ask their partner to also use a condom every time they have sex.

3. **True**   Most spermicides can be put into the vagina up to one hour before sex.

4. **False**   After you put spermicide in once, you **cannot** have sex as often as you would like in 24 hours. You must add more spermicide before each time you have sex.

5. **True**   Rinsing out the vagina after sex does wash away spermicide before it can kill all of the sperm.

   It is okay to take a shower or bath after you have sex. If you want to rinse the vagina, you need to wait at least 6 hours after the last time you had reproductive sex.

6. **C, E**   *Film* and *suppositories* are two spermicides that must melt in the vagina before you can have sex. It may take up to 20 minutes for them to melt.

   If you use foam, jelly, or cream, you can have sex right after you put the spermicide in the vagina.

Go on to the next page.

7. One possible side effect of using spermicides is an allergy to the spermicide. The allergy can cause skin rashes, itching, burning, or redness in or around the vagina or penis. Patients who are allergic to the spermicide can change brands or try using a different type of spermicide.

8. Here are things that some people like about using spermicides:

   - They cause few health problems.
   - They can be found at most drugstores.
   - They can be put in up to 1 hour before having sex.
   - You only use them when you need them.
   - They help lubricate during sex.
   - They can be used with many other methods.

Remember, what some people like about a method, other people might not like. Every patient is different.

Emergency Contraception (EC)

What you can do if your birth control method fails

This section is mostly written as though you were talking to your patients. It gives you an idea of how to explain Emergency Contraception (EC) in a way your patients can understand. This section also has notes written directly to you, as the health worker. Those "health worker notes" look like this one.

EC gives you a second chance to prevent pregnancy.

Emergency Contraception (EC) is a way to keep from getting pregnant even after sex. If you have sex without using a birth control method or if your birth control method fails, you can still try to prevent pregnancy by using EC. EC works in two ways to prevent pregnancy after unprotected sex. You can:

EC and Teens

All over the United States, it is legal for teens to get confidential family planning services. Find out what your health care site's policy is about providing EC to teens without parent or guardian permission.

> ▶ Take an EC pill orally (swallow it) within 3-5 days. For the progestin EC pill try to take within 3 days.

> ▶ Have an IUD placed in your uterus within 5 days.

The sooner you use EC, the better your chances of not getting pregnant.

How do EC pills work?

There are two ways to use emergency contraceptive pills (ECPs):

> ▶ A single pill is packaged for emergency contraception.

> ▶ There are some birth control pills you can take in special doses (multiple pills are swallowed).

Other names for EC Pills...
- ECP or ECPs
- oral EC
- plan B
- morning after pill

ECPs work by delaying ovulation (keeping an egg from leaving an ovary) while sperm may still be alive in the tubes. If there is no egg to meet with sperm, you can't get pregnant.

ECPs will *not* stop implantation of a fertilized egg and will *not* stop a pregnancy that has already started. It is *not* an abortion pill and does not cause an abortion. Oral EC will not harm you or the baby if you are already pregnant.

EC Pills and Weight Concerns

Q: Do EC pills cause weight gain?

A: No.

Q: If a user is overweight, does ECP still work?

A: Yes, but higher weight may reduce the effectiveness of ECP. Ella is more effective than Plan B versions for those who are overweight. Some health care providers may recommend overweight patients take a double dose of oral EC to increase the chances of preventing a pregnancy.

How well do EC pills work?

ECPs work well to prevent pregnancy, when used the right way. They are good to use in an emergency.

If you take an ECP that has ulipristal acetate in it (sold under the name of Ella):

You have a 62-85% chance of preventing pregnancy by taking Ella. For maximum effectiveness, wait 5 days to start on-going hormonal birth control after taking Ella.

If you take an ECP that has only progestin in it (like Plan B, Next Choice, After-Pill or My Way):

You have a 52-100% chance of preventing pregnancy by taking a progestin-only EC pill.

If you take ECPs that have both estrogen and progestin in them (taking birth control pills in special doses):

You have a 56-89% chance of preventing pregnancy by taking specific doses of combined hormonal pills.

In other words, if 100 patients used ECPs perfectly after each act of unprotected sex in a year, between 0 to 15 of them may get pregnant.

How do you use EC pills?

Teach your patients these steps so they can use EC pills correctly.

Taking EC Pills

Be sure your patients know that they must *swallow* the pill or pills.

1. **Talk to a health care provider or pharmacist about getting an EC pill or pills.**

   They will decide which type of ECP is best for you. Get the pill or pills as soon as you can within 3-5 days of having unprotected sex.

   ▸ Progestin-only EC pills (Plan B and generic) are available without a prescription to anyone of any age.

   ▸ Some health care providers may give you ECP in advance to keep on hand for when you need it.

2. **Take the EC pill or pills as soon as you can after having unprotected sex.**

   The health care provider, pharmacist or pill packaging will tell you how many and what type of pills to take. You may be told to take 2 doses or a single dose. Take yours exactly the way you are instructed to.

3. **Call your health care provider or pharmacist right away if you vomit within an hour after you take the first dose.**

   You may need to take another dose of pills right away. Do not take any extra pills.

4. **Make a follow-up appointment if you need to.**

   You should set up a visit with your health care provider if:

   ▸ You don't have a regular birth control method.

   ▸ You don't have a normal period within 3 to 4 weeks after taking the ECP. You may need a pregnancy test at this time.

   ▸ There is a chance you could have gotten an STI.

> **Using contraception after ECPs**
>
> Patients who take the Ella (ulipristal) EC pill must wait 5 days after taking it to resume or start a hormonal birth control method and then use a back-up method or abstain from sex for another 7 days.

Are there any side effects?

Some patients may have some of these side effects for a day or so after taking emergency contraceptive pills:

▸ **Upset stomach or vomiting** The upset stomach is usually mild and may last for a day. It is more common with EC pills that have estrogen or ulipristal in them.

▸ **Changes in your period** Your period might be earlier or later than usual. It could be lighter or heavier than usual.

▸ **Dizziness**

> **Upset stomach**
>
> The provider may order a medicine to prevent upset stomach. Or your patient can buy a medicine at a drugstore. They can ask the pharmacist what to take.

What about complications and warning signs?

ECPs do not cause any complications.

Are there any precautions?

EC pills are safe for most patients. They will not harm you or your baby if you are pregnant or breastfeeding.

Make sure your patient understands.

Before your patients leave, you will want to make sure they understand what they need to know about ECP. Some of these questions may help.

Things you can ask your patient:

▸ Tell me what you know about emergency contraceptive pills.

▸ How do EC pills work?

▸ If you choose to use oral EC, when do you need to take the pill or pills?

▸ How would you get an EC pill or pills?

▸ When might you need to take a pregnancy test?

▸ What might be the most difficult thing for you about using ECP?

▸ How would you get around that problem?

▸ What type of regular birth control method will you use?

Learn More About All EC Methods:

www.cecinfo.org

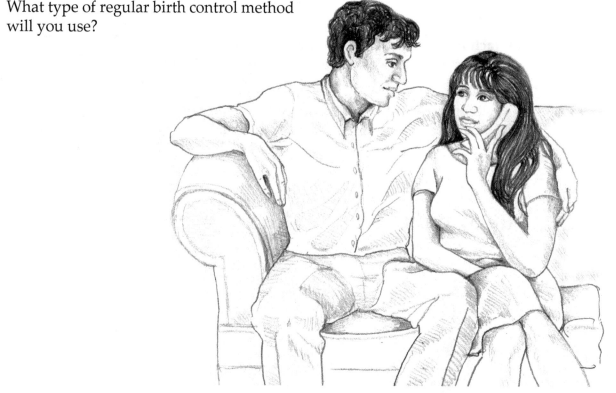

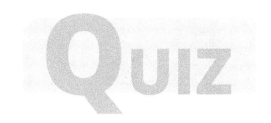

EMERGENCY CONTRACEPTIVE PILLS

Directions: Circle the best answer.

1. Which of the following statements about EC pills is true?
   a. EC pills are taken after having sex to try to prevent a pregnancy.
   b. EC pills must be taken within 3-5 days after unprotected sex.
   c. The sooner EC pills are taken, the better the chances of not getting pregnant.
   d. All of the above

2. How do EC pills help stop a potential pregnancy?
   a. They keep any egg from leaving an ovary by delaying ovulation.
   b. They dislodge any fertilized eggs from the uterus.
   c. They stop an established pregnancy early on.
   d. All of the above

3. When can someone get EC pills?
   a. Some providers give patients EC pills before they need them. That way, they will have them when and if they ever need them.
   b. Anyone can get EC pills when they come to the health care site within 5 days after having unprotected sex.
   c. Never
   d. Both A and B

4. Which of the following is a side effect of using EC pills?
   a. Upset stomach or vomiting
   b. Changes in periods
   c. Dizziness
   d. All of the above

Check your answers on the next page.

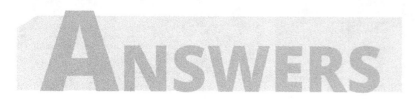

EMERGENCY CONTRACEPTIVE PILLS

Check your answers.

1. **D**   All of the above. All of the following are true about EC pills:
   - EC pills are taken after having sex to try to prevent a pregnancy.
   - EC pills must be taken within 3-5 days after unprotected sex.
   - The sooner EC pills are taken, the better the chances of not getting pregnant.

2. **A**   EC pills ONLY work by keeping the egg from leaving an ovary. If there is no egg to meet with sperm, there can be no pregnancy. If an egg is already fertilized by sperm or implanted in the uterus, the EC pill will have no effect.

3. **D**   Both A and B. Some health care providers give patients EC pills before they need them so they have them on hand in an emergency. Usually a patient is given the EC pills when they come to the health care site within 5 days after having unprotected sex. Remember, progestin ECPs can also be bought over-the-counter now.

4. **D**   All of the above. Upset stomach or vomiting, changes in periods, and dizziness are all possible side effects of EC pills.

How do IUDs work as EC?

The copper intra-uterine device (IUD) or a 52 mg progestin IUD works mainly by keeping the sperm from getting to the egg (it stops fertilization). If an egg has already been fertilized, the IUD will keep it from attaching to the lining of the uterus (it stops implantation). It is not an abortion. It will not stop an existing pregnancy.

How well do IUDs work as EC?

When you talk to your patients, talk to them about how well the IUD works as EC (how effective it is).

The copper IUD or a 52 mg progestin IUD work extremely well as emergency contraception. They are also excellent to use as a regular birth control method. So after you have a copper IUD or a 52 mg progestin IUD placed for use as EC, you can keep using it as your regular birth control method.

The copper IUD or a 52 mg progestin IUD is 99.2% effective as EC.

That means that if 100 patients use an IUD as EC, only 1 (and probably none) of them may get pregnant in a year.

How do you use an IUD as EC?

Teach your patients these steps to get an IUD placed.

1. **Get an appointment with a health care provider to have a copper IUD or 52 mg progestin IUD placed.**

    You will need to have the IUD placed in your uterus (womb) within 5 days after you had unprotected sex. The sooner you have it placed, the better. The health care provider will talk with you about whether the IUD is right for you. The provider will also give you information about the advantages and disadvantages of both types of IUDs.

2. **The health care provider will place the copper IUD or a 52 mg progestin IUD in your uterus.**

   The provider uses a special applicator to put the IUD through the cervix and into the uterus. This takes just a few minutes.

3. **After the IUD is placed, you can use it as your regular birth control for up to 6 years to 12 years.**

   You can have the IUD taken out at any time for any reason. It can be taken out if you want to change your birth control method or if you want to get pregnant. It stops working right away after it is taken out of your uterus. But if you want to keep using it as birth control, the copper IUD can prevent pregnancy for up to 12 years and a 52 mg progestin IUD can prevent pregnancy for up to 6 years.

4. **Call your provider if you have any problems.**

   Call if you miss your next period, think you may be pregnant, or have any other questions.

5. **Make a follow-up appointment if you need to.**

   You should set up a visit with your provider if it is recommended.

Are there any side effects?

- ▶ **You may have brief cramping during placement of a copper IUD or a 52 mg progestin IUD.** Some spotting and mild cramping is not unusual for a few weeks after having an IUD placed.

- ▶ **Changes in your period: Copper IUD** You will still have a regular period with the Copper IUD but it might be heavier or you may have more cramps than usual. This often gets better with time.

- ▶ **Changes in your period: 52 mg progestin IUD** Your periods will be irregular and lighter and you may have spotting throughout the month. After 6 months, you may even stop having periods.

What about complications and warning signs?

Serious health problems from an IUD are rare, but some patients do get them. Here are some of the possible complications you should tell your patients about.

- ▸ **Infection or Pelvic Inflammatory Disease (PID)** This is not common and if it happens, it would be during the first few weeks after the IUD is placed. If you get symptoms of foul discharge, a fever, pelvic pain, abdominal pain, or pain with sex, tell your health care provider right away.

- ▸ **A tear or hole in the uterus or cervix** This can happen when the IUD is being placed in the uterus.

IUD Warning Signs: P A I N S

If you have any of these warning signs, call your provider or a health care setting right away.

P = **P**eriod late, abnormal spotting or bleeding. These could mean pregnancy or infection.

A = **A**bdominal or pelvic pain, pain with intercourse. These could mean pregnancy or infection.

I = **I**nfection, abnormal discharge.

N = **N**ot feeling well, fever, chills. These could be signs of an infection.

S = **S**tring missing or changed. The IUD may be out of place.

Are there any precautions?

A health care provider may advise you to use a different EC method if any of the following is true:

- You have a current infection of the uterus or fallopian tubes (PID).
- You have vaginal bleeding for no known reason.
- You have current cancer of the cervix or uterus.
- You are already pregnant.

Make sure your patient understands.

Before your patients leave, you will want to make sure they understand what they need to know about using a copper IUD or a 52 mg progestin IUD and about using an IUD as EC. Some of these questions may help.

IUDs and Weight Concerns

Q: Does using either IUD as EC cause weight gain?

A: No.

Q: If a patient is overweight, will either IUD work as well as EC?

A: Yes.

Q: If a patient is overweight, will either IUD cause medical problems?

A: No.

- Tell me what you know about the copper IUD and the 52 mg progestin IUDs.
- How does an IUD work to prevent pregnancy?
- What are side effects you may have in the first few weeks after you have an IUD placed?
- When might you need to take a pregnancy test?
- What might be the most difficult thing for you about using an IUD?
- How would you get around that problem?
- Would you like to keep using this as your birth control method?

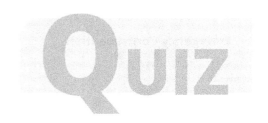

USING AN IUD AS EC

Directions: Circle the best answer.

1. Which of the following statements about using an IUD as EC is true?
    a. Patients can have a copper IUD or a 52 mg progestin IUD placed after having sex to prevent a pregnancy.
    b. A patient must have an IUD placed within 5 days of unprotected sex.
    c. The sooner a patient has an IUD placed, the better their chances of not getting pregnant.
    d. All of the above

2. How does an IUD prevent a pregnancy?
    a. It dislodges an implanted embryo from the uterus.
    b. It stops sperm from meeting with an egg.
    c. It keeps the egg from attaching to the lining of the uterus.
    d. Both B and C

3. How effective is an IUD as EC?
    a. When placed by a health care provider within 10 days of unprotected sex, it lowers the chance of pregnancy by 88%.
    b. When placed by a health care provider within 5 days of unprotected sex, it lowers the chance of pregnancy by more than 99%.
    c. When placed by a health care provider within 5 days of unprotected sex, it will lower the chance of pregnancy by 33%.
    d. When placed by a health care provider within 3 days of unprotected sex, it lowers the chance of pregnancy by 50%.

4. Which of the following is a side effect of using a copper IUD or a 52 mg progestin IUD?

   a. Tiredness

   b. Headache

   c. Spotting for a few weeks after placement

   d. Fatigue

Check your answers on the next page.

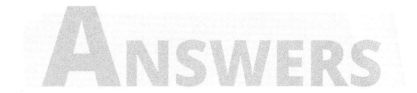

USING AN IUD AS EC

Check your answers.

1. **D**   All of the above. All of the following are true about using an IUD as EC:
   - A patient can have a copper IUD or a 52 mg progestin IUD placed after having sex to prevent a pregnancy.
   - A patient must have an IUD placed within 5 days of unprotected sex.

2. **D**   Both B & C. An IUD works by preventing the sperm from reaching an egg (stops fertilization). It will also stop a fertilized egg from attaching to the uterus.

3. **B**   When placed by a health care provider within 5 days of unprotected sex, it lowers the chance of pregnancy by more than 99%.

4. **C**   Spotting for a few weeks is not unusual after having an IUD placed. Other on-going side effects:
   - With the copper IUD, the patient will still have regular menstrual periods, they may just be heavier or crampier.
   - With a 52 mg progestin IUD, the patient will have irregular periods with spotting. Periods may be lighter and less crampy and some users may even stop having periods after 6 months.

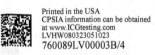

9 781736 984604